MANAGEMENT ISSUES
IN CRITICAL CARE

CAROLE BIRDSALL, R.N., M.S.N., CCRN

Staff Nurse, Critical Care
New York Hospital
Management Consultant
St. Luke's-Roosevelt Hospital Center
Doctoral Student
Teacher's College, Columbia University
New York, New York

Illustrated

Mosby Year Book

St. Louis Baltimore Boston Chicago London Philadelphia Sydney Toronto

Mosby Year Book
Dedicated to Publishing Excellence

Executive Editor: Don Ladig
Developmental Editor: Robin Carter
Project Supervisor: Barbara Merritt
Editing and Production: Carlisle Publishers Services
Design: Laura Steube
Cover Design: Julie Taugner

Copyright © 1991 by Mosby–Year Book, Inc.
A Mosby imprint of Mosby–Year Book, Inc.

All rights reserved. No part of this publication may be reproduced, stored in a retrieval system, or transmitted, in any form or by any means, electronic, mechanical, photocopied, recorded, or otherwise, without prior written permission from the publisher.

Printed in the United States of America

Mosby-Year Book, Inc.
11830 Westline Industrial Drive
St. Louis, MO 63146

Library of Congress Cataloging-in-Publication Data

Management issues in critical care / [edited by] Carole Birdsall
      p.   cm.
   Includes bibliographical references and index.
   ISBN 0-8016-6071-8
   1. Intensive care nursing—Management.   I. Birdsall, Carole.
   [DNLM: 1. Administrative Personnel. 2. Critical Care—organization and administration. 3. Personnel Management.   [WY 154 M266]]
RT120.I5M35   1991
362.1´73´068—dc20
DMLM/DLC
for Library of Congress   90-13680
                                                                                                               CIP

GW/GW/RRD   9 8 7 6 5 4 3 2 1

To my mother
Gloria Curran Wallace
*for her strength, direction, and caring
over many years of sharing and being.*

CONTRIBUTORS

JO ANNE BENNETT RN, MA, CNA
HIV Clinical Nurse Specialist
New York, New York

CAROLE BIRDSALL RN, MSN, CCRN
Staff Nurse, Critical Care
New York Hospital
Management Consultant
St. Luke's–Roosevelt Medical Center
New York, New York

MARY-MICHAEL BROWN RN, MS, CCRN
Nursing Coordinator Cardiovascular Surgical Unit
Georgetown University Hospital
Washington, D.C.

SHARON J. CONNOR RN, MSN, CCRN
Coordinator of Chapters and Director of Education
American Association of Critical Care Nurses
Newport Beach, California

NICOLETTE FIORE-LOPEZ RN, MA, CCRN
Assistant Director of Nursing
New York University Medical Center
New York, New York

MARIE FOLK-LIGHTY RN, MSN, CCRN
Clinical Nurse Specialist
St Joseph's Hospital Health Center
Syracuse, New York

NANCY J. GANTZ RN, MBA, CNA
Manager Critical Care Units
Good Samaritan Hospital & Medical Center
Portland, Oregon

PATRICK E. KENNY RN, MSN C, CNA
Divisional Director of Nursing
Warminster General Hospital
Warminster, Pennsylvania

KATHLEEN KLOCK RN, BS, CEN
Administrative Supervisor
St. Joseph's Hospital Health Center
Syracuse, New York

JEANNE S. LATIMER RN, BSN
Nursing Quality Assurance Coordinator
The Graduate Hospital
Philadelphia, Pennsylvania

BARBARA LEEPER RN, MN, CCRN
Cardiovascular Clinical Specialist
Humana Hospital
Dallas, Texas

JANET MACKIN RN, MSN
Director Nursing Education
St. Luke's/Roosevelt Hospital Center
New York, New York

BONNIE S. McCANDLESS RN, MS
Director AACN Certification Corporation
American Association of Critical Care Nurses
Newport Beach, CA

MARLAINE (SPARKI) ORTIZ RN, MS, CNA
Instructor Staff Development & Nursing
Strong Memorial Hospital & University of Rochester
Rochester, New York

SUSAN G. OSGUTHORPE RN, MS, CCRN, CNA
Veterans Administration Medical Center
Salt Lake City, Utah

KATHLEEN E. POWDERLY RN, CNM, MSN
Assistant Director Division of Humanities in Medicine
Assistant Professor of Nursing
State University of New York
Brooklyn, New York

SARAH J. SANFORD RN, MA, CNAA
Executive Director
American Association of Critical-Care Nurses
Newport Beach, California

SUSAN CRAIG SCHULMERICH RN, MBA, MS, CEN, CNA
Director Home Health Agency
Montefiore Medical Center
Bronx, New York

MARY JANE SPUHLER-GAUGHAN RN, MSN
Assistant Director QA Program
The Graduate Hospital
Philadelphia, Pennsylvania

GEORGITA TOLBERT WASHINGTON RN C, MSN, CCRN
Critical Care Clinical Nurse Specialist
Holston Valley Hospital & Medical Center
Kingsport, Tennessee

DONNA SCULLY WATTS RN, CCRN
Former Coordinator Critical Care Nursing Education
UCLA Medical Center
Los Angeles, California

KATHLEEN DALEY WHITE RN, MS, CCRN
Director Critical Care Institute
University Hospital
State University of New York
Stony Brook, New York

GAYLE R. WHITMAN RN, MSN
Director Cardiothoracic Nursing
Cleveland Clinic Hospital
Cleveland, Ohio

Consultants

KATHLEEN BLANCHFIELD, RN, MS
Director of Nurse Development, Evengelical Health Systems, Oak Brook, Illinois

LAURA CHICKERING, RN, MA
Nursing Supervisor, Missouri Baptist Medical Center, St. Louis, Missouri

MARIA ANNE CONNOLLY, RN, MSN, CCRN, PhD Candidate
Professor of Nursing, Governors State University, University Park, Illinois

LYNNE HUTSON DANEKAS, RN, MSN
Cardiovascular Clinical Nurse Specialist, Edward Hospital, Naperville, Illinois

MARY P. FITZGERALD, RN, MA, CCRN, CEN
Assistant Director of Nursing, Doctor's Hospital, New York, New York

MARY B. GALLAGHER, RN, MSN, CCRN
Nursing Supervisor, Critical Care Division, Bryn Mawr Hospital, Bryn Mawr, Pennsylvania

EDWINA A. McCONNELL, RN, PhD
Independent Nurse Consultant, Madison, Wisconsin

JANICE PIAZZA, RN, CCRN
Director, Critical Care, Mercy Hospital, New Orleans, Louisiana

LOIS SCHICK, RN, MBA
Clinical Director, Surgicare One, Saint Joseph Hospital, Denver, Colorado

BRENDA K. SHELTON, RN, MS, CCRN, OCN
Critical Care Clinical Nurse Specialist, Johns Hopkins Oncology Center, Baltimore, Maryland

ROBERT SMITH, MPA
Administrative Assistant, New York University Medical Center, New York, New York

SANDRA SPERRY, RN, MA
Vice President for Nursing, Beekman Hospital, New York, New York

SARA J. WELLS, RN, MN
Director, Acute Care Services, Lankenau Hospital and Medical Research Center, Philadelphia, Pennsylvania

PREFACE

In the current cost-conscious economic environment, one thing is certain: ongoing change. As hospitals and other health care delivery systems continue to evolve in the 1990s, nurse managers and practitioners who want to be nurse managers require practical information written by experts who manage critical care units. This book is written for nurse managers who need a ready reference to make effective, meaningful change in their units. In addition, many practitioners who want to move up into management can use the book to plan their careers as managers. The authors of each chapter are experts in their fields and have practical leadership and management experience. All were selected because of their experience and willingness to share their knowledge.

The original concept for this book emerged from a continuing education program presented by the New York City Chapter of American Association of Critical-Care Nurses (AACN). This program was developed to address current management concerns. It became obvious that a reference book was needed to help managers succeed in the changing practice environment.

ORGANIZATION

Management Issues in Critical Care is organized into three units of 21 chapters. **Unit I, Developing People Skills**, includes an introductory chapter on planning a successful career and four chapters that identify different key concepts needed by managers to provide a working environment that fosters team work. Chapter 1, **Career Development**, provides an overview of planning and making the right moves to move up in management. Chapter 2, **A Climate for Caring**, introduces the concept that the manager is pivotal in creating a positive work environment. Chapter 3, **Facilitating Job Satisfaction**, builds on this concept and identifies behaviors that allow the nurse manager to enhance the working environment. **Performance, Time, and Energy**, Chapter 4, provides specific tools that can be used by the manager to streamline job responsibilities. Chapter 5, **Fostering Participative Management**, introduces techniques that are used to involve staff in the process of effective management. Finally, **Collaborative Practice**, Chapter 6, identifies how this joint mode of providing care is operationalized using managed care and incorporating principles to facilitate discharge planning.

Unit II, Developing Managerial Skills, addresses specific aspects or topics unique to management. Chapter 7, **Standards of Care**, provides an overview of the use of standards of care as a basis for nursing practice. **Quality Assurance and Risk management**, Chapter 8, demonstrates the actual application of nursing theory to a model that is used to monitor and evaluate significant aspects of care. Chapter 9, **Patient Classification**, provides an overview of the different classification tools in current use and suggests ways the nurse manager can use existing tools to justify staffing and budget. Chapter 10, **Twenty-Four Hour Staffing**, identifies the different types of staffing patterns used and includes information on tying staffing to classification. **Competency-Based Orientation**, Chapter 11, addresses the need to move away from traditional orientation programs as they are too costly and identifies specific reasons for moving to a competency based system. Chapter 12, **Career Ladders**, explores the options available to the nurse manager when considering implementation of career ladders as a mechanism of reward for professional practice. Chapter 13, **Nurse Intern Program**, discusses the actual process and results used to successfully deal with a nursing shortage. The **Role of the Clinical Nurse Specialist**, Chapter 14, provides the reader with specific actions that facilitate maximal benefits of delineating the role of a clinical nurse specialist in a unit.

Unit III, Developing Administrative Skills, introduces the manager to concepts that are part of nursing administration, and ends with a chapter that looks to the future in critical care. Chapter 15, **Benefits of Evolving Technology**, suggests ways a manager can easily incorporate the demands of growing technology in unit practice. **Strategic Planning**, Chapter 16, provides specific steps that can be used to start this process. Chapter 17, **Budgeting Concepts**, introduces the terms and elements used in budgeting while Chapter 18, **Analyzing and Forecasting Budgets**, develops these skills for the manager by providing tables and examples that demonstrate application. Chapter 19, **Labor Relations**, provides an overview of the elements of labor relations and suggests ways a manager can work with a labor union through specific examples that use contract language. **Ethical and Legal Considerations**, Chapter 20, introduces the legal decisions relevant to critical care practice and identifies the types of ethical dilemmas facing managers. Chapter 21, **On to the Future**, predicts the type of sophisticated communication systems that will be part of the critical care manager's world in the future and suggests ways the manager can grow and learn with anticipated change.

Each of the 21 chapters can be viewed as a separate entity, for each covers a topic completely. However, the organization of the chapters allows the reader to build a wide body of knowledge in a particular area if all of the chapters in a unit are read in sequence. And finally, if the book is read in its entirety, each chapter builds on the knowledge of the previous chapters and provides an overview of the minimal skills needed to manage critical care units. For most of the chapters, a case study is used to demonstrate the way theory can be applied in practice. The format for each case study varies to allow the individual style of the author.

ACKNOWLEDGEMENTS

The editor wishes to acknowledge the contributors who put forth energy and commitment to make this project a reality. An additional word of thanks is given to the reviewers who took time to read it and make such helpful suggestions to improve content and style. Special thanks to the past and current Board Members of the New York City Chapter of AACN who encouraged me along the way. Special thanks also to Jo Anne Bennett who continues to be a mentor in every way and to Nikki Fiore-Lopez who always lends an ear. Lastly I want to thank my editors Don Ladig and Robin Carter at Mosby–Year Book for their patience, direction, and help.

Carole Birdsall

CONTENTS

UNIT I	DEVELOPING PEOPLE SKILLS
1	**Career Development, 3** Nicolette Fiore-Lopez RN MA CCRN
2	**A Climate for Caring, 21** Georgita Tolbert Washington RN C MSN CCRN
3	**Facilitating Job Satisfaction, 39** Bonnie McCandless RN MS Sharon J. Connor RN MSN CCRN
4	**Performance, Time, and Energy, 55** Carole Birdsall RN MSN CCRN
5	**Fostering Participative Management, 69** Marlaine (Sparki) Ortiz RN MS CNA
6	**Collaborative Practice, 83** Susan G. Osguthorpe RN MS CCRN CNA

UNIT II	DEVELOPING MANAGERIAL SKILLS
7	**Standards of Care, 99** Sarah J. Sanford RN MA CNAA
8	**Quality Assurance and Risk Management, 113** Jeanne S. Latimer RN BSN Mary Jane Spuhler-Gaughan RN MSN
9	**Patient Classification, 131** Carole Birdsall RN MSN CCRN
10	**Twenty-Four Hour Staffing, 155** Susan Craig Schulmerich RN MBA MS CEN CNA

11	**Competency Based Orientation,** 169	
	Janet Mackin RN MSN	
	Donna Scully Watts RN CCRN	
	Carole Birdsall RN MSN CCRN	
12	**Career Ladders,** 189	
	Marie Folk-Lighty RN MSN CCRN	
	Kathleen Klock RN BS CEN	
13	**Nurse Intern Program,** 205	
	Kathleen Daley White RN MS CCRN	
14	**Role of the Clinical Nurse Specialist,** 221	
	Barbara Leeper RN MN CCRN	
UNIT III	**DEVELOPING ADMINISTRATIVE SKILLS**	
15	**Benefits of Evolving Technology,** 239	
	Mary-Michael Brown RN MS CCRN	
16	**Strategic Planning,** 259	
	Nancy J. Gantz RN MBA CNA	
17	**Budgeting Concepts,** 271	
	Carole Birdsall RN MSN CCRN	
18	**Analyzing and Forecasting Budgets,** 287	
	Gayle R. Whitman RN MSN	
19	**Labor Relations,** 309	
	Patrick E. Kenny RN MSN C CNA	
20	**Ethical and Legal Considerations,** 331	
	Kathleen E. Powderly RN CNM MSN	
21	**On to the Future,** 345	
	Jo Anne Bennett RN MA CNA	

Unit I

Developing People Skills

Chapter 1

CAREER DEVELOPMENT

Nicolette Fiore-Lopez

A successful career is the result of careful planning. Many aspects of career development can help critical care managers reach long-term goals. This chapter will discuss useful techniques for planning and developing a career in critical care nursing management. Case studies will be used to demonstrate some of the key points discussed in this chapter.

DEVELOPING OR REVISING A CAREER GOAL

The first job as nurse manager can provide a valuable first step in developing career goals. Career planning is a conscious decision of the prospective nurse manager to set out in a reasonable direction and to establish an associated timetable. A thorough self-assessment of long-term personal goals must be completed. One must decide whether nursing is a job or a career. Vestal[15] clarifies the difference: a job involves specific role expectations, a career results in upward mobility. Not all staff nurses are interested in careers. Some have important personal goals that take precedence. These nurses may choose to travel, raise a family, or pursue non-job-related interests. They have short- or long-term personal goals that are not related to a nursing career.

Once the goal to have a career in critical care management has been set, the qualifications necessary to reach this goal must be determined. This can be accomplished in a variety of ways. One of the more common ways is to speak with someone already in a management position. In addition, it may be worthwhile to check the classified section of local newspapers and nursing journals, because advertisements for nursing positions usually state the required qualifications.

Next, a plan and a timetable for obtaining the necessary experience is developed. For example, if a master's degree and three to five years of line management experience are the qualifications needed in a particular geographic area, the staff nurse should seek both graduate study and a line management position. Knowing the number of years of experience needed helps when constructing a timetable for the career plan.

The kind of experience one has can be critical to future success. For example, in some institutions the job of nursing staff educator is considered strictly a staff position. Acceptance of a critical care nursing staff educator position may impede progress on the career plan timetable. Although the experience may enhance managerial ability in the long run, it is not considered line management experience and later may put the staff nurse at a disadvantage, compared with job applicants who do have line management experience. It is prudent to pursue line management experience, which is possible in a variety of settings.

Moving too quickly toward a career goal prevents the development of a good management foundation; therefore, a *realistic* timetable for the career plan is needed. The staff nurse who knows that not everyone develops at the same pace understands that development may not be uniform. In fact, development occurs at different points in a career. Timetables can be revised when necessary, but taking on a position without adequate preparation can lead to failure.

All parties involved in any endeavor benefit by accurately predicting potential job success. Adequate support mechanisms are important, and include a comprehensive orientation period, follow-up goal-setting between employer and employee, and periodic verbal and written performance reviews. Peers, superiors, and structure of the organization all contribute to employee success.

FINDING THE RIGHT JOB

A good *job fit* between employer and employee is the result of several factors. For example, the employee feels valued by the employer. The employee feels he has been well prepared for the job through past experience and on-the-job training, and the organization supports his endeavor. A good job fit enables the individual to feel positive about the work experience if the individual is competent and works in an environment that supports personal goals.[15] As growth and development occur, career issues arise. Therefore, job fit should be continually assessed. As time passes, the unit size or type may no longer offer the challenge it did in the beginning. Experiences fostering professional growth may now be too limited. Assessment should be ongoing.

Identifying Career Opportunities

How does one identify career opportunities? The more traditional places to look include classified advertisements and professional recruitment agencies. In addition, professional organizations and word of mouth are sources that are often useful.

Classified advertisements and professional recruitment agencies are intended to sell the prospective employee on the available job. Their sales pitch usually tends to emphasize the positive aspects of a position. Therefore, it is wise to use all available contacts and networks to discover as much as possible about the location and position *before* submitting a letter of application. Some key questions to ask are: Why did the previous person who held the job leave the position? How long was she in the position before leaving? How long has the position been vacant? Are there potential candidates in-house? Is the job "as advertised"?

Job openings found through professional organizations and word of mouth are often accompanied by more realistic information that helps in deciding whether to submit a letter of application. The job application process is a two-way street. Just as the employer may choose not to hire an applicant, the applicant may choose not to accept a position offered by the employer.

Considering Career Moves

Once a career plan is established, the nurse should periodically reflect on the progress made. The key to success is knowing when it is time to move on. When learning or upward mobility has ceased, there are generally three options available. The first is to remain in the present position, which may be a very comfortable place to be as change always carries an element of risk. Although it is very easy to maintain the status quo, the nurse manager who chooses this option accepts that professional growth will not occur as rapidly as planned. This may prove frustrating as time goes by.

A second option in seeking upward mobility is to look for a position in a different clinical area of the same institution. This option entails some trade-offs. First of all, if critical care has provided a satisfying career thus far, do you wish to change from this specialty focus to broaden your management experience? Secondly, would you feel comfortable as the nursing director of a specialty area that is clinically unfamiliar? The management philosophy of the nursing department plays a pivotal role in this decision. For example, if the clinical expertise of the nursing directors is not emphasized, and the subordinates who make up the management team possess excellent clinical expertise, applying for this position may be desirable.

Finally, choosing a position in critical care at a different institution is a viable option. This may be a difficult choice, because when people are satisfied with their workplace, they tend to develop a strong institutional loyalty that makes it hard to leave. However, remaining in critical care while advancing your position may be more important than your loyalty.

Mentors

Mentoring occurs when a seasoned professional identifies potential in an individual and uses his or her wealth of knowledge and experience to foster that individual's growth and development. Mentors can be sought out or mentors may find their "mentee," or novice. Some mentoring relationships begin consciously, others develop over the course of time.

Generally, a mentor understands upward mobility and often can guide the novice through the prepatory phases. Mentors are usually active in professional nursing organizations and can show novices the benefits of active involvement, and they encourage participation by introducing the novice to others in the group. This involvement enhances professional development, and it provides new members for the organization.

Career Advancement

If one is interested in career advancement, one must seize opportunities that arise. Price, Simms, and Pforitz[13] found in an exploratory study of nurse executives that 83 percent had not planned their advancement, but instead had taken opportunities that passed their way. Positions that are not considered "glamorous" can be used as stepping stones in career paths, especially if other people in the position desired have held these positions in the past.

The most common unglamorous positions are those in shift management, and they are unglamorous because of their inherent hours. Setting a specific time limit makes the position more appealing, and the professional rewards of achieving personal goals often offset the difficulties.

Preparing for the Job Interview

CASE STUDY

Two weeks ago, you submitted a letter of application and your curriculum vitae to two different hospitals for a nurse manager position. The first position is in a unit of a large metropolitan hospital across town, and the second is in the unit where you have been employed as a staff nurse for the past three years. Both positions are in 12-bed cardiac units. Both interviews are next week. What should you do to prepare for your interview?

For a successful interview, the first thing to do is perform a self-evaluation.[14] Through self-evaluation, accurate and effective assessment of past and present achievement provides the building blocks of future development. The questions that a prospective nurse manager needs to ask include:

- Why did I choose nursing as a profession?
- Why did I choose critical care nursing as a specialty?
- How have I demonstrated leadership and professional growth in each of the positions that I have held?
- Can I articulate at least one accomplishment for each position that I have held?
- Were job changes made for "progressive experiences" or were they lateral moves made for personal reasons?
- How do I keep current and broaden my knowledge in critical care nursing?
- What is my ultimate career objective?
- How is my present job contributing toward my career objective?
- What is my self-concept of my nursing and leadership potential?
- Have others supported this perception?

The second step in preparation for an interview is to list questions you have about the institution and the unit. If you can find answers to the more basic questions before the interview, not only will you save time, you will also enable higher-level questions. A career-minded individual answers the following questions *before* being interviewed:

- How many beds are there in the institution?
- What is the occupancy rate?
- What is the medical and nursing hierarchical structure?
- What is the method of nursing care delivery? Is it uniformly practiced throughout the institution?
- Is the professional nursing staff unionized? Is there a union for the nonprofessionals?
- What is the nursing vacancy rate? What was it each of the past two years? What is it in critical care? in your unit? What contributes to the nursing shortage in this institution?
- Are agency nurses used in the institution? in critical care? in your unit? What is the ratio of full-time staff to agency nurses?
- What is the type of orientation program available?
- What types of ongoing staff development are available?
- Are there specific in-house programs for critical care?
- Do nurses float from unit to unit?

The third step of the interview preparations is to develop a list of questions pertaining to the actual job itself. This list should go above and beyond contractual sorts of things (i.e., job title, salary, and benefits).[9] Start by asking about the role of the staff nurse in the unit, and then about the role of management. Questions that provide a better understanding of how nurses at the bedside are perceived include:

- What is the philosophy of the nursing department?
- Is there centralized or decentralized decision making?
- To what extent is there staff nurse participation in management decisions?

Management role questions include:

- Where is this position on the organizational chart? Who reports to me and to whom do I report?
- What will a typical shift be like for me?
- What types of support staff are available (i.e., secretaries, unit managers, patient transport/escort, computers)?

The Interview

Take the day of the interview off so you can devote your full attention to the interview. Your appearance is important to the first impression given to a prospective employer. However, be sure that appearance is not the *only* impression left with a prospective employer. It is recommended that business attire be worn.

Sufficient preparation fosters confidence before the interview process. Remember that the interview is an important information source for both the interviewer and interviewee.[14] Questions and responses of the prospective employer and employee enables both of them to arrive at an informed decision.

Generally, the interviewer may ask any question that pertains to the applicant's suitability for the job. It is within the interviewer's legal rights to ask about the applicant's previous employment. Questions such as "Why are you leaving your present position?" or "What types of references would I receive from previous employers?" are appropriate. The interviewer may also ask about the applicant's sick time pattern.

Any question that discriminates against any potential hire is illegal.[14] Questions that should not be asked by the interviewer and which you have no legal obligation to answer include:

- In what year were you born?
- What are the ages of your children?
- Do you plan to have more children?
- What are your child care arrangements?
- Do you plan to move?
- What is your marital status?
- What are the surnames of each of your parents?
- What church/synagogue do you attend?
- Where do you do your banking?

If one of these questions is posed by the interviewer, be direct and state that the question is an illegal one and one that you are not required to answer. If the interviewer feels that it is within her rights to ask the question, either party may choose to end the interview. However, if the interviewer admits to a mistake, the interviewee should accept the apology and allow the interviewer to proceed to the next question.

Selecting the Right Unit

Once the field of hospitals is narrowed to two, how does one choose the best unit? Vestal[15] suggests making a list of positives and negatives for each position by rating the size and location of the institution, job content, colleagues and superiors, opportunities for advancement, and financial and benefit package. Accept a position at the hospital where the list of positives and negatives best meets personal goals and desires. Of paramount importance is the awareness of how each position would benefit the career path.

FUNCTIONS OF NURSE MANAGER

CASE STUDY

> You have accepted the position of nurse manager in the unit where you have been employed for the past three years. At a leadership meeting, you participate in a discussion about hiring practices. For the past two years only nurses with at least one year of medical or surgical experience have been hired for this unit. Having been a former new graduate in critical care, you believe that new graduates with no previous full-time graduate experience could do well with the proper support. You would like to change the hiring practice because of the limited number of available experienced staff. Your supervisor asks if you are willing to chair an ad hoc committee to explore hiring practices. You agree to this.

Hiring Practice

The nurse manager must clearly delineate the characteristics of new graduates who do well in critical care. Generally, seek out applicants who have actual nursing exposure gained through a student preceptor program, or through licensed practical nurse or nurse aide experience. In addition, look for applicants who can clearly articulate their reasons for choosing critical care nursing.

The support of the staff education department is needed during the orientation process so the needs of the new graduate are met. A *preceptor program* is frequently utilized as a method of orientation. Assimilation of new graduates is facilitated by having one consistent preceptor rather than multiple "buddies." The problems encountered by new graduates during orientation are predictable and should be anticipated by the educator in charge of orientation in order to deal with them effectively. For example, the orientee's fear of being alone during a cardiac arrest can be alleviated simply by reassuring all orientees that they will not be alone in the unit.

The support of the nursing staff is crucial to effective orientation and integration of new graduates. If staff have never been involved in the orientation of new graduates to critical care, immediately begin small group discussions to determine their needs. For example, a special program to train preceptors may be warranted that outlines the things the new graduate must know. Encourage staff to draw positive parallels from their own experience as new graduates. Seek out the most supportive staff members and carefully plan staff meetings so that at least one of them is present to influence the discussions positively. Many successful critical care nursing staffs blend new graduates with experienced practitioners; they often work harmoniously as a team and are open to change.

Retaining Staff

Nursing staff retention has been and continues to be a top priority for nursing departments in institutions of varying size. Fain[3] and Kramer and Schmalenberg[6,7] have chosen to use the characteristics identified by Peters and Waterman[10] in their book *In Search of Excellence*. In comparing nursing excellence to the best-run companies in the corporate community, the assumption is made that nursing excellence will attract and retain excellent nurses. Institutions that have no difficulty attracting and retaining staff fall into the category of institutions of excellence.

The use of in-house transfers can help institutions improve staff retention. Sometimes, however, poor performers are just shuffled around, rather than counseled to seek employment elsewhere, because the hospital does not want to lose another nurse. In institutions of excellence, a transfer is a reward for good performance.[6,7]

Another common staff retention strategy is financial remuneration. Staff retention is enhanced when salary is competitive within the geographic area. However, this does not mean the salary must be the highest in the area. At many institutions of excellence, clinical ladders or credentials tied to performance, rather than longevity, are used as the bases for salary increases.[6,7]

In light of the nursing shortage, Marquis[8] identified the "revolving door syndrome," which is characterized by nurses' increasing dissatisfaction as awareness rises that jobs are plentiful. Consequently, retention becomes even more difficult. Marquis suggested that strategies enhancing recruitment, interviewing, and selection should improve retention.

Staff input in the interview process is invaluable. It is beneficial to have prospective employees spend time alone with senior staff members so that questions regarding day-to-day unit operations can be answered from the staff's perspective. This provides the prospective staff member with a more realistic idea of the commitment made by accepting the offer of employment in the critical care unit. Furthermore, the senior staff member will have the satisfaction of involvement in the interviewing process.

The nurse manager plays an important role in staff retention.[11] All practitioners have known nurse managers who are great role models, as well as some who are the antitheses of what role models should be. Cox,[2] talking about nurse managers, asked, "Does the head nurse grow staff or control staff?" To be effective, the nurse manager should understand the needs of all staff members so that the appropriate management approach to each situation is chosen.

Reducing Turnover

Prestholdt and colleagues[12] said that reducing nurse turnover is challenging because attrition is not caused by any one factor. They found three factors that are predictors of resignation: attitude, social pressure, and moral commitment. In addition, four categories of beliefs about the consequences of resigning or staying were identified: nursing practice, alternative options, work environment, and economics. Quite simply, nurses stay at institutions where they like their jobs and feel they have control over their practices. Nurses are most satisfied when their jobs are challenging, interesting, and meaningful.

Institutions that retain staff have certain characteristics including a spirit of teamwork and cooperation that begins at the top. Immediate supervisors are in touch with all staff members, and instill in them not only a sense of self-worth but a sense that the work they do is integral to the smooth functioning of the unit. Nurses feel there may be no other institution that will treat them better interpersonally or financially. Nurses want to come to work because their experience there brings them personal satisfaction—it is not just a job.

Levels of Nursing Management

There are usually three levels in the nursing hierarchy of each unit. The first level is a position that encompasses eight-hour responsibility and accountability that is often referred to as *shift management*. Traditionally available solely on evening and night shifts, they recently have also been established on the day shift. The titles given this role include *charge nurse* and *assistant head nurse*.

The second level in nursing management is a position historically referred to as *head nurse*. Many institutions, in an effort to be more progressive, have changed the title to *clinical supervisor, patient care coordinator,* or *nurse manager*. Second-level management positions include 24-hour responsibility and accountability for a discernable unit of patients and staff. In critical care, this is usually a specific unit such as coronary care or surgical intensive care.

The third level of nursing management usually carries the title of *director, assistant director,* or *associate director* of a defined group of nursing units. The group of critical care nursing units usually comprises all of the institution's intensive care units; occasionally, however, some subspecialties are excluded: the emergency department, the postanesthesia care unit, the neurosurgical unit, and the pediatric intensive care unit. The third-level nurse manager generally reports to the director or vice president of nursing. The director of critical care is responsible and accountable for initiating institutional goals, and implementing and evaluating long-range goals that concern all of the units. The director delegates the responsibility for activities to be achieved to the various nurse managers.[4]

For example, at a department meeting, the vice president of nursing asks all clinical directors to explore case management as a method to help with recruitment and retention. To operationalize this plan, the third-level nurse manager (the critical care clinical director) is ultimately responsible for development and implementation, and so she clearly delineates the activities needed to achieve each goal, and delegates the responsibility and accountability for each activity to nurse managers.

Leadership Styles

Many leadership styles have been described; often quoted is McGregor's Theory X and Theory Y. Theory X views employees as generally indolent, irresponsible, and in need of close supervision; Theory Y views employees as motivated, concerned, creative, and desirous of an optimal degree of control over the workplace.[4] One can view leadership styles as a continuum with an employee-centered style on one end, and a task- or goal-centered style on the other. Effective leaders achieve an appropriate balance on this continuum. Ongoing self-evaluation of leadership style and fit within the unit structure fosters a sense of belonging and makes goal achievement clearer.

The nurse manager can make significant contributions to change.

CASE STUDY

> As a new nurse manager you recognize that the task of time planning could be shared with staff, who you believe would be motivated by their greater degree of control. You have proposed to your superior that you pilot a system of self-time-planning for your staff. She gives her approval.

Before beginning to make this change, self-assessment is important. What should be the initial thoughts of the nurse manager? It would be appropriate to reflect on how the director allows each nurse manager to plan her own time. Ask if this approach can be used by the staff. What types of constraints are present? What is the rationale for each constraint? What is the purpose or goal of self-time-planning?

If the nurse manager finds that the director's guidelines for self-time-planning work, they could be the model for developing staff self-time-planning. If, however, the nurse manager believes the director's guidelines are not helpful or specific enough, is it because her management philosophy differs from that of the director? If so, do they complement each other, resulting in the "best of both worlds" for the staff? Or are they in direct conflict? Can staff live with this direct conflict of management philosophies?

Often teamwork is facilitated when there is mix of personality types with different leadership styles. The best chosen subordinates may be those who complement the manager's leadership style. On these units where there is a mix, managers and subordinates will all be found working harmoniously toward a common goal with a great deal of job satisfaction.

Managerial Job Types

Mintzberg's study of managerial job types helps one to understand the role of the nurse manager and the director of critical care within the context of the organization.[5] Kirsch adapted Mintzberg's eight types to describe nurse managers: Contact Person, Political Manager, Entrepreneur, Insider, Real Time Manager, Team Manager, Expert, and New Manager[5].

The critical care nurse manager who creates a name for herself and the institution she represents by being highly visible within professional organizations and the community can be considered a *Contact Person.* The *Political Manager* is usually savvy about key figures and is the person often selected to negotiate sensitive issues related to critical care or to the institution as a whole. The trailblazing critical care nurse manager is an *Entrepreneur.* She is only interested in initiating or implementing change and will feel frustrated if thwarted in her efforts. The critical care nurse manager with a strong institutional allegiance is an *Insider.* Because of her tenure she often possesses a wealth of information about the policies and procedures in place and the strengths and weaknesses of other individuals. The *Real Time Manager* is the critical care nurse manager who tries to have input into every task and committee. Although appropriate in head nurse and assistant head nurse positions, this managerial type is problematic when found in higher levels of more centralized structures. Because critical care requires coordination of groups of highly skilled experts, the *Team Manager* is very important. The *New Manager* wants to establish a territory and work on a personal project.

Knowing this, the nurse manager could ask the following questions: Which of these managerial types and functions are used by the director? Which are used by the nurse manager? Are there any not used? Does this detract from the smooth functioning of the unit?

Ideally, the job types of the director and manager are complementary. For example, if a New (nurse) Manager wishes to implement a project, the director might act as a Political Manager to obtain administrative approval for it. Likewise, the Entrepreneur (nurse) manager who wants to use her critical care nursing staff in a community-based project will need the support of her superior–the Contact Person to implement this project successfully.

Managing Staff

One of the most important functions of the nurse manager is setting the tone or workplace philosophy for the unit. Setting the tone or workplace philosophy must be deliberately planned and executed; it should not be allowed to happen by chance.[1]

CASE STUDY

As the nurse manager of a 12-bed cardiac care unit, you have noticed that the number of medical patients admitted to the unit is increasing. The nursing staff is becoming more and more dissatisfied with this situation. The medical director has stated that this trend will continue into the foreseeable future because of the shortage of medical critical care beds.

This nurse manager should first carefully examine her own attitudes about medical patient admissions to the cardiac care unit. The nurse manager's explicit and implicit attitudes affect the staff's attitudes. Then the nurse manager should address the staff's attitudes in a direct and positive manner.

The next consideration is the staff's knowledge base. Is the staff's reluctance to have medical patients in the cardiac care unit related to their lack of knowledge of medical patients' nursing care needs? Does the staff feel that medical patients are not as "exciting" to care for as cardiac patients? Address this issue through nursing rounds and/or patient care conferences. It may be worthwhile to employ a multidisciplinary approach or clinical experts to enhance the educational opportunity.

Fostering Excellence

Fostering excellence, part of setting the tone or workplace philosophy is a major responsibility of the nurse manager.[1] This is commonly accomplished through role modeling. To be a role model the critical care nurse manager must be an expert clinician.

CASE STUDY

As the nurse manager of the cardiac intensive care unit, you have been notified that the hospital has just been approved to perform cardiac transplants. How will you prepare the staff for this new challenge?

Preparation includes identifying all aspects of needed resources, such as educational plans, personnel, and equipment. All of these must be in place before the first cardiac transplant patient arrives in the unit. Throughout the planning phase and into the execution phase, it is imperative that the nurse manager become aware of all the nursing care needs of cardiac transplant patients, so the staff can have all the available resources necessary for delivering excellence in patient care. Once the program begins, it is the responsibility of the nurse manager to carefully monitor the signals indicating a need for practice changes as the staff gains experience. The goal remains constant: to promote excellence in patient care.

Certification and education, career ladders, and nursing research foster excellence in patient care.[1] The cost of certification and educational endeavors should be reimbursed and time off should be allowed. Certification in critical care nursing (CCRN) is administered through the American Association of Critical Care Nurses Certification Corporation. Support for this is easily achieved. For example, those critical care nursing departments that sponsor a core curriculum review program in preparation for the certification examination demonstrate their commitment to excellence.

Educational endeavors include continuing education, which can be obtained through in-house and outside conferences, as well as formal education, where staff may be pursuing baccalaureate, master's, or doctoral degrees in nursing. For those staff members who attend continuing education in critical care nursing, forums can be designed that promote sharing of new knowledge and allow designing changes in current nursing practice based on this new knowledge. The critical care nurse manager can negotiate a work schedule with those in degree-granting programs to allow fulfillment of school and work obligations.

Many institutions have clinical or career ladders that recognize excellence in patient care by granting different titles, greater responsibility, and higher salaries—all of which encourage nurses to remain at the bedside. Nursing career ladders may have anywhere from three to six levels with generic practice criteria clearly delineated for each level. Experience should be a prerequisite for promotion, not a criteria. The critical care nurse manager fosters clinical ladder movement for the staff and works with senior staff who are interested in a career ladder move.

To make the evaluation process more objective, specific competency-based criteria for promotion are needed for each specialty. These criteria are based on the established department practice standards. The critical care nurse manager involves staff in the formulation of criteria for each level of the career ladder. Once criteria are established, a program to inform all staff is instituted.

Participation in nursing research is becoming an integral part of nursing departments that strive for excellence in patient care. "Research" includes applying research findings to nursing practice, identifying potential research areas, participating in the research, developing research projects, and writing grants. Some institutions have a full-time nurse researcher that acts as a resource and clearinghouse for all nursing areas. Others have agreements with local nursing schools to provide expert advice on nursing research. The critical care manager, regardless of the setting, is responsible for keeping current in research findings and methodology to be able to assist the staff in applying results to their practice.

NURSE MANAGER IN CRITICAL CARE

The nurse manager is one of the most vital links within the critical care nursing department structure.[1] The critical care nurse manager is the clinical expert in the unit for common patient problems. It is her responsibility to ensure that safe, high quality nursing care is delivered to each patient by her expert understanding of each patient's nursing care needs. The nurse manager knows the resources available to the staff that are needed to update their knowledge, refine their skills, and prepare them for competent management of unusual patient care problems.

The nurse manager must also be thoroughly familiar with each staff member's abilities. This is accomplished through direct observation, peer review, patient or family feedback, and review of nursing documentation. The nurse manager remains highly visible to staff and patients with planned and unplanned time for clinical interaction.

Knowledge of patient care needs and staff capabilities enables the critical care nurse manager to perform the important function of making patient assignments. Some managers choose to delegate this task. Carefully planned assignments that match patient care needs with staff strengths contribute to excellence in patient care.

The nurse manager's primary goal is to ensure that all the equipment and supplies necessary to allow staff to deliver excellent nursing care are plentiful and accessible. Second, the nurse manager makes sure all appropriate equipment is available, well maintained, and in proper working order, and develops mechanisms that provide around-the-clock service (or back-up equipment). Finally, the hospital ancillary personnel's responsibilities in the critical care unit must be clearly delineated in well-defined job descriptions that are developed with some nursing input, even for personnel in nonnursing areas such as building service, dietary, and respiratory care. To enhance smooth integration with nursing and help solve mutual problems, the critical care nurse manager must develop good working relationships with her counterparts in each of these ancillary departments.

The nurse manager represents the unit favorably within the institution by carefully selecting staff members of nursing and interdisciplinary committees, and by providing a positive voice in decisions about activities and policies that directly affect the unit. For example, the unit should have input into infection control policies and quality assurance activities. Staff meetings with the medical director of the unit are planned and coordinated for maximum communication. Interdisciplinary collaboration with respiratory therapy, dietary, and social services can be beneficial.

Managing Critical Care Nursing Professionals

Over time, critical care nursing is probably one of the most labor-intensive and knowledge-intensive nursing subspecialties.[1] Because some of nursing's brightest and most assertive professionals are drawn to critical care, the challenge of managing a staff of knowledgeable professionals is exciting.

The nurse manager assists the staff in achieving high-quality patient care by appropriately using motivation, delegation, and direction. Motivation is a subjective internal force that cannot be created; it can only be increased by appealing to the employee's pride or sense of professionalism.[1]

CASE STUDY

You are a critical care nurse manager who wishes to develop the documentation of case management. Your goals include (1) Each patient will have a patient-specific care plan developed and updated by his or her case manager, and (2) the patient's response to the care plan will be documented by each nurse assigned to the patient. How will you engender staff motivation?

First, the nurse manager helps the staff determine workable, relevant care plans. Begin by holding a patient care conference in which staff assist the case manager in developing a patient care plan for a particularly challenging patient. Once the staff has seen that care plans are workable and relevant, they will begin to think about developing care plans for their own caseload.

Next, the nurse manager may wish to reward outstanding care plans. This can serve a twofold purpose: to enhance the staff member's sense of pride, and to provide a role model for others. The nurse manager may wish to establish objective criteria with the staff for the Care Plan of the Week award. Each week the case manager whose care plan best meets the criteria wins the award.

Barnum and Mallard[1] stated: "Delegation consists of several elements: what gets delegated, to whom, how it gets delegated, and how it is monitored or controlled." As management is often described as "getting the job done through others," effective delegation is a crucial management function.

The most common and the most concrete form of delegation is the job description—it contains all of the elements associated with delegation. However, it is the *uncommon* forms of delegation that are the most challenging to the critical care nurse manager because all of the elements must be clearly defined. The most common pitfall in effective delegation is the inability to articulate all elements clearly. For example, although nurse managers have 24-hour accountability and responsibility, they traditionally have worked 8-hour day shifts. Thus, shift managers are delegated the responsibility of following through on those changes initiated by the nurse manager.

Communication

Effective management requires excellent communication skills. The universal communication model consists of a *sender* who encodes a *message* that is sent through a *medium* or *vehicle* to the *receiver*. Each part of this chain is crucial to effective communication. The sender begins the chain by setting the goal that communication will take place. The next link in the chain is the development of a message that will achieve the goal of communication. Once that is established, the appropriate vehicle for the communication is selected. And, finally, the message is received, and a response, if indicated, is made.

COMMUNICATING WITH SUPERIORS
CASE STUDY

    As the nurse manager you want to establish a support group for the families of the patients in the unit. The nurse manager makes an appointment to discuss the idea with the director.

The effectiveness of the sender's message is influenced by her positive and negative personal biases: Why was the idea initiated? How will the staff be involved in this endeavor? Who can complete a literature search on family support in critical care? Does any staff member have previous experience in this area?

The next step in this communication is to encode the idea using an appropriate medium to convey the message. In this example, verbal communication will allow the nurse manager to be most effective. The nurse manager enhances the effectiveness of the verbal presentation by including a written plan of action.

The director of critical care is the receiver of the communication. The director also brings positive and negative biases: What has been the previous experience with this manager? Are ideas carefully thought out and creative? How much support will the nurse manager need? In addition, as the receiver of communication, the director provides the head nurse with solicited and unsolicited feedback. If the manager submits a written plan of action, the director may find that this facilitates the provision of written, as well as verbal, constructive criticism.

COMMUNICATING WITH PEERS AND COLLEAGUES
CASE STUDY

The critical care nurse manager wants to institute a unit dose system similar to systems on other nursing units.

The importance of communications with other nurse managers cannot be overemphasized. As a sender of communication, the critical care nurse manager must first gather information from nurse managers on other nursing units about their unit dose systems. Second, the critical care nurse manager meets formally and informally with the staff regarding their needs in a unit dose system.

After receiving approval from the director, the nurse manager finally meets with pharmacy management to devise a system both will find workable. There is often much written and verbal communication between the critical care nurse manager and the pharmacy manager as the system is planned, instituted, and evaluated. Mechanisms for ongoing evaluation of the system are crucial. The critical care nursing staff provides feedback on how the system is working so that the nurse manager can continue to have open dialogue with pharmacy on tailoring a system that meets the staff's needs.

COMMUNICATING WITH PHYSICIANS

The critical care nurse manager can be a highly visible role model for the staff in nurse/physician communication. For example, a staff nurse approaches the manager and states she believes her patient needs a Swan Ganz catheter for better fluid balance management. The staff nurse asks the manager for advice on approaching the physician. The manager helps the nurse gather all pertinent information, including recent medical and nursing research that supports her opinion. The manager suggests the most appropriate forum to air these views, rehearses the key points with the staff nurse, and supports her when she addresses the physician.

COMMUNICATING IN GROUPS

The most common group interaction for the critical care nurse manager is staff meetings. For the new critical care nurse manager this may be one of the more intimidating aspects of the job. The box below lists some basic guidelines for staff meetings.

GUIDELINES FOR STAFF MEETINGS

- Hold staff meetings at regular intervals
- Have staff generate agenda items
- Encourage staff to chair staff meetings
- Limit meetings to one hour
- Post minutes in a timely manner.

Most critical care nurse managers meet with their staff once a month. The date should be planned far in advance so that scheduling can accommodate attendance. Because it is not possible for the entire staff to attend every staff meeting, care should be taken to ensure that there is a rotation of staff who are not able to attend the staff meetings.

It is worthwhile for the critical care nurse manager to post the agenda prior to the meeting and then allow the staff to add agenda items. This helps organize the staff agenda. To promote leadership development in the staff, the critical care nurse manager encourages staff to chair the meeting. The method for choosing the staff chairperson will vary, but any method agreed upon by the critical care nurse manager and the staff fosters involvement.

A time limit of one hour for each meeting may be set to avoid time waste associated with longer nonproductive meetings. If practice/policy change is discussed, ample time for reading the minutes should be given before implementation of the change.

Another opportunity for the critical care nurse manager to participate in group communication with the staff is the development of unit-based quality assurance activities. The nurse manager or designee chairs the unit's committee. In this capacity, the nurse manager oversees all of the unit's quality assurance activities. In addition, the critical care nurse manager represents the unit in the central nursing department's quality assurance activities. This ensures that the unit's interests are served by any central quality assurance decisions.

CONCLUSION

In this chapter the reader has been given techniques for developing a career plan. Information about exploring options, finding the right unit, working with peers and superiors, and using communication skills were identified. Career goals are more readily met by those nurse managers who choose to establish career plans.

REFERENCES

1. Barnum BS and Mallard CO: Essentials of nursing management: concepts and contexts of practice. Rockville, Md., 1989, Aspen Publishers, Inc.

2. Cox SH: Retention of staff: the head nurse connection, Current Concepts in Nursing 2(5):3-7, 1988.
3. Fain JA: Nursing excellence—lessons from America's best-run companies, Nursing Forum 22(4):153-156, 1985.
4. Hardy OB and McWhorter RC: Management decisions: new challenges of the mind, Rockville, Md., 1988, Aspen Publishers, Inc.
5. Kirsch J: The middle manager and the nursing organization: human resources, fiscal resources, Norwalk, Conn. 1988, Appleton and Lange.
6. Kramer M and Schmalenberg C: Magnet hospitals: part I, institutions of excellence, Journal of Nursing Administration 18(1):13-24, 1988.
7. Kramer M and Schmalenberg C: Magnet hospitals: part II, institutions of excellence, Journal of Nursing Administration 18(2):11-19, 1988.
8. Marquis B: Attrition: the effectiveness of retention activities, Journal of Nursing Administration 18(3):25-29, 1988.
9. Muir J: Hiring and firing: the ins and outs, Nursing Times 82(32):38-40, 1986.
10. Peters TJ and Waterman RH Jr: In search of excellence, New York, 1982, Harper & Row.
11. Prescott P and Bowen S: Controlling nursing turnover, Nursing Management 18(6):60-66, 1987.
12. Prestholdt PH, Lane IM, and Matthews RC: Predicting staff turnover, Nursing Outlook 36(3):145-147, 1988.
13. Price SA, Simms LM, and Pforitz SK: Career advancement of nurse executives: planned or accidental? Nursing Outlook 35(5):236-238, 1987.
14. Swansburg RC and Swansburg PW: Strategic career planning and development for nurses, Rockville, Md., 1984, Aspen Publishers, Inc.
15. Vestal K: Management concepts for the new nurse, St. Louis, 1987, JB Lippincott.

Chapter 2

A Climate for Caring

Georgita Tolbert Washington

Managing a critical care unit involves more than following rules, regulations, policies, and procedures. The creative and innovative critical care nurse manager enlists the assistance and support of the nursing staff to create a caring environment. Communication tools, negotiation concerns, retention emphasis, safe and competent patient care, family involvement in patient care, physical environment, and staff caring for each other are the components of a climate for caring explored and developed in this chapter. To illustrate key points, a case study is included at the end of the chapter. It involves the staff's identification of a unit concern, their exploration and development of ideas related to the concern, and the nurse manager's use of management techniques to assist the nursing staff's resolution.

IDENTIFYING UNIT NEEDS

Managing a critical care unit begins with determining what is needed to function effectively. Patients, families, and staff require a caring, nurturing, supportive environment. Providing a caring climate can have a positive influence on all people in the area.

The critical care manager must first assess the behavioral characteristics of the staff by identifying personality types, maturity levels, and motivating factors that influence their behaviors. With this assessment, the nurse manager can predict staff behavior and anticipate their responses.[5]

Both age and opportunity contribute to the maturity level of each individual, which is assessed in terms of experience. If the factors that motivate staff to perform are understood, they can be applied to help achieve established unit goals.

The personality composition of the unit staff can be learned through communication. Planned staff meetings facilitate information transfer between manager and staff. Informal staff meetings with flexible agendas make it easier for staff to express their ideas and thoughts. The informal approach allows the staff to talk about their needs, and shows them that you value their individual contributions. Rigid, formal meetings with strict agendas may stifle and discourage free expression.

The nurse manager's observations can be very informative. Staff conversations often disclose unidentified needs. Monitoring personalities in action helps discovery of individual strengths and weaknesses, identifies how well staff interact among themselves and with others, and helps predict how individuals will function in a variety of situations.

Identify informal leaders. These persons usually initiate or direct most of the unit non-patient-care activities, which can be either constructive, such as presenting inservices, or destructive, such as perpetuating gossip. These leaders are those whose opinions are sought most often by their peers and whose practices are most often followed.

If the staff helps decide what is necessary to have a productive and efficient critical care unit, they may take more interest in creating a climate for caring. In addition to staff input, patient and family input is important. Discharge surveys of patients and families can help identify what would make critical care admissions less anxiety-producing. (Staff should help develop these surveys.) The manager shares both the positive and the negative survey responses with the staff, because this feedback encourages growth and change.

Discussions with other nursing managers and leaders reveal outside perceptions about the unit. Often those not directly associated with the unit can contribute constructive, objective suggestions. The manager can weigh these and initiate change based on suggestions congruent with unit goals. The perceptions of external observers are important tools for assessment of the unit image.

Effective communication is bidirectional. The manager and staff must be able to speak with and listen to each other. All staff have something to offer and are encouraged to express themselves. The nurse manager's action on the staff's ideas demonstrates the value the manager places on these ideas.

Communication from the manager is effective when purposeful, authentic, valid, and reliable. Therefore, planned meetings and ongoing verbal interaction are needed. The manager's visibility on the unit is very important. Managers who are always in the office or at meetings miss interacting spontaneously with the staff. Staff mailboxes, unit communication books, organized bulletin boards, and timely performance evaluations help keep the lines of communication open,[11] as do posted office hours and an open door policy. A suggestion box allows a central collection point for (anonymous) spontaneous ideas. If unit evaluations are included in orientation manuals, problems, needs, and ideas of the new employees who have fresh, different perspectives can be identified.

MAKING ASSIGNMENTS

Patient acuity, staff experience and individual strengths, available resources, and learning experiences for staff growth are considered when making patient assignments. Combining these considerations with staff preferences, care continuity and patient needs requires the nurse manager's good judgment and decision making.

An assignment that gives the most critically ill patients only to the experienced nurses limits the practical learning opportunities of less experienced nurses, and contributes to overload and burnout of the more experienced nurses. Instead, *buddy* two nurses with two patients. When a less experienced nurse is assigned to a more critically ill patient, and an experienced nurse is given a lighter assignment, the experienced nurse can act as a preceptor and resource person to the less experienced nurse. This will increase the knowledge base of the entire nursing staff and build the confidence of less experienced staff. Staff new to the unit or just recently out of orientation also require special consideration. Expose them to controlled learning as their confidence increases by assigning a preceptor or buddy. Careful planning precludes overload, burnout, and resignation before the new nurse learns the system.

When making assignments the nurse manager considers both logistics and the unit's physical layout, so that each nurse remains in a specific geographical area. This facilitates patient monitoring and meets patient needs. This type of planning is best in units with glass windows, walls, or curtains between patients. When dealing with open units, the nurse manager must consider the sight lines and the distance between patient and supplies so the nurse is never too far away from her patients.

When patient needs dictate, float nurses are used in the unit. Plan carefully so that the float nurse is assigned to the most stable patients. Care of the critically ill is difficult enough without nurses' having to work in unfamiliar areas. Assigning a resource person to assist the float nurse with unusual routines or procedures helps ensure quality patient care.

Consider infection control when making assignments. If possible, septic patients should not be assigned to a nurse who is also caring for postoperative or very debilitated patients. Even when isolation precautions and handwashing protocols are strictly followed, nosocomial infections do occur. Therefore, it is best to assign separate nurses to these different kinds of patients. Well thought out assignments show patients, staff, and physicians that you care.

DECISION MAKING

A critical care nurse manager must have good judgment and good decision-making skills. As an experienced practitioner, the manager knows that the staff will observe, evaluate, and comment on the decisions she has made. Therefore, the manager is always expected to demonstrate the best technique, to use critical thinking, and to be able to defend her position on issues. Accepting accountability for the consequences of these decisisions goes with the responsibility of leadership.[7,8] Learning the skills needed to make the right decisions takes time.

The manager sets priorities, goals, and objectives based on the needs identified with the staff. Then the manager and the staff implement plans to reach these goals. Use logical, fact-based reasoning in making decisions; they should be made intellectually, never emotionally. Some decisions can have a negative influence on the staff and the unit. You must be aware of this to develop good decision-making skills. Accepting negative results, reevaluating the plan, and moving ahead will engender growth, which should be expected whenever unsatisfactory results are identified.

At certain times, decision making can be very difficult, and timing is of the essence. When is the right time to approach a nurse or physician about their professional conduct, lack of patient follow-up, or personal practices that interfere with job performance? Should nothing be done? Although deciding not to act is an option, any identified problem has already been noticed by others who will then judge your response to the problem. A manager cannot be intimidated by this, but can address problems in a timely fashion.

In human interactions, there will always be someone who disagrees with a decision. Although sometimes effective management and popularity are mutually exclusive, the manager should still explain the rationale of her decision to those who disagree. Having made the decision does not mean that no rational alternative can be considered. The effective manager always remains open to modifying her decisions.

Facilitate decentralized decision making. Decentralization encourages decision making at lower management levels. Staff-level decisions that are supported and encouraged by the nurse manager raise morale, which promotes professional growth, enhances personal satisfaction and increases the quality of patient care. This may happen without increasing costs.

Staff who serve as charge nurses often feel insecure about the decision-making aspects of the role. A manager can prevent this anxiety by establishing helpful guidelines for behavior. Teach staff to collaborate on tough decisions. When two staff nurses fully discuss a problem and agree that a decision is correct for patients in a particular set of circumstances, the manager should fully support that decision. This eliminates the fear of making a bad decision, shows that you expect the staff to work together, and tells them that when you are gone, they are capable of making good decisions. This also has a positive effect that denotes caring.

NEGOTIATION

Skillful negotiation is an art that the nurse manager learns and hones. To do it well, you must collect the facts needed to argue convincingly. Needs identified in the unit assessment must be stated clearly and directly. A proposal outlining the plan to implement a program lends credibility to the manager's position. Negotiations can be used to find a common ground between the unit's and the organization's needs.[1]

Unit manager–peer communication often results in negotiation, when one manager tries to think as the other manager might think considering the request from the other point of view. Both points of view are equally important.[10] Therefore, when managers agree on the same basic goals, they expect give-and-take between themselves. Successful negotiation usually results in concessions, but both parties will consider it worthwhile if the results benefit both.

At times, for example, bargaining with staff is necessary; extra staff are needed for an increase in patient census or acuity. A day off or a more favorable shift may be given for working unexpectedly when needed. However, the considerate nurse manager remembers that undue pressure to work overtime may meet the immediate need, but can destroy the staff's belief that the manager cares. The manager avoids this by always asking if it is convenient to work the additional shift; if not, she goes on to the next person. Reasonable requests for overtime are met more fully by staff who believe the manager cares about them and recognizes their right to meet personal needs.

NETWORKING

Within the nursing department itself, the nurse manager is responsible for creating a network that facilitates positive interchange. The image of the unit within the institution is influenced beneficially by interactions between unit staff and other nursing personnel. The nurse manager seeks out opportunities to exchange ideas with other department leaders when department structure permits.

Often the education department is a separate department that assists the unit with orientation and staff development. Formally acknowledging the education department's role and praising their contributions is a good practice. The education department helps meet educational needs. Let the department know what these needs are; perhaps existing programs can be revised, or new programs developed.

The nurse manager and education department manager may be able to devise some creative methods to help staff grow. For example, they could find some way to provide time for education and development during the times that patient acuity and workload are increasing. Instructors could give programs in the unit, instead of having staff leave the unit for classes. A committee of staff nurses assembled to give educational presentations on their own units might stimulate growth. The education department's expertise would be used in the teaching plan and developmental material, and the regular instructors would give moral support during the presentation. Presentations could either be given at scheduled intervals or be taped so they can be played back on all shifts. The result of this support is help in meeting staff educational needs and hospital requirements.[12]

If the critical care nurse manager encourages participation in the staff's self-development, the critical care unit has the potential to be a model that encourages other units' participation in educational development, and that assists the education department in achieving its goals and objectives. The unit could develop a reputation for caring within the hospital as word spreads about the peer support.

Similarly, the nurse manager assesses the unit's working relationship with other units that exchange patients with the critical care area. Concern for the Emergency Department (ED), awareness of their special problems, and attempts to accept patients as quickly as possible will set the tone of caring between the units. When the critical care unit cannot quickly accept a patient because of a unit problem (such as a cardiac arrest), the ED staff in turn is more inclined to understand and be patient. This is especially true if the manager expects her staff to inform the ED of the problem, apologize, and then contact the ED as soon as the transfer is possible.

In the surgical critical care unit, the relationship with the Post-Anesthesia Care Unit (PACU) is important. Most areas have developed transfer times that facilitate smooth patient transition. The critical care nurse manager needs to spend time with the PACU staff to understand the routine demands placed on that staff by the Operating Room (OR).

Medical-surgical floors also require attention. Premature transfer to the unit may result from fear of dealing with the critically ill. This fear is also why nursing staff are often reluctant to accept a long-term critical care transfer. Discuss these problems with the medical-surgical nurse manager. Explore the potential of having the critical care staff as part of the code response team, or offer to teach tracheostomy care to a new medical staff nurse. After giving report to the floor nurse who will be caring for the transfer patient, accompany the patient to the new floor and introduce patient, family, and nurse. This enhances continuity of care. This also bolsters the confidence of the patient and family. By taking a supportive, helpful position, the manager sets the expectation for the staff and conveys a caring message to non-critical-care staff.

ANCILLARY SUPPORT

Marketing the critical care area to ancillary services so they will provide services involves creativity. The critical care area deserves their very best, timely efforts, as do all nursing units. To encourage good working relationships, explain how they have helped the unit. Ancillary departments should understand that the critical care unit does not compete with the other units for services, but does require timely responses.

Quality patient care is everyone's primary goal, and to accomplish this, everyone must work together. Everyone must be motivated to perform at their best.

Ancillary departments will do this if there is a collective commitment to the organization, the manager, the patient, and to themselves. All departments working together ensure successful patient services. Those who take pride in their work can motivate others. A commitment to quality care is most apparent in employee performance appraisals and in results of patient care. The product of fast, appropriate, efficient service performance motivates staff and reinforces caring behavior.[4]

Interdepartmental education makes critical care needs better understood. If other department managers understand that critically ill patients need constant, intensive attention, their departments will have more patience when the nurse cannot leave the bedside immediately to answer the phone. Speaking with these ancillary department managers and inviting their firsthand observations benefits the working relationships between departments.

The nurse manager can help the other departments serve the critical care unit by telling them what is needed and by suggesting how to achieve the objectives. It would be wonderful if this friendly help would just appear, but realistically, it has to be solicited and cultivated. To do this, the nurse manager interacts with others off the unit.

Taking time to get acquainted with each ancillary department manager is a nurse manager's responsibility. Learning the goals of each department and offering to work together to reach mutual goals will begin the spread of the caring climate. Enthusiasm about unit activities generates outside interest in them.

As time progresses, persons in other departments become allied with the unit. The more numerous and diverse the allies, the better. Consider working relationships with librarians, social workers, dietitians, respiratory therapists, clinical engineers, physical therapists, financial officers, clinical nurse specialists, and any other persons or departments that can help the unit achieve its goals.

It is easier to get other department managers to help the critical care unit reach its goals of timely, efficient patient care if they are given immediate credit and appreciation for their patient care contributions. Written acknowledgements of work well done, and recognition of and conversations with non-nursing employees who are regularly assigned to the unit help create a friendly, caring atmosphere.

Potential problems can be avoided if the nurse manager explores the problem of management of the critically ill patient during transport to another department for diagnosis. By reaching out and offering clinical expertise when needed, and by discussing care coordination with diagnostic and therapeutic services, you express your concern for both patient and staff. Issues that can be addressed include transportation needs, airway maintenance, location and content of code carts, code management, isolation requirements and management of human excrement. Understanding the ancillary departments' problems and sharing this knowledge with staff enables the manager to troubleshoot and to avoid potential problems. Knowing that the Magnetic Resonance Imaging (MRI) room has no registered nurse, that Radiology does not have a bedpan hopper, or that Radioisotopes has no code cart results in better coordinated care. Alternative arrangements can be made. Together, the nurse manager and the department manager may be able to have hospital administration remedy their problems.

Brainstorming sessions with other department managers often result in ideas for increased productivity and effectiveness. For example, the critical care nurse manager might explain that a change in patient population has affected the type of supportive services needed. The manager should assess the services required and identify needs that are not being met. Consider the employees and departments that are involved in obtaining supplies, which might be difficult to acquire. Spend time discussing possible changes with that manager. Lab results, late diet changes, laundry restocking, resuscitation bags, and isolation gowns are equally important to unit staff. The manager is responsible for resolving these problems.

The effective nurse manager recognizes the expertise of ancillary departments. The respiratory therapist knows much more than the average staff nurse does about ventilator management. The critical care manager knows and appreciates this, and seeks out ways to involve both departments in rewarding practice. Shared inservices, patient care conferences, and timely thank-yous demonstrate the commitment to caring.

Inviting the laboratory manager to the unit to see the urgency of *stat** potassium results helps both departments improve blood collection, labeling, transport, and result acquisition. Exploring the potential for a special satellite laboratory for critical care provides the manager with greater understanding of the laboratory's goals and objectives. In a similar way, communicating a belief that a blood transfusion is equated with organ transplantation gives appropriate recognition to blood bank technicians, especially if nursing staff tend to be cavalier about transfusion policies and procedures.

Involve the pharmacy in medication issues. Ask for input regarding the acquisition, storage, and administration of medications. Review the code cart, check out the medication refrigerator together, and discuss the way intravenous solutions are prepared, if this is done in the unit. Talking about emergency medication needs is fruitful, especially for the patient. Sharing often invites creative change that leads to long-term improvement in services.

Suggesting the need for an on-site clinical pharmacist, a satellite pharmacy, an intravenous admixture program, or a way to get timely pharmacokinetic information results in thought-provoking questions and answers about systems and services. If physical space is an obstacle, individual unit service in a central pharmacy is still possible. If a specific group of pharmacists is responsible for the critical care staff's drug education, and is associated with that one specific area, their sense of caring is likely to increase. As a bonus, staff spend less time procuring medications and more time learning about the effects of medications.[13]

---

* Abbreviation for *statim* (L): at once, immediately.

Having regularly assigned environmental services personnel facilitates a neat unit, because they are more familiar with the physical layout and routines of the unit. Expansion of services to other areas, such as responsibility for eliminating used needle containers, stocking gloves, emptying laundry bags, and cleaning equipment, can occur only if the department managers are aware of the need for these services, and recognize the environmental personnel's contribution to the unit.

A unit-assigned transportation aide, regular deliveries of laundry several times a day, and around-the-clock services helps make caring for the patient the nurse's primary focus. Regular deliveries of supplies to the unit, or a 24-hour Central Supply service contributes to uninterrupted patient care. If the nurse manager supports the delegation of non-nursing functions to ancillary personnel, the ancillary department heads will need little coaxing to take on responsibility for their own services.

THE CARING ENVIRONMENT

The nurse manager is responsible for the care, for the policies and procedures utilized in that care, and for the environment in which that care takes place. This responsibility can be met by budgeting necessary personnel and equipment, making provisions for the effective operation of the personnel and equipment, and facilitating an environment for optimal patient care. Recognizing that patients are hospitalized for nursing care, the manager uses the knowledge of the critical care unit, of types of procedures, and of complications and expected outcomes to develop an approach to meeting those care needs.

Building a solid, knowledgeable, strong nursing staff will almost always ensure the best patient care possible. For this to occur, the nurse manager retains the present staff and helps them grow. Appropriate ongoing staff education and recruitment to replace nurses lost to attrition is necessary.

Factors such as pay and benefits, standards of patient care, scheduling, the level of respect for nurses, administrative support, and opportunities for career advancement are all important in the recruitment and retention of nurses. However, the current nursing shortage and the lack of qualified nursing personnel predicted for the near future will affect hospital organization. Thus, the nurse manager puts more emphasis on retention than recruitment.[9]

Caring for the care giver is a primary concern that is facilitated by providing a caring environment. Caring for the nursing staff involves providing continuing education, scheduling flexibility, and assigning patients fairly, which are all important to the staff. The environment must be conducive to patient care. Thus the manager is concerned with the physical layout at the bedside, temperature control, noise level, cleanliness, and infection control practices. This is by no means an all-inclusive list, but it gives some idea of where to begin in environmental control.

Noise can be minimized by having the staff set expectations that unnecessary noise will not be tolerated, that alarms will be answered promptly, and that all staff will stand next to the person with whom they are speaking. In new or renovated units, encourage the use of acoustic ceiling tiles, curtains, and glass or carpeted walls to decrease noise. Neutral colors and natural lighting have a soothing influence.[3] Yellow and green should be avoided if possible because these colors adversely affect the patient's appearance. A constant temperature should be maintained. The bedside and commonly used areas are kept as neat as possible. After using these areas it is expected that staff pick up after themselves. The appropriate use of gloves, gowns, masks, and goggles is encouraged.

ESTABLISHING MUTUAL RECOGNITION

Building a qualified team to care for critically ill patients is the priority of the nurse manager. The team consists of all staff members—nursing and others—providing services. Efficient team performance that leads to optimal patient care depends on cooperation. The nurse manager fosters teamwork and cooperation, and encourages mutual recognition.

Mutual recognition of staff nurses involves open-mindedness and some unselfishness. Willingness to give a pat on the back, relief in a crisis situation, and encouragement when it's needed is part of being a team player. The team does not always need a formal leader to function well, but does require members who cooperate, communicate, and negotiate with each other. The nurse manager sets the tone that facilitates this.

As professional nurses, labels such as "old staff" or "new staff," "full timer" or "part timer," "day shift" or "evenings" are not conducive to team playing. Labels are disruptive; they encourage cliques, divide staff, and defeat attainment of unit goals and objectives. The nurse manager is a role model of professionalism who refers to all staff as *critical care professionals.* People who feel good about themselves feel good about others; they take pride in what they do, are more conscientious, easier to work with, and open to new ideas.[2] Nurse managers exert a positive influence by helping elevate the self-esteem and self-concept of all staff.

Instilling the expectation that co-workers support each other is a very important element in the management of a critical care unit. Staff thrive on camaraderie. Trust, support, and helpfulness make a unit run smoother. Ideally, no undercurrents of animosity or unprofessionalism jeopardize patient care or unit functions. Support and recognition from the nurse manager encourages reciprocal action from the staff. When staff know they have the full support of the manager, each individual contributes fully to the unit's growth and sense of caring. By promoting positive feelings of self, patient care improves.[2]

Mutual support builds a staff alliance that fends off outside forces which could disrupt the unit's mission. Often positive reinforcement comes from peers and co-workers. This is a crucial support system for nurses. Demoralization that leads to lowered self-esteem and diminished self-confidence can result if peer support does not exist. The amount of support needed depends on the staff nurse's existing sense of self-esteem, control, and confidence.

Staff follow when the leader provides a model of professional caring. Desired behaviors should receive positive reinforcement. Recognize individual accomplishments and share them with the entire staff to encourage continuation of the same effort. Teammate and peer acknowledgement is rewarding, and also instills a sense of personal pride and goodwill. Awards such as Nurse of the Month (with the choice of extra time off or a special luncheon) are best initiated by the nurse manager after the staff decide they want to do this. Given today's nursing shortage, high stress, and rising patient acuity, consistency, support, and demeanor of the manager may be the factors that help reduce nursing turnover in the unit.[6] With a united and supportive staff, facing any crisis is easier.

Recognition for a job well done is satisfying to all people. The nurse manager learns to use verbal acknowledgement as a reward to motivate desired behavior. Patients and families are very receptive to staff who provide humanistic care. Practitioners who are rigid in practice, adhere to all rules, and focus only on the tasks that need doing, are not providing humanistic care. Because the manager is responsible for seeing that tasks are done in a timely fashion, skill is needed to balance individual approaches to care and efficient practice. When the nurse manager expects staff to provide quality patient care, staff rise to these expectations.

Staff expect themselves to provide quality patient care, but sometimes the system gets in the way. Staff nurses cannot deal with system problems directly, but the nurse manager can. By verbally recognizing humanistic care that is centered on meeting patient or family needs, and by demonstrating this care of staff by handling system problems, the nurse manager establishes a precedent for the staff to follow.

GUEST AND EMPLOYEE RELATIONS

Ideally all hospital employees have some degree of "people skill" and can maintain a positive, professional attitude when dealing with people. However, on occasion this professionalism fails. The nurse manager demonstrates a commitment to positive working relations by assuming that all people entering the unit are guests, and that all staff are expected to treat these guests with courtesy and kindness. This behavior gives the impression of a nurturing and caring environment. "Guests" includes other staff, non-nursing personnel, volunteers, visitors, and clergy.

Nurse managers set the tone for this behavior and are obligated to confront those who do not project a positive, professional attitude. Although differences of opinion still occur, an apology and a smile may diffuse unacceptable situations. The nurse manager must follow-up these situations so they can be prevented in the future. Keep in mind that there are some situations in which the apology and smile are not warranted. There may have to be an agreement to disagree.

When staff are expected to behave professionally and courteously, enhanced self-worth may ensue, and the manager can expect that these staff will speak highly of the unit's working environment. When satisfied with working conditions, staff tell family, friends, and patients, and this enhances the image of the unit.

During times of critical illness, both the patient and family need every support system available. Support begins with information and family education. Knowledge about the illness and the interventions necessary helps relieve fear and anxiety.

In an elective admission to the critical care unit, specific information about the environment and the treatment is very helpful to patient and family. Introduction to some of the staff and a tour of the unit is ideal and should help dispel some of the myths that the patient and family may harbor. Ideally, a staff member—preferably the nurse who will be caring for the patient—volunteers to give the tour. Unfortunately, it's often hard to say which nurse will be assigned to that patient.

In the event a preadmission tour is not possible, enlist the aid of the clinical nurse specialist, social worker, or volunteer to give the tour. When available, videos, tapes, or programs are also helpful. When the admission is emergent, small bits of information are easiest for the family to absorb.

When a prolonged patient stay is anticipated, the nurse manager expects the staff to explore the family's plans regarding housing, meals, and the vigil often associated with critical illness. Sometimes family members need "permission" to leave the hospital even for a short time, and a plan may need to be drawn up to tell family members to leave the hospital to rest themselves. Assure the family that telephone information is available to a designated family spokesperson twenty-four hours a day. Nurse managers support families by assigning staff so patients receive continuity of care. With a high acuity level and 12-hour shifts, this may be problematic, but assigning the same nurse to a patient facilitates rapport and continuity of care.

When nurses are sensitive to the family members' needs, it really helps the family through a difficult time. The nurse manager's support of the staff nurse—who is supporting the family—eases many difficulties encountered when caring for severely ill patients. Sharing and collaboration are needed from all team members. To alleviate some anxiety, observe the patient while his or her nurse is talking with the family.

Although the environment can be overwhelming, a neat, clean bedside, respectful treatment of the patient and family, and as much privacy as possible during visiting hours have a positive impact on the family. By encouraging the family to touch the patient, hold the hand, or stroke the forehead, you can alleviate much fear.[14] When the culture of the family and patient permits, the nurse manager expects the staff to demonstrate this high-touch skill. By encouraging patience, understanding, courtesy, and honesty for all family-staff interactions, a climate for caring is enhanced.

Care of the family is essential to the total care of the patient. When a member of the family system is ill, the system does not function as it usually does. In a caring climate, family members are encouraged to be a part of integrated care. Integrated care has many aspects, including care of the family, family involvement in planning and implementing patient care, coordination of services for the patient, and as much patient involvement in self-care as possible. Involvement in the care plan helps the family continue to operate as a support system and facilitates discharge planning.

A family member should be allowed to assist with care activities if the patient requests it, or if the family requests it and the patient consents. Examples of this kind of care include assisting with a bath, grooming, nourishment, incentive spirometry exercises, placing a support pillow with turning, or giving the patient a cool cloth for his head. The nurse manager encourages staff to establish guidelines for these activities.

Involving the patient in self-care is condition dependent. All conscious patients should be encouraged to participate in their own care in any way they can, unless this is medically contraindicated. Patient participation is achieved by giving the patient choices. If the patient can answer verbally or by gesture which direction she wants to turn or whether she prefers her bath now or later, she can gain a sense of some control. Although it is sometimes easier, quicker, and less frustrating to do these for the patient, if the patient is encouraged, she can regain the independence that leads to an optimal level of health.

The staff must be careful to be as consistent as possible with each patient and family. Family care activities should be coordinated with visiting hours to avoid random traffic through the unit. They should be balanced with unit activities to avoid disrupting unit functions (which are secondary to the family's psychosocial needs). The nurse manager encourages staff behavior that integrates patient care.

Visiting Hours

Many critical care units have policies that restrict visiting hours. Structured visiting hours allow staff to plan and complete care and to prepare the patient for visitors. However, a very strict visiting policy is stressful and leads to friction between staff and family, creates noncompliance with the policy, and may not meet patient and family needs. If staff are aware of this stress, they can adjust the rules when circumstances change, to allow more frequent or less frequent visits, or eliminate one visiting period. Within written guidelines, the critical care nurse manager lets the staff adjust policy when patient and family needs dictate, and supports these adjustments. This caring attitude of the nurse is remembered when an exception to the rule is allowed.

With staff input, the nurse manager may be able to experiment with a variety of visiting policies to find one that works best for the unit. Policy variations include coordinating visiting hours with the attending physicians' rounds so the physicians can speak with family members after rounds, and adjusting the time for visiting to suit each family.

CASE STUDY: ADJUSTING VISITING HOURS

> The head nurse of a 18-bed medical-surgical intensive care unit for the past two years is gregarious and well liked on the unit. Under her leadership, the unit has emerged as a star within the hospital. There is little turnover, staff work well together, and a climate for caring prevails. However, visiting hours are limited to four 15-minute blocks spread over twelve hours, and are tightly monitored by security. The unit has a comfortable, spacious family lounge, and many families sit for hours waiting to visit their loved one. One staff nurse feels that this policy is too limited and wants to expand the hours. She speaks to the head nurse who encourages her to develop a plan to change the visiting hours.

The staff nurse who is questioning the visiting hours is an informal leader. In planning for change, she confers with her peers and asks how they feel about the visiting policy. The majority of the staff agree that the hours are restrictive. A small group of volunteers state that they are willing to work on a project to change the visiting hours. This task force develops a plan to survey attitudes of staff, visitors, and patients about visiting times, and agrees to make recommendations for change. These actions display a high level of maturity because the nurses are planning with little direction from the nurse manager.

Their first plan of action is to survey the entire staff for suggestions about visiting hours, giving everyone an opportunity for input into the project. The most common suggestions in rank by preference are:

- Every two hours for fifteen minutes
- Every hour around the clock
- Individual contract with family

For the next two weeks, visitors in the waiting room are surveyed about their preferences. A volunteer spends two hours each day helping visitors fill out a questionnaire about visiting times. During this same time period, patients who are able to answer questions complete the same questionnaire with staff help.

Patients' visiting hour preferences are as follows:

- At random
- Every two hours for thirty minutes
- Every hour
- Every half hour

Visitors' visiting hour preferences are as follows:

- Every hour
- Every four hours
- At nurse's convenience
- At random

Every 2 Hours for 30 Minutes	Family contract for visiting hours
Advantages	*Advantages*
Increased frequency for family visits	Family convenience
Interim time for patient rest and care	Better family compliance
Easily remembered by the family and patient	Family has some control
Interim time for family rest	Less friction over hours
Better traffic control	
Schedule allows for planning	
Disadvantages	*Disadvantages*
May disturb patient rest	Random traffic in the unit
Rigidity of schedule	Takes time to agree
	Infringe on privacy of other patients

Reviewing the surveys, staff decide to explore visits every two hours for thirty minutes, and individual family contracts. A pilot project is developed to test the feasibility of the new visiting hours. Each policy is to be tested for two months, and then reevaluated.

Communications to physicians, administration, and security are coordinated by the head nurse, which demonstrates visibility of nursing management and leadership and open communication lines. Each patient and family member is given a printed sheet with a brief overview of the pilot, listing the hours and policy currently undergoing evaluation. A form for comments is provided and a box for the forms is kept in the lounge.

After the two-month trials, the staff and participating families are asked to evaluate the results. These forms are summarized by the task force and presented at a staff meeting for discussion. Staff identify several advantages and disadvantages of both methods. The box summarizes these results.

In reviewing the advantages and disadvantages, the staff decide to adopt the visiting policy of every two hours for thirty minutes between 7:00 A.M. and 11:00 P.M. Visitation during the night is permitted for labile patients. Individual consideration of family needs is continued.

Visitation can be a source of contention and friction between staff and visitors. By encouraging staff to solve these problems on their own, the manager helps ensure that staff comply with policy while providing less restrictive visiting hours.

The nurse manager helped the staff develop leadership skills and caring attitudes and actions. From their observations, staff identified a need, communicated with each other in staff meetings, and interacted with families. Attempts to reduce stress with less restrictive visiting hours may have improved guest relations. Interdepartmental cooperation with security, physicians, and administration was fostered while trying to care for the whole family system. These actions and attitudes demonstrate their striving for a climate for caring.

CONCLUSION

This chapter identified and discussed specific behaviors that the nurse manager uses to develop leadership skills and manage staff in a caring environment. Communication, assessment techniques, and the art of negotiation helps the critical care nurse manager build a climate for caring. In so doing, the nurse manager uses all the available resources to ensure that the unit is perceived in a positive way within the framework of the hospital. By encouraging staff to participate actively in decision making, the manager facilitates a caring environment that promotes quality patient care.

REFERENCES

1. Bradford D and Cohen A: Managing for excellence, New York, 1984, John Wiley & Sons.
2. Brooker C: Positive strokes in leadership, Nursing Management 19(6):64H-64P, 1988.
3. Fein IA: Critical care unit design: environmental and psychosocial considerations. In Fein IA and Strosberg MA, editors: Managing the critical care unit, Rockville, Md, 1987, Aspen Publishers, Inc.
4. Garfield C: Peak Performers: the new heroes of American business, New York, 1986, William Morrow & Co., Inc.
5. Hersey P and Blanchard K: Management of organizational behavior: utilizing human resources, ed 4, Englewood Cliffs, NJ, 1984, Prentice-Hall, Inc.
6. Katzin L: Great head nurses, American Journal of Nursing 89:42, 1989.
7. Mackay H: Swim with the sharks without being eaten alive, New York, 1988, William Morrow & Co., Inc.
8. Massie JL: Essentials of management, ed 4, Englewood Cliffs, NJ. 1988, Prentice-Hall, Inc.
9. Neathawk R, Dubuque S, and Kronk C: Nurses' evaluation of recruitment and retention, Nursing Management 19(12):38-45, 1988.
10. Rambaud R: Justification through negotiation, Nursing Management 18(7):79-80, 1987.
11. Spicer J and Macioce V: Retention: sound communication keeps a critical care staff together, Nursing Management 18(5):64A-64F, 1987.
12. Sutcliff SA: Nurse-to-nurse staff development, Nursing Management 20(1):73, 1989.
13. Sylvan L: Developing satellite pharmacies for critical care units. In Fein IA and Strosberg MA, editors: Managing the critical care unit, Rockville, Md, 1987, Aspen Publishers, Inc.
14. Urban N: Responses to the environment. In Kinney MR, Packa D, and Dunbar S, editors: AACN's clinical reference for critical-care nursing, ed 2, New York, 1988, McGraw-Hill Book Company.

SUGGESTED READINGS

1. Bean J: Decentralizing of nursing management, Nursing Management 17(6):68-70, 1986.
2. Daley L: The perceived immediate needs of families with relatives in the intensive care setting, Heart & Lung 13:231, 1984.

3. Friedman V: Purchasing hi-tech equipment: the rules of the game. In Fein IA and Strosberg MA, editors: Managing the critical care unit, Rockville, Md, 1987, Aspen Publishers, Inc.
4. Girard N: Marketing yourself as a CNS. In Menard S, editor: The clinical nurse specialist, New York, 1987, John Wiley & Sons.
5. Jones B: Rewarding bedside nursing, Nursing Management 17(8):43-46, 1986.
6. Knaus W, Draper E, Wagner D, and Zimmerman J: An evaluation of outcome from intensive care major medical centers, Annals of Internal Medicine 104:410, 1986.
7. McConnell CR: Making upward communication work for your employees: process and people with emphasis on people, Hospital Topics 66(2):23-27, 1988.
8. Peters T and Waterman R: In search of excellence, New York, 1982, Harper & Row Publishers.
9. Stanfill PH: Participative management becomes shared management, Nursing Management 18(6):69-70, 1987.

Chapter 3

FACILITATING JOB SATISFACTION

Bonnie S. McCandless
Sharon J. Connor

This chapter is about relationships—those essential relationships that are the foundation of a satisfying work environment. These include relationships of mutual trust, a relationship to the job itself, and interpersonal relationships. When any of these relationships are strained, job stress occurs and job satisfaction decreases. Figure 3-1 depicts the possible consequences of job stress on retention and turnover. The nurse manager is responsible for identifying the symptoms of job stress, and for developing strategies to deal with it effectively, so that the negative consequences of turnover are avoided, and retention is ensured. The best strategy is to provide a working environment that reduces job stress and promotes job satisfaction and retention.

This chapter begins by describing job-related stress and its profound effect on job satisfaction. Although a certain amount of job stress is inherent in the practice of critical care nursing, prolonged high levels of stress lead to job dissatisfaction and turnover. However, dealing with stress effectively can lead to job satisfaction.[11] The elements necessary for establishing and maintaining a satisfying work environment are discussed and specific strategies are offered to enable the manager to create a great place to work.

No one particular management theory is the panacea to managerial woes. Although such theories as Maslow's Hierarchy of Needs, McGregor's Theory Y, Ouchi's Theory Z, and Hersey and Blanchard's Situational Leadership all offer

```
                        Job stress
                            |
                            v
   Job satisfaction  <------------->  Job dissatisfaction
         |                                    |
         v                                    v
      Retention                            Turnover
```

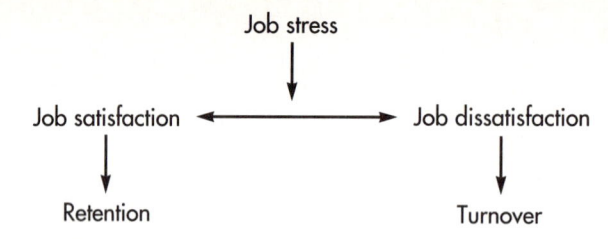

FIGURE 3-1. Consequences of stress on staff satisfaction.

useful models of management and leadership, a more basic and fundamental approach to management includes the following concepts: treat people with respect; give them a say in what they do; and communicate, communicate, communicate. Research has demonstrated that not all managers behave in this way. To implement a management philosophy that uses this approach, the nurse manager needs to understand the relationship between stress and satisfaction.

UNDERSTANDING STRESS

People respond to different stimuli. Stress is a type of stimuli most commonly thought of as an event *impinging* on the person. *Stressors,* or stress stimuli, range from internal drives, such as hunger, to external universal events, such as wars. Life is filled with stressful experiences that arise from personal responsibilities. These experiences can include dealing with a sick pet or having an argument with a family member. Each person's perception of a stressor is unique. Perception, however, is an intellectual process that is enhanced by personal growth and new knowledge.

Lazarus and Folkman[17] stated:

> Psychological stress is a particular relationship between the person and the environment that is appraised by the person as taxing or exceeding his or her resources and endangering his or her well-being.

Figure 3-2 identifies Selye's physical manifestations of stress.[23] Note that this process as described by Selye can be compared to a cascade. If the stressor is not alleviated, the symptoms involve more and more body systems, and their effect on the person becomes more destructive.

Stress in the Workplace

Stress in the work environment can often lead to burnout on the job. *Burnout* is characterized by physical, emotional, and spiritual exhaustion. Bailey[1,2] described burnout as "a process that involves the loss of concern with whom one is working." Research has demonstrated that job stress results in emotional exhaus-

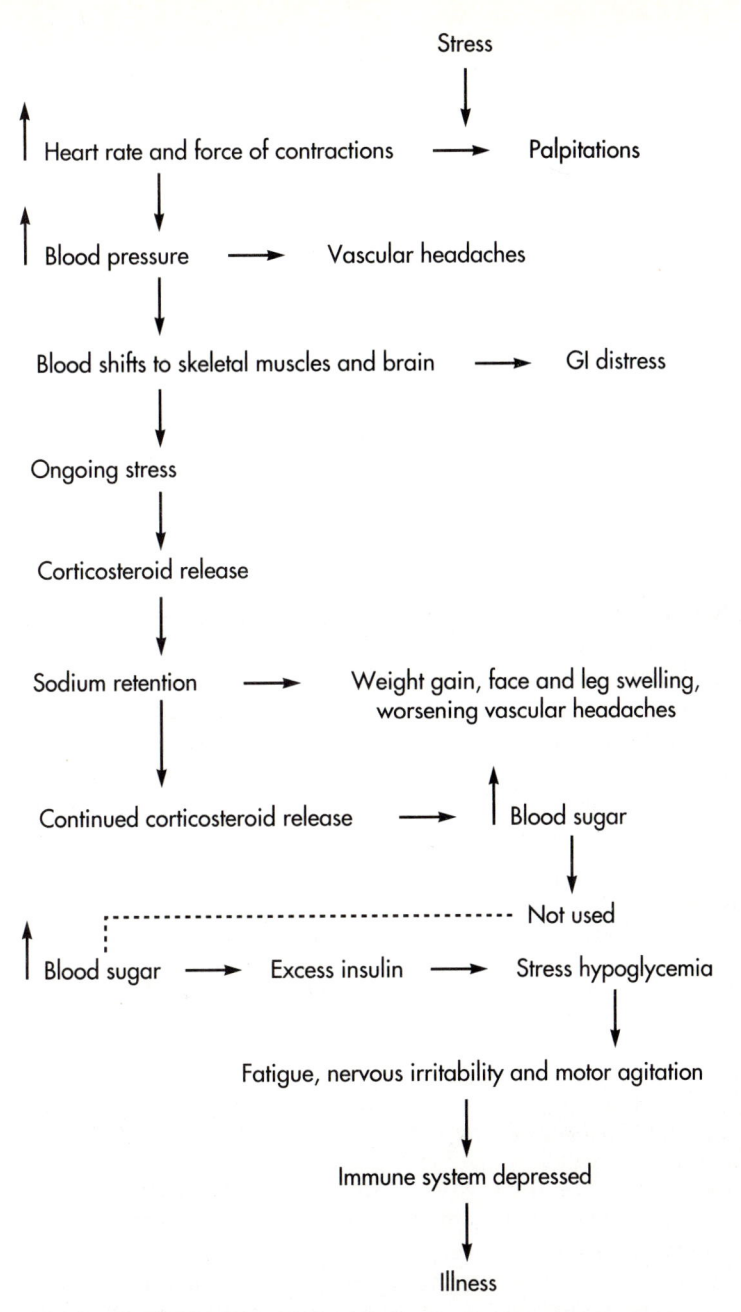

```
                              Stress
                                │
                                ▼
↑ Heart rate and force of contractions ──→ Palpitations
                │
                ▼
↑ Blood pressure ──→ Vascular headaches
                │
                ▼
    Blood shifts to skeletal muscles and brain ──→ GI distress
                │
                ▼
        Ongoing stress
                │
                ▼
    Corticosteroid release
                │
                ▼
    Sodium retention ──→ Weight gain, face and leg swelling,
                │              worsening vascular headaches
                ▼
    Continued corticosteroid release ──→ ↑ Blood sugar
                                              │
                                              ▼
         ┄┄┄┄┄┄┄┄┄┄┄┄┄┄┄┄┄┄┄┄┄┄┄┄┄┄┄┄┄ Not used
         ┆
↑ Blood sugar ──→ Excess insulin ──→ Stress hypoglycemia
                                              │
                                              ▼
              Fatigue, nervous irritability and motor agitation
                                │
                                ▼
                    Immune system depressed
                                │
                                ▼
                             Illness
```

FIGURE 3-2. Selye's physical manifestations of stress. *(Adapted from Selye, H: The Stress of Life ed 2 New York, 1976, McGraw-Hill, p. 203.)*

tion, low morale, helplessness, hopelessness, and other forms of frustration that contribute to job dissatisfaction and job turnover.[7] Job burnout may be manifested by fatigue, frustration and anger, negative self-concept, lack of enthusiasm, and a feeling of entrapment.[14]

The nurse who is feeling frustrated and helpless, and who is therefore suffering from job-related stress, may experience anger. Anger is a behavior that protects against helplessness, and is an alternative to anxiety.[16] However, anger in the work environment is not socially acceptable. Frequently, a stressed employee may turn the anger inward and become depressed. Many stress-related physiologic responses occur and often manifest in absenteeism. Levering[18] put a price tag of $150 billion in annual losses to American industry because of stress-connected absenteeism, reduced productivity, and medical fees. He cited the National Institute of Occupational Safety and Health: "Lack of control over one's work [is] a major factor in work-related stress, which contributes to hypertension, heart disease, ulcers, and depression."

Satisfaction involves a simpler process than stress does. Satisfaction results when needs, expectations, or wishes are met, and manifests itself as a positive feeling associated with anticipation. Satisfaction occurs when the outcome fulfills the expectation. Several studies of job stress in nursing provide insight into the relationship between stress, satisfaction, and the work environment. Packard and Motowidlo[21] found that high stress resulted in job dissatisfaction; and Browner[7] found that sources of job stress did not stem from problems associated with patient care, but from the employees' inability to control other critical aspects of their work.

For the critical care nurse, stress may come from work itself, environment, equipment, emotional demands of patients and their families, conflicts with physicians, administration and supervisors, other health care team members, other critical care nurses, inadequate staffing, and work overload.[19] Note that this last study includes demands of patients while the previous study[7] stated this was not so. The contradiction may or may not be significant.

Hinshaw, Smeltzer, and Atwood[13] looked at retention and reported:

> The major stressors to be buffered were lack of team respect and feelings of incompetence, while the primary satisfiers were professional status and general enjoyment in one's position, which correlated significantly with the ability to deliver quality nursing care.

Another source of stress in the work environment is the perception that supervisors are nonsupportive. In the authors' experience, this perception is often the deciding factor in staff resignations.

Steffer[25] looked at stress among intensive care unit nurses and found that interpersonal relationships were the most frequently reported sources of stress and the second most frequently reported sources of satisfaction. In other words, interpersonal relationships were extremely important: positive relations lead to satisfaction while negative experiences lead to stress. Keane, Ducette, and Adler[14] studied stress in critical care nursing. They found that "nurses who were more committed to their job, who felt more in control of their job, and who felt challenged by their job were less burned out."

Bartz and Maloney[5] provided a profile of the intensive care nurse most likely to experience burnout. Five demographic variables significantly correlate to burnout: (1) burnout is greatest for young workers and lowest for older workers; (2) those with less education experience less burnout; (3) males experience more burnout in the form of depersonalization and emotional exhaustion than females; (4) burnout is greater for military nurses than civilian nurses; and (5) the longer an intensive care nurse is in nursing, the less likely it is for burnout to occur.[5]

Note the controversy in these last two studies. Keane, Ducette, and Adler[14] suggested that commitment is a positive factor, while Bartz and Maloney[5] stated less burnout occurs with less education. These two concepts are somewhat unclear: critical care nurses are usually well educated, committed, and challenged by their work. The seemingly unclear reports about job stress in nursing are difficult to explain. However, all studies seem to indicate that some personal characteristics and job stressors lead to feelings of lack of control. These feelings result in job stress.

Employees, including managers, initiate and control their own actions in a satisfying work environment. At the same time, the objectives and priorities of the organization must be accommodated. However, control denotes participation—having an active voice in how the job is done. In an environment controlled by a multitude of rules, this opportunity is not given to the employees. Job stress results because control over self no longer exists.

Coping Strategies

Fortunately, systems can be put into place to reduce stressors. Learning to recognize personal stressors and responses to stress facilitates a person's ability to have stress work for them. Gramling and Broome[11] reported on a Pediatric Intensive Care Unit (PICU) staff who, after a stress assessment meeting, planned a stress reduction program. They identified their stressors and discussed self-diagnosis of burnout. Compartmentalization and prioritization were two methods they used to deal with stress. *Compartmentalization* refers to being able to separate personal and professional life. *Prioritization* may reduce stress by identifying tasks and separating high-priority from low-priority tasks. "Stress reduction has implications for improved patient care, improved job satisfaction for nurses, and a reduction in staff turnover."[11]

An additional method used by the PICU staff to deal with stressors was self-talk revision. *Self-talk* refers to the way one thinks about one's behavior. For example, thinking about the job and saying to oneself "I *must* be the perfect nurse" sets up unrealistic expectations that add unnecessary stress to goal achievement. The PICU staff found the program for stress reduction beneficial.

They believed that "an ongoing and mutually respectful relationship between staff members and nursing administrators" is very necessary.[11]

A study by Kelly and Cross[15] found that nurses use coping strategies such as "drawing on past experiences, talking over a problem with others, and basing an action on understanding of a situation." These nurses recommended the following stress-reducing strategies to improve coping behaviors:

> An increase in staff numbers, more training in the knowledge and skills area, improved communication between medical and nursing staff, and better communication between nurses and nursing administration.

Learning to manage stress effectively is important to nurses' well-being. Those things that are stressors and the responses to them must be recognized. Once they are identified, active stress reduction is possible.

One method of managing stress is through relaxation exercises. "The overall purpose of relaxation meditation is to relieve muscle and mental tension and to induce quieting responses."[2] Stress can also be released through physical activity or exercise. Aerobic exercise can decrease muscle tension and mental tension. Sensible eating habits that result in a sound nutritional status go hand in hand with physical exercise.

There are a number of psychological responses to stress that may lower the stress level. Bailey[2] stated the more common responses: disengagement or giving up, avoidance, detachment or aloofness, denial, and humor. All of these except humor are negative responses. An astute nurse manager identifies the negative behaviors and looks for the source of stress in staff when they occur.

A key concept in well-being is that "individuals need to assume responsibility for their own well-being and strive to move forward on the well-being continuum."[2] Following sound health practices is a highly effective way to deal with stress. Stress reduction activities can be thought of as either physical or mental. The physical activities provide a mechanism to achieve the mental perspective. The mental perspective can then be moved to the final step for stress reduction—communication.

DEFINING A SATISFYING WORK ENVIRONMENT

Promoting job satisfaction among nurses is important for three reasons. Numerous studies indicate that job dissatisfaction has a causal relationship to turnover, resulting not only in instability in the work environment, but also in escalating costs to the institution. Job satisfaction is also related to effective job performance. Creating job satisfaction among nurses has positively affected patient satisfaction. Research findings also suggest that patients' satisfaction with the care they receive and patients' compliance with treatment are adversely affected when nurses are dissatisfied.[27]

Job satisfaction is important in its own right. When satisfaction exists, staff demonstrate a greater commitment to the job, as well as to the institution, and they have a feeling of pride in what they do. Thus, it is incumbent upon the nurse manager to work with her staff to develop an environment that enhances professional growth and, ultimately, job satisfaction. Creating a great place for employees and employers to work is an important goal of any organization. What are the essential elements of such an environment?

Levering[18] interviewed executives to determine their opinions about what makes a great place to work. Their answer: the nature of the relationship between the company and the employees. Levering then interviewed hundreds of employees and concluded that a key quality of good work places is the distinctive ways in which people work and relate to each other. When asked to characterize good work places, employees consistently talked about their relationships with their supervisors, with the organization, and with other employees. The idea routinely expressed was that *people get along with each other*.

It is clear that nurse managers must give time, thought, and energy to developing relationships with employees. There is not a manager worthy of the title who would not like to hear *this is a great place to work*. The time spent creating an environment that fosters this attitude is time well spent. To begin, identify the relationships in an organization, and, on a smaller scale, in the unit that promote a positive work environment.

Essential Relationships

Three primary relationships occur in the work place that describe the essential qualities of a great place to work. First and most important is the *relationship of mutual trust* between employer and employee. Trust is the defining characteristic of a good work place. Second is the *relationship to the job* itself. In other words, employees, including supervisors, feel a sense of pride in what they do. Third, is the *interpersonal relationships* that occur among the employees, including managers. Within a satisfying work environment, a sense of camaraderie prevails. Each person feels part of a friendly community where people help each other grow personally and professionally.

Although these three relationships are somewhat interdependent, one can affect the other two. It is also possible that one relationship is good, while the others are not. For example, employees may feel pride in what they do but may not trust the nurse manager. Others may not enjoy their particular job, but think the hospital is a good and fair employer. In addition, if there is not a sense of camaraderie with the people on the job, it is difficult to find satisfaction with the job itself. On the other hand, if a trusting, respectful, and fair relationship exists between the staff and the nurse manager, relationships with others are facilitated and job satisfaction is enhanced.

Trust

Trust cannot be established overnight, nor does it exist naturally in the work place. It evolves. Once established, it requires constant attention and care. So basic to this notion is the concept that underscores all employment relationships: communication at an interpersonal and group level.

Communication, which can be defined as sending, receiving, and validating information, is circular and involves feedback. Feedback, whether positive or negative, is integral to communication. Managers are expected to be open to negative feedback and to be willing to pursue it as an opportunity for change.

A mechanism that allows for and ensures open, bidirectional communication is crucial to the development and maintenance of trusting relationships. The need for consistent communication is such a simple managerial concept, yet ineffective communication accounts for the majority of problems within an organization. Constant, consistent, open communication involves a serious commitment and an extraordinary amount of time and energy. It is not enough to convey information; one must be sure that the information has been perceived as intended. When information is conveyed and communicated by the nurse manager, the receiver perceives the message and responds directly to the manager, who follows through to be sure that message was interpreted correctly. Direct communication between manager and employee is not always the problem. If a communication is sent by one staff member to another staff member, the nurse manager must keep the feedback loop open so that staff can question and clarify any information that troubles them. Follow-through is the key to ensuring effective communication. Lack of follow through is consistently cited by employees as a source of frustration.

Effective communication can be thwarted for many reasons. Information is a source of power in all organizations. Those who restrict information may enlarge their power base at the expense of others. Limited information is typical of a hierarchical organizational structure. Sometimes, those at higher levels of the hierarchy do not trust those on lower levels to make the right decisions. Unfortunately, such thinking is self-defeating.

Levering[18] cited Earl Wantland, president of Tetronix:

> In general, the highly planned, hierarchical approach to business doesn't work. Each person, no matter where they are in the hierarchy, only knows so much, and that's not near enough. If you push everything through a hierarchy, you're going to be missing important elements of what it is that you're dealing with, because of the natural filtering process that goes on whenever information is passed along. Some people have skills in management, but that doesn't make them the most knowledgeable person about any particular issue that comes up. So it's very important that we have an open enough atmosphere here so that we can bring knowledge to whatever issues we are dealing with—and to let the information flow in a fairly free and fluid form.

The way information is handled affects the sense of community and interdependent relationships. When information is restricted, rumors fly and power structures are created. Knowledge and understanding are essential to enable each individual to participate fully and contribute to the work itself. Mutual trust is dependent on communication. Without mutual trust, there is no cooperation, no credibility. Therefore free-flowing communication facilitates group work.

Self-perception has a tremendous influence on the effectiveness of communication, as well as on the relationships developed with others. Effective leaders have high enough self-esteem to engage in sharing and supportive relationships. The nurse manager with a positive perception of self communicates this to others, thus also increasing their self-esteem. Douglass and Bevis[8] found that effective leaders in the helping professions felt *a part* of others rather than *apart* from others, adequate, trustworthy, wanted rather than ignored, and worthy rather than overlooked and discounted. These are all positive attributes that enhance effective communication. The nurse manager sets the stage for effective communication within the work environment. Although it is an awesome responsibility, it provides unique opportunities to create an environment where the foundation is mutual trust and respect; where creativity and unique ideas are encouraged and rewarded; and where change is seen as an opportunity for growth rather than as a catalyst for dissent.

The following managerial principles, if translated into practice, foster an environment of trust and open communications: accept honest mistakes; criticize up and praise down; and broadly share information. Briefly defined, accepting honest mistakes does not mean that the nurse manager ignores accountability. Instead, the manager's goal is to get people to learn from their mistakes. When a manager criticizes up, there is a chance of problem resolution from those above the manager in the organization. However, the nurse manager must remain willing to listen to complaints and take action to rectify problems. On the other hand, the nurse manager gives credit where credit is due; the manager acknowledges the contributions of others and praises employees appropriately.

Sharing information broadly helps employees make informed decisions. The manager knows that when information is restricted, it becomes distorted and people begin to mistrust each other. When people do not understand something, they are less likely to contribute fully and enthusiastically.

People are naturally skeptical and will question the motives and intentions of others. Most people are very careful about placing trust in others. Effective managers act in ways that gain the confidence and trust of employees, and then work to maintain them. Levering[18] stated that trustworthiness is demonstrated by patience and consistency, openness and accessibility, willingness to go beyond the conventional relationships with employees, delivery on promises, and sharing the rewards of mutual effort equally. The box below identifies strategies that can be used by the nurse manager to promote trust with her employees.

> **STRATEGIES TO PROMOTE TRUST**
>
> ■ Implement a scheduling system coordinated by staff nurses themselves (self-scheduling), thus challenging them as accountable professionals.[9,22]
>
> ■ Foster group cohesiveness and teamwork by using methods that assure the development and maintenance of effective group communication.
>
> ■ Increase contact between nurses and non-nursing administrators in order to improve attitudes toward administration by inviting non-nursing administrators to nursing staff meetings.
>
> ■ Directly address morale issues. Ask employees, "What would make you happier about working here?" Discuss the responses and involve the staff in identifying workable action plans to implement needed changes. Follow-through on identified and perceived problems is critical to preserving your credibility. Morale can be improved by simply showing your staff you are listening and interested.

Levering[18] cited Ewing Kaufmann, founder of Marion Laboratories and co-owner of the Kansas City Royals baseball team: "Treat others . . . the same as you would want to be treated . . . as an individual, with integrity, trust, and honesty."

Pride

Job satisfaction is directly related to one's attitude about one's work. When all staff say their work is *more than a job* rather than *just a job,* there has been success in fostering a positive working environment. Work is one of the principal means through which life becomes meaningful. People often define their personal identities through work. It follows then that work must have meaning and that people need to perceive that they can and do make a difference. In addition, it is important for people to feel ownership of and responsibility for the work they do.

Delegating responsibility and accountability is critical. For the most part, people seek responsibility. Responsibility implies control over one's work, and control relates to power. Without a sense of control, it is almost impossible to take much satisfaction in the work itself. Most studies cite lack of autonomy as a major source of job dissatisfaction. In fact, to a great degree, the nurse's professional self-image is dependent on a sense of autonomy.

Work has an important social dimension as well. Work has meaning when the employee believes that the work is a valuable contribution to society; this is particularly true of nursing. The importance of establishing an environment where individuals will know their work has meaning cannot be understated. Feeling proud of what is done and with whom it is done makes people at good

> **STRATEGIES TO PROMOTE PRIDE IN THE JOB**
>
> ■ Develop better defined nursing roles within hospital organizations. Clearly defined channels of communication and administrative accountability must be documented in written job descriptions and organizational policies.
>
> ■ Provide a support system that fosters positive self-concepts. Be aware, however, that effective leadership depends on one's own positive self-concept.
>
> ■ Provide and encourage recognition for a job well done. Implement a performance appraisal system that encourages creativity and risk taking when dealing effectively with problems.
>
> ■ Implement a clinical ladder program to evaluate and reward clinical practice.[4]

work places say that they have more than a job.[18] The box above identifies strategies that promote pride in the job that can easily be implemented by the nurse manager. As managers, creating an environment that encourages staff to say "I am more than just a nurse" fosters that sense of pride and ownership necessary in a positive working environment.

Interpersonal Relationships

Within any work environment, systems of interpersonal relationships exist between the employee and the organization, between the employee and the job itself, and between the employee and other employees. These relationships overlap and may define just how satisfying that work environment can be. Interdependent relationships within satisfying environments include caring about the organization, the job, and other employees. Each individual must feel valued. Long-term commitment to the organization, the job, and other employees produces unity and camaraderie. This helps the manager understand why good employers have higher productivity.[18]

Levering[18] stated that friendliness is a distinguishing characteristic of a satisfying work environment. Informal talking or socializing is accepted by the organization as a relationship builder between all employees. Informal networking or visiting may serve as a relaxed form of socialization.

To promote a satisfying work environment, socializing should not be restricted to one's peers. Such an environment is not conducive to a social hierarchy; people of all ranks mix. Thus, an interpersonal relationship between all employees develops. There is mutual respect for each other.

In an atmosphere of mutual respect, individuals with positive interpersonal relationships engage in healthy competition rather than in destructive power struggles. A person's work can then be evaluated by its effect within the organization rather than its effect on someone's power base. In a satisfying work environment, backstabbing and other negative behaviors do not fit. The essential criteria for this environment are a sense of community, operationalized as teamwork, and employees working toward a common cause. In a satisfying work environment, this teamwork is highly valued. Employees are rewarded for cooperating with others. Successful team workers develop strong positive relationships with other team members. Job satisfaction results.

Successful interpersonal relationships are built on fairness. Fairness means that neither the employer nor the job take advantage of the employees, who are treated consistently. Most individuals have a highly trained sense of injustice. People easily sense relationships built on favoritism, bias, inequity, or manipulation. Fairness requires a great deal of energy and commitment from the organization, the managers, and the employees. It must be present within every interdependent relationship. Within a relationship, when an individual does not feel as if they are treated fairly, there is great risk that negative behavior such as backstabbing or sabotage will occur. Managers are aware that preventing this negative behavior is important.

Levering[18] cited Bill Gore, the founder of the firm that makes Gor-Tex, as stating:

> The most destructive thing that I know about in enterprises is unfairness or perceived unfairness. People can forgive mistakes if there's a sincere effort to try to be fair. But deliberate unfairness destroys the communication, the cooperation, and all of the things that are necessary for successful teamwork.

The successful nurse manager must most often do the right thing rather than most often do things right.

The concepts of commitment, camaraderie, mutual respect, teamwork, and fairness are also found in both Herzberg's Two-Factor Theory and Ouchi's Theory Z. Herzberg believed that the major satisfiers—achievement, recognition, the work itself, responsibility, and advancement—must balance the dissatisfiers. Herzberg's dissatisfiers included administrative policy, poor working conditions, problems in one's personal life, unnecessary supervision, and negative interpersonal relationships.[26] The box below identifies strategies to nurture interpersonal relationships that can help foster job satisfaction. It is within management's power to offset the dissatisfiers and encourage the movement toward job satisfaction.

Theory Z contends that both job satisfaction and job quality depend on a collaborative work style.[26] Employees must be trusted and consulted on matters affecting them and the product. The product of nursing is health care delivery to those unable to care for themselves. Theory Z is worth considering, "because at its center lie truths about the kind of behavior which should characterize the relationship between all employees and employers."[10]

In summary, the degree of job satisfaction attained from a work environment involves three distinct but overlapping relationships: the relationship of mutual respect or trust between employer and employee; the employee's sense of worth

> **STRATEGIES TO NURTURE INTERPERSONAL RELATIONSHIPS**
>
> ■ Develop and implement patient care strategies to reduce role strain in the critical care environment.
>
> ■ Provide opportunities for nurse-physician interactions, or networks, to strengthen the professional relationship between them.[6]
>
> ■ Redesign orientation programs to include transition programs that use preceptors or mentors. Programs that focus on professional role development and skill acquisition by providing consistent feedback over a longer period of time have been shown to improve job satisfaction and subsequent retention.[12]
>
> ■ Explore alternative care delivery methods such as case management or managed care. Involve the staff in identifying ways to improve efficiency.[3] Increasing nurses' participation in efficiency improvement and cost reduction results in a greater sense of teamwork.
>
> ■ Institute guest relations programs that focus on strategies to improve guest relations rather than teaching staff nurses how to be nice to patients and visitors.[3]

or pride related to the job itself; and the interpersonal community relationships or teamwork among all the employees, including managers. In other words, trust, pride and teamwork. A successful manager recognizes that people have individual differences and that job satisfaction is enhanced when people are treated with respect, given a say in what they do, and treated fairly.

STRATEGIES TO ASSURE SUCCESS

Research findings indicate that the work environment is a primary reason for attrition among nurses.[4] Studies have documented that nurses leave their jobs and the profession because of conditions in the work setting.[24] How does the nurse manager create an environment that decreases stress, enhances job satisfaction, and thus improves retention?

Given the nursing shortage, retention of experienced nurses is essential to the success of health care organizations. In 1988, the Office of the Inspector General, Department of Health and Human Services, examined thirteen hospitals that had successfully reduced nurse turnover and vacancies to find the secret to their success. They found management committed to nursing and nurses, strong nursing leadership, and competitive salaries and benefits. The innovative strategies that promoted positive work environments included matching the number of beds to the number of available nurses, salaried versus hourly wages, joint practice committees between physicians and nurses, career ladders, self-scheduling, delegation of non-nursing tasks, and use of clinical nurse specialists to provide professional and personal support to bedside nurses.[20] The nurse manager is responsible for strategies that promote a positive work environment.

CASE STUDY: Increasing Job Satisfaction

As an experienced critical care nurse manager of a 10-bed cardiothoracic unit, you were recently confronted with the resignation of a disgruntled nurse who stated in the exit interview that the working environment in the open heart unit was oppressive, and that true professionals would not be able to derive any job satisfaction from being there. Although you recognize this is one employee's opinion, you also realized the comment deserves further evaluation. First you read the 1988 report out of the Office of the Inspector General, Department of Health and Human Services. Next you develop a tentative plan to assure your unit is in fact a great place to work. You focus on strategies to promote trust and pride, and strategies that enhance interpersonal relationships.

Knowing that staff involvement is vital to the success of any plan, you introduce the concept of job satisfaction and present the list of tentative strategies (boxes on pages 48, 49, and 51) at a unit staff meeting. You ask the staff to discuss the ideas and to be prepared to provide input and feedback at the next unit meeting.

The staff are excited about the plan and the suggested strategies. At the staff meeting, the plan and strategies are prioritized into short- and long-term goals, and target completion dates are set. The staff want immediate success and choose a short-term strategy that focuses on grand rounds.

The medical and nursing grand rounds that began four years ago had ceased when staff was short and interest had decreased. An article by Bream and Shapiro[6] about interaction leads you to believe that grand rounds would provide opportunities for nurse-physician interactions, which would strengthen the professional relationships between them. You include this topic as a suggested strategy. The staff think that resuming grand rounds would be beneficial, and they form a task force to work out the details. You coach the task force and encourage all staff to communicate openly about their progress. As you watch your staff work together on this project, you can clearly see the trust, the pride, and the positive interpersonal relationships that are valued in satisfying work places.

CONCLUSION

Job stress is inherent in the practice of critical care nursing, but it does not have to lead to job dissatisfaction and turnover. Nurse managers have the basic ingredient necessary to create a great place to work: a commitment to caring. Effective nurse managers care enough about their co-workers to provide an environment that strengthens the relationships of trust, pride, and teamwork.

A manager cannot create this environment alone. The relationship between manager and employees must be a partnership in which everyone works toward common goals and makes valuable contributions. Levering[18] said it well: "The concept of the workplace as a partnership carries with it the element of mutual respect, a fundamental characteristic of a great place to work."

REFERENCES

1. Bailey JT: Job stress and other stress-related problems. In Claus KE and Bailey JT, editors: Living with stress and promoting well-being, St. Louis, 1980, CV Mosby Co.
2. Bailey JT: Taking charge of your stress and well-being. In Claus KE and Bailey JT, editors: Living with stress and promoting well-being, St. Louis, 1980, CV Mosby Co.
3. Baird JE: Changes in nurse attitudes: management strategies for today's environment, Journal of Nursing Administration 17(9):38, 1987.
4. Barhyte DY: Levels of practice and retention of staff nurses, Nursing Management 18(3):70, 1987.
5. Bartz C and Maloney J: Burnout among intensive care nurses, Research in Nursing and Health 9(2):147, 1986.
6. Bream T and Shapiro A: Nurse-physician networks: a focus for retention, Nursing Management 20(5):74, 1979.
7. Browner C: Job stress and health: the role of social support at work, Research in Nursing and Health 10(2):93, 1987.
8. Douglass LM and Bevis EM: Nursing management and leadership in action, ed 3, St. Louis, 1979, CV Mosby Co.
9. Elliott TL: Cost analysis of alternative scheduling, Nursing Management 20(4):42, 1989.
10. Flynn R: The nurse manager and the art of Japanese management, Nursing Management 18(10):57, 1987.
11. Gramling L and Broome M: Stress reduction for pediatric intensive care nurses, Clinical Nurse Specialist 11(4), 1987.
12. Hamilton EM and others: Effects of mentoring on job satisfaction, leadership behaviors, and job retention of new graduate nurses, Journal of Nursing Staff Development 161:July/August 1989.
13. Hinshaw AS, Smeltzer C, and Atwood J: Innovative retention strategies for nursing staff, Journal of Nursing Administration 17(6):8, 1987.
14. Keane A, Ducette J, and Adler D: Stress in ICU and non-ICU nurses, Nursing Research 34(4):231, 1985.
15. Kelly F and Cross D: Stress, coping behaviors and recommendations for intensive care and medical surgical ward registered nurses, Research in Nursing and Health 8(4):321, 1985.
16. Lawrence R and Lawrence S: The nurse and job related stress: responses, Rx, and self-dependency, Nursing Forum 23(2):45, 1987/88.
17. Lazarus R and Folkman S: Stress, appraisal and coping, New York, 1984, Springer Publishing Co., Inc.
18. Levering R: A great place to work, New York, 1988, Random House, Inc.
19. McCrane E, Lambert V, and Lambert C: Work stress, hardiness and burnout among hospital staff nurses, Nursing Research 36(6):324, 1987.
20. Office of Inspector General: Hospital best practices—nurse recruitment and retention, DHHS Pub No OAI-03-88-01121, Washington, DC, 1988.
21. Packard J and Motowidlo S: Subjective stress, job satisfaction and job performance of hospital nurses, Research in Nursing and Health 10:253, 1987.
22. Ringl KK and Dotson L: Self-scheduling for professional nurses, Nursing Management 20(2):42, 1989.
23. Selye H: The stress of life, ed 2, New York, 1976, McGraw-Hill Book Co.

24. Sowell RL and Alexander JW: Role issues, job satisfaction and unit of assignment, Nursing Connections 2(2):19, 1989.
25. Steffer SM: Perception of stress: 1800 nurses tell their story. In Claus KE and Bailey JT, editors: Living with stress and promoting well-being, St. Louis, 1980, CV Mosby Co.
26. Strader M: Adapting theory Z to nursing management, Nursing Management 18(4):61, 1987.
27. Weisman CS and Nalhanson CA: Professional satisfaction and client outcomes, Med Care 23:1179, 1985.

SUGGESTED READINGS

Bregan MA and Mueller CW: Nurses' job satisfaction: a longitudinal analysis, Research in Nursing and Health 10(4):227, 1987.

Geiger JK and Davit JS: Self-image and job satisfaction in varied settings, Nursing Management 19(12):50, 1988.

Holmes SW: Managing the stress of primary nursing, Nursing Management 18(3):62, 1987.

Longo RA and Uranker MM: Why nurses stay: a positive approach to the nursing shortage, Nursing Management 18(7):78, 1987.

Mann EE and Jefferson KJ: Retaining staff: using turnover indices and surveys, Journal of Nursing Administration 18(7,8):17, 1988.

Roedel RR and Nystrom PC: Nursing jobs and satisfaction, Nursing Management 19(2):34, 1988.

Winker CK: Care for the care givers, Nursing Management 18:49, June 1987.

Chapter 4

Performance, Time, and Energy

Carole Birdsall

Being a nurse manager in a critical care unit in the current economic environment is difficult. Words like *cutback, limited resources, short staffing, productivity,* and *efficiency* are heard daily in acute care hospitals. The emphasis on doing more with less has never been greater, although the rewards for managing a unit well are less clear. In several states, staff nurses' salaries have increased so much, they are higher than those of first-line nurse managers. Recently the classified section of the *New York Times*[12] listed 65 advertisements for staff nurses; the highest salary advertised, $53,435. While the demand and salaries for staff escalate, nurse manager positions suffer from attrition. Often these positions remain vacant or are filled with less skilled individuals, the only ones who want them. For example, in the same issue of the *New York Times*,[12] there were 18 other advertisements for managerial-level registered nurses; this represents about 22 percent of the total ads. Alas, salaries for these positions were not advertised.

In addition to the monetary discrepancy, there are other difficulties with management-level jobs. The nurse manager stands with her feet in two worlds—that of practice and that of management. Balancing takes courage and know-how. Why then do practitioners take management-level jobs? McBride[11] described nursing administration as a natural process resulting from maturation within the profession. In other words, as practitioners gain experience in nursing, they see that those in management exert a greater influence on the whole. Thus, career-minded nurses choose management positions to improve patient services. This chapter provides the career-minded nurse with ways to create personal rewards for a job well done. It also identifies the effect of the nurse manager's performance on staff, and how the nurse manager can use time and energy to enhance her own performance and, subsequently, the staff's performance. A case study illustrates how to apply this information to practice.

MANAGING TIME

Using time well is difficult for many people. The perceptions people have about time affect the way they use it. For children, time seems to stand still; for adults, time flies. Tappen[14] stated that "time is finite and the effective manager must make the best use of the time available." To achieve professional goals, the efficient use of time is of paramount importance to a nurse manager in a critical care unit. Tappen's phrase, *the tyranny of time,* evokes thoughts about the amount of time we have on earth, the amount of time we have already used up, and the amount of time we have remaining. The nurse manager's goal is to maximize the efficient use of time to ensure that staff, unit, and personal goals are achieved.

Time management can be streamlined. A time log helps the manager stay on target. Keeping a time log involves using calendars, schedules, and tick files. Every manager needs a calendar to schedule tasks, projects, and meetings. The calendar can organize personal and professional dates, or it can be used exclusively for unit events. The nurse manager reviews the calendar each morning to see what needs to done and to set daily objectives. By scanning the scheduled meetings, thinking about the tasks that need doing, and noting the project due dates, the nurse manager can plan the best use of her time. Adding unit plans to the calendar ensures that all goals are considered in daily planning.

In addition to a calendar, many managers use a list of things that need to be done to remind them of incomplete, outstanding tasks. To be really effective, the nurse manager must think about and create a workable list. In fact, several lists that separately cover personal, unit, and professional tasks may be better. Although a list of lists may be a bit compulsive, the smart nurse manager uses whatever does the job. For many, satisfaction of crossing out a completed task is very rewarding and is the incentive to start a new task.

All activities can be categorized and put on a time line. The manager efficiently approaches and completes each activity before moving on to the next one. Activities should be divided into bite-size tasks, or the system won't work. For example, if the nurse manager has line authority for 25 staff members, a listed activity that says "do performance evaluations" will be overwhelming. Think the problem through. There are twelve months of the year, so two evaluations per month would be reasonable. If there are evaluations overdue, split this task into manageable pieces. In a hospital where the professionals are not unionized, but the ancillary help are, the manager might decide to do the professional evaluations first and then start the ancillary staff evaluations. Union contract mandates annual reviews; therefore, once the professional evaluations have been completed, the incentive to comply with union regulations ensures that *all* evaluations will be done in the next year.

A tick file is a reminder system that works backwards: To use a tick file, mark the date the task is due on the calendar. Then divide the task into four to six manageable pieces. Put these pieces in reverse order and then mark off due dates for each piece backwards from the final due date. As time passes and as each item in the tick file appears on the calendar, a visual reminder appears, hinting the project's due date is getting closer. The nudge received by the nurse manager who views the calendar daily makes the tick file effective. Dividing the task into manageable pieces prevents the manager from feeling overwhelmed.

The manager organizes time to reduce interruptions and avoid recurrent crises, and completes tasks as quickly as possible, considering accuracy and neatness. If the manager needs supportive data to complete a task, she writes this as a step on the "to do" list. Thus, the data are available when the manager is ready to complete the task.

Most managers need to plan time to address large-scale projects and difficult tasks. A two-hour period can be set aside on the same day every week—not during peak times when interruptions, staff questions, and external interactions are expected. One day a month can be reserved for paperwork. Staff should know in advance what day that will be, and on that day, the manager should vary her clothes (wear street clothes, for instance), her starting time (come later than usual), and her routine (avoid report). When units are well managed, the nurse manager has the luxury of dedicating a whole day to completing nonroutine tasks.

ORGANIZING WORK

Organizing work includes dealing with paper efficiently and using a reliable filing system. Paper, especially mail, should be handled only once. For example, a memo from Pharmacy should be dealt with immediately. If this means responding, the nurse manager writes the response then. If it means a staff communication, the nurse manager writes the memo then. Otherwise, later, when the manager must respond, she doesn't have to waste time shuffling papers to find the original memo. Immediate responses shave minutes off of a busy schedule.

Automate many repetitive tasks to really save time. This is the communication era: Critical care leaders and managers are expected to be computer literate. Computers organize work, retrieve data efficiently, and facilitate moving in and out of tasks. For example, a computer with a good printer can save time looking for the right forms. Once a form has been developed on the computer, it can be printed easily. In general, if a form is used once a month or more, automate it—don't just copy it. Copying it means you have to keep track of it.

Avoid *crisis quicksand;* that is, when the manager runs and reacts to every major and minor crisis. This is a big time waster. Let staff deal with day-to-day crises commensurate with their experience and skill. The manager provides support, information, and resources as needed to help staff resolve problems. Occasionally select a day-to-day crisis to resolve quickly and efficiently, thereby demonstrating effective leadership and management skills.

To avoid wasting time, do something constructive; don't just talk, worry, or complain about what needs to be done, do it. A good manager explores the average work day and identifies the barriers to effective time use—barriers such as reality distortion, breakdown of plans, and true work overload. Perhaps too much time is spent socializing. When there are lists of many uncompleted tasks, the realization that many of these tasks would take only a few minutes becomes the impetus to complete them. Personal strategies include giving up the routine, looking at what is available to achieve goals, accepting the reality of changes in the unit, and working with staff to create an environment that fosters collegiality.

Once the calendar, tick file, and lists are being used, start working on goals. List your personal goals, then goals identified by your supervisor, and then staff and unit goals. Combine these into one master list and develop a plan that allows work on more than one goal at a time. Be sure to include all entries on the master list. After a while, evaluate how many of these goals have been met. Unit goals, part of the strategic plan, demonstrate unit growth. However, personal goals are equally important. And finally, it is always prudent to meet your supervisor's goals. The day-to-day ability to juggle all of these goals gets easier *once they are recognized*. Use selective attention—choose the focus that ensure that your actions effect desired outcomes.

Unfortunately, the process of making a master list of goals shows how impossible it is for one person to do so many tasks. What we want to do doesn't equal what we think we should do, nor what we are capable of doing. Before adopting numerous goals, evaluate your leadership and management skills.

> Wowk[16] suggested investing time in goal setting with team members. By defining what, how, and when needs to be done and *by whom* results can be measured. Team input into goals is paramount before final adoption.

SELF-APPRAISAL

Self-appraisal is not easy. An inaccurate self-perception results in poorly focused plans for personal growth and improvement. Although seeing yourself as others see you is difficult, this self-awareness will enhance your leadership ability. However, be aware of the limits of your authority and the need to clarify your role. To do well as a nurse manager, desire is not enough. The effective nurse manager must be committed to being a proactive leader, eliminating personal rigidity, insuring participatory governance, and developing staff by delegating responsibility for decision making. Most importantly, the nurse manager grows and develops with a role.

Begin the self-appraisal with the nurse manager job description, and develop a tool by condensing the crucial elements of the job description until they fit on one sheet of paper. This list should be a fair overview of the job. Use a 10-point scale, where a score of 1 means that the task was not done at all, 5 means that the task was 50 percent done, and 10 means that the task was completed. Label the months on twelve columns to the right. Each month, use the scale to rate personal performance. A sample of a working list is shown in Table 4-1. Over time, you will identify areas that need work from patterns and trends. By using the calendar, lists, and tick files, you will achieve your goals, which are seen as markers that demonstrate growth.

To acquire additional leadership and management skills, you may need graduate study or continuing education courses. Nurse managers are active in professional organizations and often take advantage of annual meetings and conventions to enhance their skills. The nurse manager considers all skills that make her role easier as personal goals. For example, computer literacy is a desired skill. Start by talking with in-house people who use computers. Decide whether the computer would be most useful at home or at work. Explore the possibility of getting a computer on the capital budget. Buy a computer. Once a computer is available, plan to acquire computer skill over time.

Each manager hopes for success and fears failure. However, proactive managers do not let this fear immobilize them. Anxiety is normal when something new is attempted. This anxiety is often referred to as healthy stress; it provides energy to overcome the fear of failure. Managers who are always complacent and comfortable in their roles are not trying hard enough. McBride[11] said,

> It is naive to think that you will rarely make mistakes. But if you rarely make the same mistake twice, you are likely to contribute solidly to your field. To learn from mistakes and find ways for others to avoid making the same ones is characteristic of professional leadership.

A nurse manager and effective leader lives by several rules. Share uncertainty about different aspects of the job with others. Embrace errors you or others make, and use them to direct future growth. Respond to failure—yours and others'—by stating that we are not perfect and that the perfect world does not exist. Learn to listen, not just to the words, but to the meaning of what is said. Self-assess to enhance interpersonal skills and improve knowledge. And finally, be prepared to face your personal Waterloo. If you are not out there leading, trying, experimenting, and risking, you are not being proactive.

Good managers realize they can't let excuses get in the way of success, and they also refuse to let other people's hang-ups interfere. Kriegel[9] said that a leader doesn't let the "Yeah, buts" get in the way, but uses the "Can dos" to go

Table 4-1. NURSE MANAGER SELF-EVALUATION

Communication with
  Staff
  Physicians
  Ancillary departments
  Patients
  Families
  Supervisor

Staff
  Evaluation — 2 per month
  Promotions
  Development coordination with instructor
  Discipline — review sick- and late-time patterns

Environment
  Morale
  Motivation
  Participatory decision making

Budget
  Development
  Control
  Cost effective & efficient care

Staffing
  Relationship to Patient Classification
  Adequate
  Overtime reviewed

Meetings
  Staff
  Supervisor
  Standing Committees

Organizational Responsibilities
  Infection Control
  Standards of care
  Writing relevant policy and procedure
  Unit–based Quality Assurance
  Analysis of unit incident reports

where she wants to go. Keep in mind that as a nurse manager you also have rights. As a contributor to the unit's overall goals, the manager needs personal satisfaction from a job well done. Unfortunately, the daily praise, thank-yous, and recognition bestowed on staff by the nurse manager often does not come the manager's way. Leadership responsibility is recognizing that the manager often does without compliments and pats on the back. Over the long haul, the manager of a successful unit derives job satisfaction in different ways.

The nurse manager uses critical thinking skills, including openness and self-awareness. In addition, if she analyzes her beliefs and practices that relate to the way she thinks she manages the unit, and examines the way she actually does manage the unit, she will keep growing and learning. Remember, the effective leader sets daily goals, uses her knowledge and skills to help achieve those goals, communicates well up or down the ladder, and is action-oriented and energetic. Know yourself. Identify your motives, your desired achievements, your potential, and your leadership style you use to exert power and influence on staff. About careers, McBride[11] said,

> Escalating responsibilities may not be something you embrace without reservations. I believe it is important throughout your career to give a high priority to handling your own stress. Too many nurses pay insufficient attention to their own needs . . . and get strangled by job pressures. . . . Nurses do not always realize that self-presentation is important (not just in the sense of dressing for success); the stressed never impress.

End your monthly self-appriasal with how you handle stress and find ways to deal positively with stress.

SELF-ESTEEM

The nurse manager's self-esteem is pivotal to unit success. A belief in self is tightly tied to success. The way you look and feel when you come to work affects others. The nurse manager who faces staff each day and only sees "a sinkful of dirty dishes" will not have the motive, time, or energy to succeed. Maslow's hierarchy states that physical needs, safety and security, belongingness and love, and self-esteem are necessary before self-actualization is possible. The nurse manager helps herself and staff move toward self-actualization daily. If she makes a decision to start each day by focusing on helping herself and staff build self-esteem, the foundation for success would become stronger.

People need to feel achievement to increase their self-esteem. The nurse manager acts as a catalyst; with interpersonal skills and persistence, she helps staff reach a high level of self-esteem by giving them positive feedback. This support prepares them for maintenance of a high level of real self-esteem. In an environment where they feel cared for and where nurtured morale is high, staff are likely to become more self-motivated and put more effort into achieving patient goals.

The nurse manager can immediately use daily praise to improve the unit. Consciously seek a care provider—nursing or non-nursing—who is doing a good job and praise their work. Soon staff will expect the manager to recognize and reward meaningful practice.

STAFF APPRAISAL AND DISCIPLINE

New managers often have difficulty with *performance appraisals.* Identify personal fears and don't let them get in the way. Base comments in evaluations on realistic performance standards. Change in behavior will not result if these standards are written poorly or if they are meaningless to the staff. Use active verbs when telling staff behavior expectations. If the evaluation form requires a long handwritten narrative, consider forming a task force to revise it. The ideal evaluation form outlines performance expectations, contains mostly check-offs, and is easily completed. Develop meaningful key phrases to express patient-centered behavior and performance that result in quality care. In the evaluation, use these phrases with anecdotal notes on each staff member's performance to reward good nursing practices. Over the course of a year, anecdotal records show growth and change. As a rule of thumb, write an anecdotal record daily as praise is given to staff. Most people easily remember negative events; thus these don't need to be documented. However, do not wait for the annual review to deal with repetitive negative behavior[1]. Write the final form of the evaluation immediately; do not waste time writing a draft. Express goals in measurable terms and follow problems up in a timely fashion.

Most nurse managers dislike disciplining staff. Discipline staff when necessary but do not constantly focus on the negatives. The manager who links learning with experience and who nurtures leadership skills usually finds that little discipline is necessary; this behavior also develops staff's potential. When staff are learning new practices, the manager doesn't criticize staff, but encourages them to accept small defeats with humor. The manager teaches staff that autonomy is desirable. Professional staff need self-direction to achieve self-actualization. Striving for staff autonomy helps insure the manager's personal success.

POSITIVE BEHAVIORS

To inspire confidence in staff, the nurse manager behaves calmly, receptively, pleasantly, and sensitively when interacting with staff, patients, families and other personnel. It is also extremely important that the leader develop feelings of affection for those who are working with her to achieve mutual goals. This affection occurs naturally when the nurse manager accepts people as they are and recognizes that most people want to do a good job. Certain behaviors of the manager benefit the unit. The ability to negotiate is crucial, because "win-win" situations are necessary. Accommodating the individual needs of staff, families, or others who provide care to patients is affirmed by staff. The unit leader who can smooth and soothe ruffled feathers can be extremely effective.

These behaviors are related to nonverbal communication skills. The nonverbal component of communication is greatly significant to message transmission. Nonverbal skill is the ability to decode and interpret other's perceptions and feelings accurately.[10] The whole message is influenced by conscious and unconscious actions. Nonverbal cues are interpreted as spontaneous, accurate, and truthful.[2] Effective nonverbal communication has occurred when the receiver agrees with the intent of the sender's information; the message is specific, its conveyance rapid; and the face is a focal point that transmits emotion.[1,3,4,15]

An effective manager understands the power of nonverbal communication and recognizes that nonverbal messages have a greater impact on the receiver than the corresponding verbal statements. Cues and facial expressions are read unconsciously and consciously, and people respond to what they read. Nonverbal messages are perceived through the eyes and supplemented by hearing and touch[5]. The manager who cares remains open and uses body position and appropriate touch to signify openness to communication; she knows the power of a smile and uses it endlessly to enhance staff self esteem.

Make it easy to complain about unit problems, and then do something about them. If you can't resolve the problem, inform the staff and your supervisor. As long as the problem affects the unit, keep trying different approaches and bringing it to the forefront of other's minds. Provide staff with continuous feedback when problems aren't resolved. The manager considers staff-identified problems important.

VALUING STAFF

Weddle[13] recommended that companies put all of their staff in the asset column of the organization. He, of course, is referring to measuring the value of employees. This is achieved by the nurse manager who sets standards, rewards staff when standards are met, and demonstrates that employees are valuable assets to the unit.

The nurse manager has a great advantage over staff, because she can use what is already known to build on unit success. Knowledge about leadership theory, motivation, mentoring, marketing, people power, and risk taking are part of the manager's repertoire. Weddle[13] said,

> We are undergoing a shift from an industrial age to an information age that is forcing us to reassess the way we appropriate resources. . . . People take on an increasingly critical role. And people, as they collect information, master their jobs, and acquire new skills, increase in value with time.

We are moving into a decade where the contribution of nursing will be recognized. Knaus and colleagues[8] reported lower mortality rates in critical care units where communication between physician and nurse was good. More recently, Hartz and colleagues[6] found

> The hospital characteristics most strongly associated with a lower mortality rate were related to the training of medical personnel. . . . A higher percentage of nurses who were R.N.'s were associated with a significantly lower mortality rate.

Literature in nursing abounds with articles focused on nurse retention and the value placed on nurses as contributing members of the team. Addressing nurse executives, Wowk[16] said, "Think of nurses as fully functional partners and help them find an integral place in your organization." This can easily be advice to the nurse manager. These leadership skills—in addition to valuing participative interaction, knowing when to delegate, knowing how to coach others, and recognizing that all team players are important to the unit—contribute to the unit's sense of colleagiality. The nurse manager sets the stage and insures that this process occurs.

Most managers know about Management By Objectives (MBO). Experienced staff who have worked in problem units can tell you about Management By Anxiety (MBA), in which the nurse manager has rigid, impossible expectations. MBA is not desirable and managers who use it often have high unit attrition rates. The ideal nurse manager uses the technique of Managing By Walking Around (MBWA). This says it all: The nurse manager literally walks around the unit to help ensure patient care goals are met. The manager who uses MBWA is considered fair by staff, because nursing notes, flow sheets, charts, and care plans are read by the manager. The manager speaks to families, patients, physicians, and allied health care providers, and sees the kind of care delivered to patients. This manager knows firsthand what is happening on the unit and can evaluate the structure and process used to provide quality care.

The effective nurse manager builds on the staff's sense of personal worth and morale. Enhanced productivity results. Remember that staff have social and family needs. No matter how frantic the unit is, rest breaks are needed to prevent fatigue from affecting quality and to allow rejuvenation before the second half of the shift. Stress reduction in the form of humor, off-work social activities, and consulting services of the psychiatric nurse specialist may be needed periodically. The nurse manager must be able to recognize the need for these. Although it sounds trite, treating other people as you would like to be treated continues to be sound advice, and saying "thank you" goes a long way. Kelley[7] stated,

> What distinguishes an effective from an ineffective follower is enthusiastic, intelligent, and self-reliant participation—without star billing—in the pursuit of an organizational goal.

A nurse manager who creates an environment where employees know they are valued fosters effective followers.

CASE STUDY: DEVELOPING A CALENDAR

You are the newly hired nurse manager for an 8-bed surgical intensive care unit in a large metropolitan hospital. You have had six years of staff experience in critical care, but you are new to this setting and this unit. During these first three months at this job, you have had difficulty spending your time efficiently. You need a system that keeps your objectives in sight on a daily basis, but you aren't sure of the best way to do this. When you meet with your supervisor, she suggests using a large poster-size calendar for each month.

Performance, time, and energy **65**

Using a flip chart found when you moved in, you label twelve sheets with the months and then write the dates, using a Monday through Friday approach, leaving large rectangles for each date to write in everything. You mark off time for the annual Critical Care National Teaching Institute, for your two weeks' summer vacation, and the meetings you know about, such as

- Critical Care committee meetings of the medical board
- Weekly meetings with your supervisor
- Monthly hospital-wide Nurse Manager meetings
- Monthly unit-based Quality Assurance committee
- Department policies, procedures & standards monthly meetings
- Monthly staff meetings

While examining the nursing department calendar, you note the date for next year's Nurses Week celebration and cross off major legal and hospital holidays. You make a list of routine things with deadlines, such as

- Monthly time sheets
- Capital budget forms for proposed new items
- Budget development
- Monthly sick-time reports
- Overtime expenditures
- Budget review of nonpersonnel expenditures
- Two staff evaluations per month

Thinking about inservice dates you added the following to the calendar:

- Personal CPR, ACLS recertification dates
- Staff CPR (March each year), ACLS recertification (May each year)
- Personal annual accreditation and state-required reviews
- Staff annual accreditation and state-required reviews (JCAHO in April)

You plan the ideas you want to explore at staff meetings to increase staff participation in strategic planning, and add a list of these ideas to the calendar. These include:

- Support group for patients' families
- Clinical ladder
- On-site CCRN certification review course
- Revise flowsheet
- Develop policy and procedure for laser angioplasty
- Change code cart contents
- Develop collaborative practice model

On every other month, you write the ideas you want to develop later, such as

- Institute pharmacy unit dose system
- Work on staff development and the charge nurse role
- Develop patient classification system for budget analysis
- Introduce staff self-time planning
- Form a unit-based Ethics Committee

Table 4-2. NURSE MANAGER'S CALENDAR FOR ONE MONTH

MONDAY	TUESDAY	WEDNESDAY	THURSDAY	FRIDAY
2 2:00 P.M.: Policy, Procedure, and Standards 3:00 P.M.: Discharge planning rounds	**3** 10:00 A.M.: Meet with supervisor Meet with unit clerks about supplies	**4** HOLIDAY	**5** Budget analysis due Meet with charge nurse about yesterday's house staff coverage	**6** Sick time report due Post note asking for agenda items from staff
9 12:00 NOON: ICU Medical board 3:00 P.M.: Discharge planning rounds	**10** 10:00 A.M.: Meet with supervisor 11:00 A.M.: Meet with Pharmacy	**11** Call MDs regarding new capital equipment	**12** 2:00 P.M.: meet nurse managers	**13** Overtime expense report due House Staff Orientation Evaluation
16 Meet with laser angioplasty staff 3:00 P.M.: Discharge planning rounds	**17** 10:00 A.M.: Meet with supervisor	**18** 8:00–9:00 A.M. Staff meeting	**19** Call others re. clinical ladders	**20** J.E.D. evaluation for promotion
23 Time sheets due 3:00 P.M.: Discharge planning rounds	**24** 10:00 A.M.: meet with supervisor Meet with Social worker re. Mrs. C's family	**25** Ask G.D. about the CCRN exam Meet with Task Force on Flow Sheet	**26** Unit based QA	**27** M.A.L. evaluation Write Project Evaluation Report on unit dose
30	**31**	vacation through the 12th of next month		

Realizing that Friday afternoon is the quietest time of the week, you schedule two hours every Friday for paperwork and inform your staff and your supervisor that you will be holed up in your office every Friday afternoon unless disaster strikes. Finally, you realize you aren't spending enough quality time with senior staff. Communications with at least four of these staff nurses are limited to report and problem identification. You realize they must be nurtured and developed by you, so you plan formal meetings with one each month for four months. Table 4-2 is a representative sample of the nurse manager's calendar for one month. Note that each day has some notation so that the manager can develop daily objectives.

CONCLUSION

Each nurse manager decides early in her career that leadership and management are challenges worthy of effort. Success as manager of a critical care unit leads to a successful career in management, in critical care, or in upper-level nursing administration—or in all three. A manager knows she is in charge of her own destiny. A manager's performance and the staff's performance under the manager's direction are greatly enhanced when the manager uses sound management theory to foster an environment where staff are rewarded for good practice. Commitment to efficient use of time and development of systems that ensure goals are met are required. And finally, the manager realizes that energy is required to self-motivate and uses knowledge about human behavior and nonverbal communication to present a positive demeanor worthy of the title of manager.

REFERENCES

1. Druckman D, Rozelle RM, and Baxter JC: Nonverbal communication: survey, theory and research. Beverly Hills, 1982, Sage Library of Social Research, 52-63.
2. Ekman P: Emotion in the human face, ed 1, Elmsford, New York, 1982, Pergamon Press Inc.
3. Ekman P: Expression and the Nature of Emotion. In L Scherer and P Ekman, editors: Nonverbal Behavior and Communication, New York: 1984 John Wiley & Sons.
4. Ekman P and Friesen WV: Unmasking the face: a guide to recognizing emotions from facial clues, Englewood Cliffs, N.J., 1975, Prentice-Hall.
5. Gilkes MJ: On seeing eye to eye, Transactions of the Opthalmological Society of the United Kingdom 105:348-50, 1986.
6. Hartz AJ, Krakauer H, Kuhn EM et al: Hospital characteristics and mortality rates, New England Journal of Medicine 321(25):1720-25, 1989.
7. Kelley R: In praise of followers, Harvard Business Review 142-48, November–December 1988.
8. Knaus WA, Draper EA, Wagner DP and Zimmerman JE: An evaluation of outcome from intensive care in major medical centers, Annals of Internal Medicine 104(3):410-18, 1986.
9. Kriegel R: The C zone, Muir Beach, Calif., 1986.
10. Marlowe HA and Marcotte A: Non-verbal decoding. Journal of Psychosocial Nursing 44(4):8-15, 1984.

11. McBride AB: Orchestrating a career. Nursing Outlook 33(5):244-47, 1985.
12. New York Times, Classified Advertisements, Section 9, New York, (July 15):17-18, 1990.
13. Spayd E: Putting people on the balance sheet, Washington Post (May 14):H3, 1989.
14. Tappen R: Nursing leadership and management: concepts and practice, ed 2, Philadelphia, 1989, FA Davis Co.
15. Topf M: Verbal interpersonal responsiveness. Journal of Psychosocial Nursing 26(7):8-16, 1988.
16. Wowk P: Partnering: a new strategy for nursing leadership, Healthcare Executive (2):22-24, 1989.

SUGGESTED READINGS

1. Abdellah F: Evolution of nursing as a profession, International Nursing Review 19(3):219-38, 1972.
2. Fagin CM: Nursing as an alternative to high-cost care, American Journal of Nursing 82(1):57-60, 1982.
3. Jones CB: Staff nurse turnover costs: Part A, a conceptual model, Journal of Nursing Administration 20(4):18-21, 1990.
4. Lloyd B and Handy C: Careers for the 21st century, Long Range Planning 21(3):90-97, 1988.

Chapter 5

FOSTERING PARTICIPATIVE MANAGEMENT

Marlaine Sparki Ortiz

There are positive and negative aspects of all nursing work environments. On the positive side, nurses have become more like equal partners in the health care team. On the negative side, nurses still complain about the lack of communication and autonomy in their practice. Phrases like "I'm so tired of being the last one to know anything around here," and "Why didn't they ask us?" are often heard. Statements like these inform the nurse manager that it is time to look at management styles and communication patterns at the workplace. Knowledge is power, and therefore empowering.[11] A working environment characterized by open communication networks, free exchange of ideas, and an atmosphere of trust is empowering for employees. To build this environment, all employees must participate.

This chapter explores the participative management style, the implications and responsibilities of the manager in this type of environment, and the ways to foster a participative environment.

LEADERSHIP VERSUS MANAGEMENT

The nurse manager of any critical care unit is expected to be an effective leader, as well as an effective manager. The title *Nurse Manager* brings to mind several desirable attributes, such as clinical competence, knowledge, superior technical skills, trustworthiness, resourcefulness, role model, personableness, fairness, and supportiveness—words that describe leadership traits. However, the management aspect also entails some words: traditional words like plan, organize, direct, implement, and control; and new words that come with participative management, such as facilitator, communicator, enhancer, integrator, and coordinator.

Leadership and management are not synonymous. To be a leader, one must have followers. There are formal and informal leaders. Formal leaders are empowered by an organizational structure that gives them the positions and titles to lead. A formal leader may be the nurse manager, supervisor, or nursing care coordinator. Informal leaders have no formal position within an organization. An example of an informal leader is the shop steward or union delegate. These informal leaders have no formal structural authority, but they do have followship.

Managers, on the other hand, are responsible for all functions necessary for achieving the goals of the unit, service, or institution. Managers may not have leadership skills, but usually have managerial skills. If the nurse manager can identify leaders and managers who have both of these skills, she can assess herself and find which skills she has, and which skills she needs to develop. This is especially important if the nurse manager believes that a staff is only as good as its leader.

TRADITIONAL ORGANIZATIONAL STRUCTURE

Historically, hospital staff nurses have practiced under a military model; that is, a hierarchical rank with division of labor. The director of nursing was at the top of a pyramid-shaped organizational chart (Figure 5-1). Staff nurses were at the bottom of the pyramid, and, in many institutions, still are. Little communication flows through the pyramid; what does, flows only in one direction: top to bottom. Only a century ago, job descriptions for nurses were virtually nonexistent. Personal characteristics were apparently more important than job tasks. Nurses were treated as physicians' handmaidens. They were expected never to question an order, always to stand when physicians enter the room, and always to treat physicians in a godlike manner. Today nursing is a maturing profession that recognizes its members as accountable, responsible, and autonomous health-care providers. Nurses are now considered as professionals who work collaboratively with physicians and other members of the health care team.

LEADERSHIP STYLES

Over the last century, there have been several dynamic leaders at the forefront of the nursing profession. Each has had different traits and leadership styles. There is not one single leadership style that works well all the time. Each nurse manager develops an *individual* style as well.

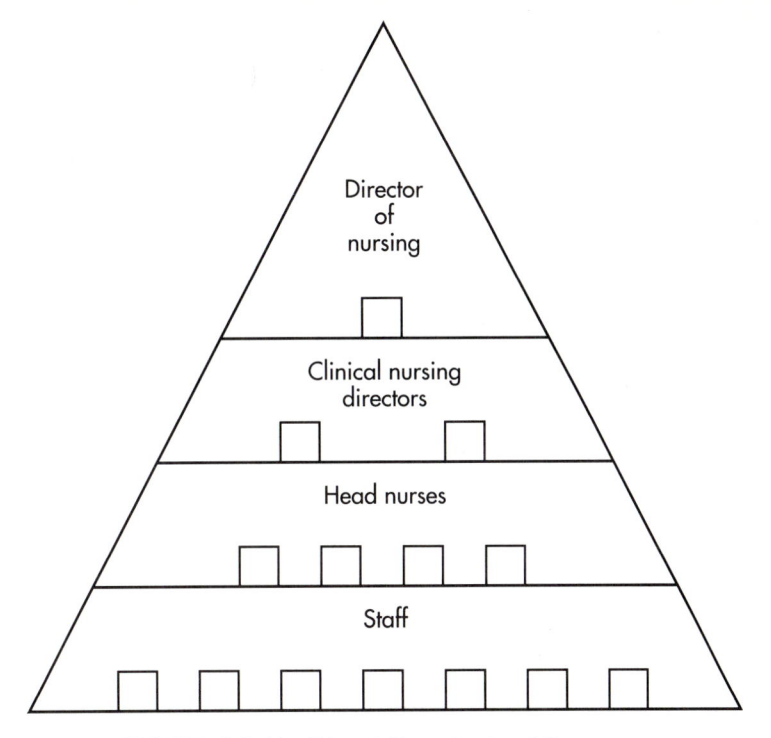

FIGURE 5-1. Traditional Organizational Structure.

Understanding of leadership begins by relating behavior to concepts that define this behavior. An *authoritarian* or *autocratic* leadership style allows no room for discussion. This type of leader "knows best," directs staff in care provision, and forbids staff participation in decision making. Many parents raise their children this way, permitting little autonomy and no power. Authoritarian styles do have a place in nursing leadership, especially during emergencies when action must be taken quickly (for example, during a cardiac arrest).

The *democratic* leader values ideas and opinions of others, and incorporates them into the decision-making process. This leader asks for group input, sets and defines appropriate limits, and then makes decisions. The *laissez-faire* manager is neither autocratic nor democratic. This person stays right in the middle, and maintains the status quo. The laissez-faire manager acts as a figurehead and makes no major decisions. Under this leader, staff are given no specific directions and staff input is not elicited or valued.

Another type of management style is called *situational* leadership. The leadership style that most closely fits the situation is used. A situational leader could use the laissez-faire style to stimulate emerging leaders among the staff, use the autocratic style during a cardiac arrest, and use the democratic style when chairing a meeting. See Table 5-1 for a comparison of leadership styles.

Table 5-1. A COMPARISON OF LEADERSHIP STYLES

CHARACTERISTIC	AUTHORITARIAN (AUTOCRATIC)	LAISSEZ-FAIRE	DEMOCRATIC	SITUATIONAL
Decision making	Alone	None made	Elicits input	Depends on situation
Group participation	None	Some	Large amount	As needed
Staff autonomy	None	Lots without support	Lots with support	Depends on us
Growth potential	None	Status quo	Lots	Varies
Times when appropriate	Emergency situations	To stimulate emerging leaders	Most times	Circumstantial

An astute nurse manager continuously evaluates her individual style by asking, What's my style? Does it change? Will it change? As a nurse manager matures in the role, change occurs; beliefs and leadership styles also change. No matter what specific leadership or management style is initially chosen by a nurse manager, staff interaction and experience will affect the leader's behavior. Over time, effective managers learn to rely upon staff participation and interaction to achieve patient, unit, or institution goals. In Maslow's hierarchy of needs, group belongingness is a lower-level need and must be achieved before self-actualization, a higher-level need, can be achieved. When staff help formulate unit objectives and goals, they gain a sense of group belongingness. Furthermore, a participative leadership style provides the manager and staff opportunities to attain higher-level needs (as defined by Maslow).

MANAGEMENT BY OBJECTIVES

The first priority of the nurse manager is to determine direction for the unit. Goals congruous with those of the organization can be more easily attained by using objectives. Objectives are used as ways to the means. For example, consider a unit goal to decrease nursing turnover. To reach this goal, an objective might be the development of a task force to find the causes of turnover and to examine staff dissatisfiers. Drucker[2], who introduced the term *management by objectives (MBO)*, stated that accomplishments (goals) can be met when objectives are used. MBO is used by nurse managers to make sure all staff know what the unit goals are. For successful goal achievement, the nurse manager and the staff work together and use MBO.

DECENTRALIZATION

In the centralized institution, control is at the top of the nursing structure; in the decentralized institution, control is at departmental, service, or unit level. In a decentralized structure, the individual nursing service (such as medicine, surgery, or pediatrics) has a director or supervisor who is ultimately accountable for that service. This accountability includes planning, budgeting, evaluating, and implementing change. Control, however, is located at the bottom of the organizational structure, and is vested in staff. Communication flows upward, downward, and sideways. Figure 5-2 represents a decentralized unit where communication flows in all directions. Note that the solid lines indicate line authority, and the dotted lines indicate the informal communication network in this organization.

Although decentralization is a significant improvement over centralized management, it is not easily accomplished. Change is slow and takes time, especially in a highly bureaucratic institution. A nurse manager understands that the participatory process is more time-consuming because the decision making is in the hands of more people. The nurse manager realizes that the advantages of this practice far outweigh the disadvantages.

Laliberty[4] said that managers in a decentralized system need the following characteristics: self-confidence, strong self-image, success orientation, good verbal and nonverbal communication skills, assertiveness, initiative, innovation, self-identification, delegation skills, the ability to foster motivation, and a caring attitude. These characteristics do not develop overnight; therefore, the nurse manager completes a self-assessment and begins working on any areas that need improvement. In the long run, acquiring these characteristics improves the quality of the management on the unit.

Decentralization leads to participatory management. It is important to be aware of the type of organization you work in—centralized or decentralized. The nurse manager in a decentralized system recognizes that unit-level changes can easily be instituted.

PARTICIPATIVE MANAGEMENT

Deines[1] stated that participative management, also known as *human relations management,* encourages each staff member's active involvement in organizational decision-making. The results of this participation are improved morale, job satisfaction, decreased turnover, and commitment to organizational goals. The change in staff behavior improves patient care. Effective managers in a participative management environment are sensitive and supportive to staff.

Sashkin[8] stated that participative management means the staff nurses within the institution have control over their jobs, have meaningful work, work collectively with other disciplines, and have real influence in goal achievement. The nurse manager insures these elements are present in the critical care unit.

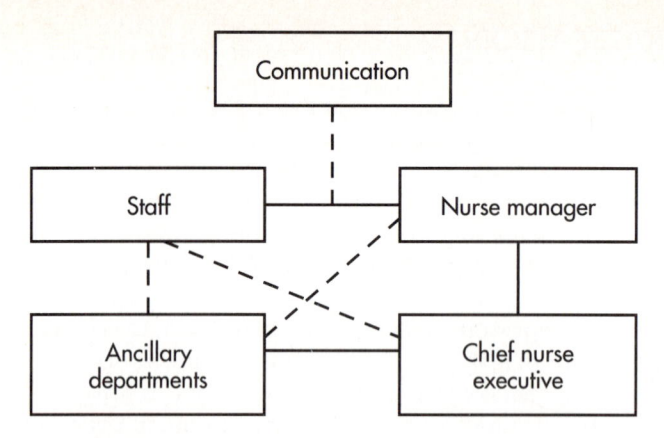

FIGURE 5-2. Decentralized Organizational Chart.

The caring nurse manager identifies what type of control staff nurses have, whether they view their work as meaningful, whether they work cooperatively, and whether they are involved in activities that lead to goal achievement. Whenever the nurse manager finds an element lacking, it then becomes a goal. The information in the box on the next page identifies managers' responsibilities in a participative environment.

Smith, Reinow, and Reid[10] equated participative management to the Japanese style of management called *Theory Z*. This theory includes concepts such as collective decision-making, work group responsibilities, and concern for employees. In this style, quality circles are used. A *quality circle* consists of a cross section of all levels of staff that meets formally to solve problems. In nursing, central committees should be organized this way. For example, the critical care committee with representatives from medicine, respiratory care, nursing management, and nursing staff can best solve problems of patient care activities.

Good communication flow is also associated with these management theories. Without clear expectations and information, employees are less productive, have less interest in their work, and have less commitment to the institution. Loyalty is enhanced by effective communication in the institution. The nurse manager is often instrumental in the success or failure of establishing a good communication network for the unit.

Characteristics of a Participative Environment

Porter-O'Grady[7] listed more features of a participatory organization: participation in developing job descriptions, roles, exceptions, and shared accountability; participation at the highest level in decision-making; participation in development of standards, policies, rules, and regulations; participation in discussions related to wage, salary, benefits, and working conditions; and the ability to make

MANAGERS' RESPONSIBILITIES IN A PARTICIPATIVE ENVIRONMENT	
Do	**Don't**
Be sensitive and supportive of staff needs.	Be uncaring and nonsupportive.
Involve staff in decision making.	Make all decisions without soliciting staff support.
Communicate, communicate.	Keep staff uninformed.
Be direct, honest, upfront.	Be discreet, untrusting, and backbiting.
Deveolp good working groups.	
Have staff participate on central committees.	Put groups together without considering personalities and productivity.
Delegate.	Represent staff on issues in which you are not directly involved.
	Assume all responsibility for everyone and everything.

changes within the organization. An organization that values their employees and encourages staff involvement is described as a participative environment; it is a decentralized organization that has autonomously functioning nursing services.[7]

The nurse manager facilitates the participative environment by ensuring that the staff participates in making unit decisions involving critical care. First, gather a task force of interested practitioners and ask them to solve one specific problem. Encourage them to develop guidelines about role responsibilities within the group, to establish deadlines, and to bring proposals back to staff meetings for input and eventual decision-making. Group participation evolves as staff experience success. The nurse manager can foster participation by giving staff time to go to the library and attend the meetings during the work shift.

Organizational Structure in a Participative Environment

A hierarchal pyramid model does not apply to the participative management environment. Conceptual structures in hospital organizations have changed and most likely will continue changing. Evidence of these changes are flattened organizational structures with direct lines of communication between all levels of staff.

Participative management involves sharing power and empowering staff. The staff are involved in the various aspects of management, and superiors have given staff the power to make decisions and help run the unit and the institution. Goals are formulated through group work; therefore, ownership and achievement are realized. Because of their involvement in these processes, staff view their jobs as more meaningful and rewarding. In this human relations approach to management, staff are viewed as individuals who contribute to organizational objectives. Employee satisfaction results in greater retention.

With a participative management structure comes shared governance. Pinkerton[6] said,

> [Shared governance is] the organizational structure that provides an environment for autonomous staff nurse practice. It is the structure . . . that accommodates professionals in a bureaucratic setting, the structure that tackles a history of subservience and dominance.

The realization of a total shared governance model in a large organization is a time-consuming process.[3,5] Nonetheless, shared governance is emerging in many institutions as a necessity in recruiting and retaining staff.

Case Study: Becoming a Participative Manager

You have just accepted the nurse manager role for a 12-bed surgical intensive care unit where you have been employed as a staff nurse for three years. The previous nurse manager, who had been there six years, had had personal reasons for leaving, but over the past six months you and other staff had noticed that she no longer listened to anyone. You had overheard someone call her "The Queen" and had realized that her behavior, which had become dictatorial, was causing staff dissonance. Your first goal is to change staff perceptions by implementing a form of participative management. In addition, you feel obligated to define your role as the unit facilitator and communicator. Where do you begin?

The nursing staff is accustomed to the leadership style of the previous nurse manager, even though she is no longer there. For insight into staff expectations, reflect on the previous nurse manager's behavior and analyze the strengths and weaknesses of her leadership and management style.

For you, the nurse manager position is an unfamiliar role in a familiar place. Many questions but few answers are evident. Because you have worked on the unit, you know the staff and are friendly with them—and there are advantages and disadvantages to this. As you assume the responsibility commensurate with the title, staff perceptions about you change. The nurse manager supervises staff. Your peer relationship no longer exists, but you want to create an environment that fosters positive peer relationships. You want staff to feel ownership, to be involved in decision making and problem solving, and to work collaboratively with all disciplines earning and giving respect and trust.

Questions to ask yourself are identified in the following box.

This initial assessment may be difficult; however, it is necessary for growth in the role. The second step includes developing personal goals, or where you want to be in 6 weeks, 6 months, 1 year and 5 years. The third step centers on staff involvement. Meet with staff individually and informally, and ask what vision they have of the unit—what problems they see—and finally, what strengths are evident to them. Make a list of the comments and suggestions you receive and post them for all to read.

Now that the initial assessment has been completed and staff input has been sought, you should hold a staff meeting to introduce the concept of a participatory environment. Define a participatory environment for staff by stating that staff will be encouraged to develop short- and long-term goals for the unit, and then to participate in making decisions about how these goals will be achieved. Not all staff will be

> **SELF-ASSESSMENT QUESTIONS**
>
> What are the strengths and weaknesses I bring to this position?
> How can I improve my weaknesses?
> What leadership style do I use? Does it work? How can I change to make it more effective?
> What type of staff work in this unit? Who are the informal leaders, rebels and role models?
> What is the climate like on the unit? Is the group cohesive? Do they function as a team?
> What are staff expectations of the nurse manager?
> What group dynamics are evident?
> Is the institution centralized or decentralized?
> Who are my support systems?

willing to do this, but most will be excited. An astute nurse manager would gain the support of informal unit leaders by involving them in this initial effort.

Adequate preparation is needed. You, the nurse manager can expect challenges and collisions with staff. Although you know that developing a true, trusting, open atmosphere is important, you also know it takes time and skill. Building is enhanced if you, the nurse manager, hand the chair to a staff member for meetings after the first one. This demonstrates the manager's trust in the staff. Staff participation does not mean giving away the power of the nurse manager role. Most seasoned managers know the more power you give to others, the broader your own power base becomes. The roots of a tree keep the tree firmly planted and growing, while the branches continue to blossom. A new manager does not develop strong roots quickly, though she may want things to happen now. Patience is important.

Once staff see how the manager manages, they will become comfortable and start to develop trust. This is when true participative management can begin to grow. Involve staff in committee work, quality assurance, and care plan review. Let staff make decisions and support these decisions. Work with staff to develop a unit philosophy of patient care. Encourage interested staff to work together and bring plans back to the entire staff for discussion and decision making. Objectives and goals naturally follow staff involvement. This is a key to participative management.

REALITY SHOCK

Schmalenberg and Kramer[9] initially coined the phrase *reality shock* to describe the feelings of the new graduate who enters the work force. When taking on a new role, the first phase is called the *honeymoon*. In this phase the individual looks through rose-colored glasses. Everything is wonderful. The new nurse manager thinks, "I have a new job with new challenges, new monetary rewards, and life is grand." The nurse manager is starting to get used to the role. All of a sudden, *reality shock* sets in. The manager thinks "Why did I take this job? Is this going to be worth it?" "I don't know anything about managing and have no business doing this!" "This is one more thing I don't know!" While in this phase, the new manager has trouble deriving benefit from sleep despite many hours in bed. Exhaustion is common, as is self-questioning about the role. Although the shock phase is traumatic, it does pass. Recognize it and, during the transition, seek support from family, friends, peers, and supervisors. By identifying this stage, the nurse manager can compensate for the lack of work-related satisfaction by socializing.

The *recovery* stage rapidly follows. Here, the nurse manager regains her sense of humor, begins to feel better about the role, and starts to move toward *resolution*. Schmalenberg and Kramer[9] described several forms of resolution. In this stage the individual finds a way to deal with the change. *Biculturalism* is an ideal way: the nurse manager brings her values to the job and integrates these values into the unit. Although bicultural individuals are risk-takers, and sometimes "troublemakers," supervisors and nurse managers know that skills will improve with time. The stages of reality shock never last forever.

Dealing with Change

Transitions are not easy for anyone. Remember the day you began your first job. Feel the anxiety, anticipation, and excitement. Was it really like you had envisioned? Many times expectations are different from actual experience. This is true for role transitions as well. In the case study, the nurse manager expected an easy transition because she came from the unit and knew the staff. However, role transition from staff to nurse manager is difficult. The nurse manager must deal with the role change. Incorporating a new manager is equally difficult for staff. Change is problematic for all people, but change does produce growth.

The nurse manager can expect her friendships with staff members to change. When the nurse manager first experiences this, it is painful. For example, the first time the nurse manager walks into the lounge and conversation stops, anxiety ensues. Be aware that there are many pitfalls to role transition—least of all is taking this type of incident personally. The realization that role transition really has resulted in a personal change makes it easier to understand that others' perceptions and responsibilities do change.

As the manager starts to exert leadership, staff begin to test her ability and knowledge by asking questions to which they already know the answers. This is normal. Accept it as part of growth, and humor staff by giving them the answers they want to hear.

The role of the nurse manager is thrilling, demanding, and often frustrating. Feeling uncomfortable about an action or intended action is common. The first confrontation, whether with staff, physicians, or families, produces sweaty palms. However, as the nurse manager works through experiences of this type, confrontation gets easier. Role transition may be difficult, but the outcome is rewarding.

THE MANAGER'S ROLE IN A PARTICIPATIVE ENVIRONMENT

Traditional unit leadership roles comprise the functions of planning, directing, supervising, and controlling. However, manager's roles are evolving. Words such as supporter, cheerleader, coordinator, and facilitator are now more appropriate in a participative environment. Educating staff, especially on issues dealing with decision making, is part of the nurse manager role. A good leader facilitates staff growth, stands by staff decisions, and when necessary, takes a stand with nonstaff personnel and represents staff concerns and problems. Furthermore, the nurse manager assures that there are effective communication paths at all levels.

Porter-O'Grady[7] said that the nurse manager assumes increased responsibilities for fiscal resources; understands the economic marketplace; focuses on problem solving with other administrative heads; fosters a closer peer relationship with staff, plans for sufficient human resources; develops the decision-making and leadership skills of the nursing staff; represents the nursing staff in problems; and manages smooth functioning, and communicates problems and resolutions.

Cheerleading was identified earlier as a role responsibility. In this era of lean staff-to-patient ratios, the nurse manager accepts responsibility for encouraging, praising, coaching, creating, laughing, rewarding, and having fun with staff. The nurse manager no longer tells staff what to do, but works with staff to achieve goals.

The focus of the job description for the nurse manager assuming these roles is on the administrative aspects. The time for change is now. Nurse managers now assume responsibility for unit budgets, collaborate with other department heads, and develop close relationships with staff. Because of the flattened organizational structure, the nurse manager works side by side with staff in problem solving and decision making. Thus the change in manager roles results from and fosters the development of a participative environment.

This new role requires taking risks. However, most managers are risk takers or they wouldn't have applied for the job. As a risk taker, then, the nurse manager tries new things, creates new ways to do things, and becomes a leader for effective change. This fosters collective participation in nursing.

UNIT AND SELF-EVALUATION

Ongoing self-evaluation is expected of all management level personnel. Self-knowledge enhances understanding of behavior and allows growth. Specific strategies that enhance the nurse manager's evaluation of herself and the unit are identified in the following box.

CONCLUSION

Participative management is not just one more nice thing to have. Participative management is necessary because it provides an environment that facilitates

> **STRATEGIES TO ENHANCE EVALUATION**
>
> Keep current by reading relevant literature.
> Facilitate participative interaction daily.
> Identify effective leader behaviors.
> Note how staff participate in the decision-making process.
> Evaluate turnover, absenteeism, and staff satisfaction on an ongoing basis.
> Assess staff expectations of the manager.
> Ask for input on a regular basis.

nurses' accountability, autonomy, and decision-making abilities—all of which ultimately enhance job satisfaction. By fostering this environment, the nurse manager helps recruit and retain excellent nurses.

REFERENCES

1. Deines E: Participative management, Nursing Management 12(11):50-53, 1981.
2. Drucker P: The practice of management, New York, 1974, Harper & Row.
3. Jones L and Ortiz ME: Increasing nursing autonomy and recognition through shared governance, Nursing Administration Quarterly 13(4):11-16, 1989.
4. Laliberty R: Decentralizing health care management, Rockville, Md, 1988, National Health Publishing.
5. Ortiz ME, Gehring P, and Sovie MD: Moving to shared governance, American Journal of Nursing 87(7):923-26, 1987.
6. Pinkerton S and Schroeder P: Commitment to excellence: developing a professional nursing staff, Rockville, Md, 1988, Aspen Publishers, Inc.
7. Porter-O'Grady T: Creative nursing administration: participative management into the 21st century, Rockville, Md, 1986, Aspen Publishers, Inc.
8. Sashkin M: Making participative management work, King of Prussia, Pa, 1988, Organization Design and Development, Inc.
9. Schmalenberg C and Kramer M: Coping with reality shock: the voices of experience, Wakefield, Mass, 1979, Nursing Resources, Inc.
10. Smith HL, Reinow F, and Reid R: Japanese management: implications for nursing administration, Journal of Nursing Administration 14:(9)33-39, 1984.
11. Sovie M: Redesigning our future: whose responsibility is it? Nursing Economics 8(1):21-26, 1990.

SUGGESTED READINGS

1. Baillie V, Trygstad L, and Cordoni T: Effective nursing leadership: a practical guide, Rockville, Md, 1989, Aspen Publishers, Inc.
2. Brooks AM, editor: Team building, Nurse Managers Bookshelf 1(4):21-26, 99-108, 1989.
3. Brownell P: The state of the art: participative management, The Wharton Magazine, pp 38-43, Fall 1982.

4. Douglas L: The effective nurse leader and manager, St Louis, 1984, The CV Mosby Co.
5. Fein IA and Strosberg MA: Managing the critical care unit, Rockville, Md, 1987, Aspen Publishers, Inc.
6. Marriner-Tomey A: Guide to nursing management, ed 2, St Louis, 1988, The CV Mosby Co.
7. McClure ML: Managing the professional nurse; part I, the organization theories, The Journal of Nursing Administration, 14:15-20, February 1984.
8. McClure ML: Managing the professional nurse;: part II, applying management theory to the challenges, The Journal of Nursing Administration, 14:11-17, March 1984.
9. Porter-O'Grady T: Participatory management: the critical care nurse's role in the 21st century, Dimensions of Critical Care Nursing 6(3):131-33, 1987.
10. Porter-O'Grady T and Finnigan S: Shared governance for nursing, Rockville, Md, 1984, Aspen Publishers, Inc.
11. Porter-O'Grady T: Shared governance: reality or sham?, American Journal of Nursing 89(3):350-51, 1989.
12. Vestal K: Management concepts for the new nurse, Philadelphia, 1987, JB Lippincott Co.

Chapter 6

COLLABORATIVE PRACTICE

Susan G. Osguthorpe

The critically ill patient either has life-threatening problems, or is at high risk for developing them.[3] Therefore, the critically ill patient requires constant multidisciplinary assessment and intervention to restore stability, prevent complications, and achieve and maintain optimal responses.[3] The expertise and skills of the different health care providers are complementary. When all health care providers work together synergistically, the quality of critical care is enhanced.[6] The critical care nurse manager is responsible for promoting collaboration with these other health care providers for an integrated approach to patient care.[2] However, most nurse managers are not sure how to achieve a critical care environment that sustains collaborative practice.

Case Study: Challenges to Collaborative Practice

You have just been selected as the nurse manager of a 16-bed surgical intensive care unit in a large university hospital. The patient population is composed primarily of cardiovascular, thoracic, and trauma patients; however, because the hospital is a tertiary referral center, there are always three or four long-term multi-system-failure patients. The house staff manages medical care, and the attending physicians (except for the cardiovascular service) do not have a vested interest in the unit. The annually appointed medical director of the unit regularly makes triage decisions with the nurse manager and charge nurses as a result of the shortage of critical care beds. Despite the nursing shortage, agency nurses are used regularly to keep all sixteen beds available. The nursing staff have a reputation throughout the hospital, particularly with house staff, for providing excellent nursing care. However, most of them have extremely aggressive communication styles and methods of managing patient care and unit situations. The shortage of critical care beds, the shortage of nurses, and the reliance on agency personnel, critical attitudes toward house staff, and the prolonged treatment of patients unlikely to benefit from further extraordinary care were identified as problems by the medical director, director of nursing, chief resident, and staff, respectively. You are charged with providing a plan of action within three months for review with these individuals.

COLLABORATION

There has recently been a resurgence of collaboration in health care with the publication of the multicenter Acute Physiology and Chronic Health Evaluation (APACHE) data by Knaus.[11] This landmark study examined the treatment and outcome of 5030 patients in intensive care units at thirteen tertiary care hospitals. Knaus, Draper, Wagner, and Zimmerman[11] said, "The degree of coordination of intensive care significantly influences its effectiveness." But what is coordination? Is it collaboration? Is it cooperation?

Before a collaborative model is developed, a working definition of *collaboration* must be established. The Styles[15] Stipulation is that "as a word gains in popularity, it loses in clarity." She defines collaboration as "working together."

Styles identified *people, purposes, principles,* and *structure* as the hierarchy of elements in collaboration. In the case study, the medical director, director of nursing, chief resident, and critical care staff are professionals with a common interest in health care and a fundamental compatibility. Their common interest is providing effective and efficient health care to critically ill patients.[15] The nurse manager who understands this can develop ground rules that relate to the values, expectations, and communications of those involved to support a collaborative professional climate. These ground rules will enable all of the health care providers to define roles, relationships, and responsibilities within a collaborative practice structure that optimizes patient outcomes and professional practice.[15]

Kilmann and Thomas[10] define collaboration in terms of the relationship between assertiveness and cooperation. *Assertiveness* is behavior that is directed to achieve one's own goals, and *cooperation* is behavior that is directed to achieve another's goals.[7,10] This relationship is illustrated in the following box.

Returning to the case study, you, as the nurse manager, review the literature on collaboration in health care to familiarize yourself with the concept. Then you begin assessing the compatibility of the critical care unit with collaborative practice as described by Ritter[14] in the box on p. 86. You meet with the medical director, the attending physicians who regularly admit patients to the unit, the director of nursing, the chief resident, and the staff nurses (individually, as well as in groups) to assess the current organizational structure, role relationships, professional issues, and patient care. As the nurse manager, you use these meetings to identify common concerns, and to educate these professionals about collaborative practice. You define collaborative practice as a planned system

ASSERTIVENESS AND COOPERATION IN COLLABORATION			
	Assertive		*Unassertive*
Cooperative	Collaboration	Parallel practice	Accommodation
	Aggressive		*Unaggressive*
Uncooperative	Competition	Tolerance	Avoidance

Adapted from Kilmann RH and Thomas KW: Developing a forced-choice measure of conflict-handling behavior: the "MODE" instrument, Educ Psychol Measurement 37: 309-25 1977; and from Clochesy JM: Relationship resulting from the interaction between assertiveness and cooperation in planning for various settings in critical care. In Cardin S and Ward CR, editors: Personnel Management in Critical Care, Baltimore, 1989 Williams & Wilkins.

through which members of the medical and nursing professions, together with other related health care disciplines, work to assure consistent, quality patient and family care.[12]

HEALTH CARE PROVIDER RELATIONSHIPS

The goal of health care is to provide effective therapeutic interventions that maximize patient outcomes at a reasonable cost. However, the actual roles and responsibilities of specific health care providers are often unclear. The physician's responsibility is the diagnosis and treatment of illness, whereas the nurse's responsibility is the diagnosis and treatment of human *responses* to (actual or potential) health problems.[4] On a day-to-day basis, however, these broad statements are interpreted differently by different individuals, and conflict often arises unless professional health care providers meet to discuss their roles in the care provided.

Returning to the case study, you, the nurse manager, plan a collaborative practice meeting with the cardiovascular surgeons outside the hospital during the evening hours. You want the meeting to be outside the hospital so that interruptions are minimized, and the environment is informal. The meeting is held at the home of one of the surgeons, and individuals bring hors d'oeuvres, desserts, and beverages to minimize the burden of hosting the meeting. The meeting was scheduled from 7:00 PM to 9:30 PM, and the agenda had been posted two weeks in advance.

At the meeting, an attending physician presents the current practice pattern preferences and last year's statistics for open-heart patients. The cardiovascular fellow briefly summarizes how nursing staff could help maximize this practice pattern and

DETERMINING UNIT READINESS	*Usually*	*Sometimes*
1. There is a willingness to collaborate in patient care by healthcare providers.		x
2. Physicians and nurses understand that each profession has unique competencies to contribute to a common goal in patient care.		x
3. The nursing staff is clinically competent and secure in making appropriate decisions.	x	
4. The nursing staff consult with the medical staff appropriately.		x
5. The nursing staff have confidence in the patient care decisions by medical staff.		x
6. The medical staff is clinically competent and makes appropriate patient care decisions.	x	
7. The medical staff consult with the nursing staff appropriately.		x
8. The medical staff have confidence in the patient care decisions of nursing staff.	x	
9. The hospital administration supports quality patient care above other considerations.	x	
10. The hospital administration accepts the nurse-physician team as the principal decision maker in patient care.	x	
11. The hospital administration will support change essential to more collaborative practice.	x	
12. The unit and hospital are committed to primary nursing.	x	
13. Physicians can readily identify their patient's nurses.	x	
14. Patients can identify their nurses as readily as their physicians.	x	
15. The unit and hospital management philosophy is participative.	x	
16. Clinical excellence by healthcare providers is rewarded.		x

Adapted from Ritter HA: Collaborative practice: what's in it for medicine? Nursing Administration Quarterly, 7(4): 31-36, 1983.

resolve postoperative care issues. Nursing staff ask several questions about therapy, and they explain the mechanics of unit triage employed during a heavy surgical schedule, when the surgeons fail to go on rounds before surgery and when they fail to write transfer orders for patients who are able to transfer that day.

You, as nurse manager, facilitate the meeting, and discuss *managed care,* a form of collaborative practice that could facilitate open-heart patient care.[5] Bower[5] described the goals of managed care:

1. To facilitate the achievement of expected and/or standardized patient care outcomes
2. To facilitate early discharge and/or discharge within an appropriate length of stay
3. To promote appropriate and/or reduced utilization of resources
4. To promote collaborative practice, coordination of care, and continuity of care
5. To promote professional development and satisfaction of hospital based registered nurses
6. To direct the contributions of all care providers toward the achievement of patient outcomes

The surgeons express concern about having a cookbook approach to patient care rather than the individualized care that patients require. You indicate that the managed-care plan would be a guide of care agreed upon by all health care providers; a guide that could be used by new house staff, new nursing personnel, other health care providers, patients, and families. The group selects a task force consisting of an attending physician, the cardiac fellow, the nurse manager, and several staff nurses to develop a draft of the managed-care plan. The task force will involve staff from physical therapy, social services, and the telemetry unit. After several reviews by the entire group, the managed-care plan is ready for a trial (see Figure 6-1).

The group and representatives from other departments continue to meet weekly to discuss patient progress, particularly of those postoperative patients who have failed to progress as expected. Open-heart surgical rounds occur around 6:00 AM each day in the critical care unit. These rounds involve primarily the attending physician, the primary nurse, the cardiac fellow, and the surgical house staff. The cardiothoracic clinical nurse specialist provides consultation for nursing staff on all patients; however, any patient who fails to progress becomes part of her formal caseload for more intensive follow-up and management. The cardiac fellow is responsible for tracking each patient's progress in the chart using a pathway progress tool (see Figure 6-2). Any health care provider can refer to the tool to discern individual patient progress and problems at a glance. It is incumbent on all health care providers to follow-up aspects of care within each specialty (see Table 6-1).

Quarterly collaborative practice meetings to discuss the overall process of managed care continue outside the hospital. As people become more comfortable with each other, the communication process becomes more collaborative and mutually supportive. Difficulties in providing care are not seen as anyone's fault, but as surmountable problems. Patients with serious complications and poor prognoses are professionally discussed and treatment goals are mutually set. Personal stress behaviors of health care providers are openly but sensitively discussed, as are barriers to effective communication and care. Mutual expectations are regularly reviewed and clarified by the entire group.

	PREOPERATIVE DAY	**DAY OF SURGERY**	**POSTOP DAY 1**
LOCATION	Admit to acute care	Operating room/ICU	ICU
VISITS BY	Cardiologist, cardiothoracic (CT) surgeon, anesthesiologist, clinical nurse specialist (CNS), physical therapist (PT), Respiratory therapist (RT)	Cardiologist, CT surgeon, anesthesiologist, CNS, PT, RT	Cardiologist, CT surgeon, anesthesiologist, CNS, PT, RT
TESTS	Complete blood count (CBC), complete electrolyte profile, protime (PT), prothrombin time (PTT), thrombin time (TT), bleeding time (?).type/cross 4 units blood, arterial blood gases (ABGs), chest x-ray (CXR). electrocardiogram (ECG), pulmonary function tests (PFTs) (?), urine analysis	Hematocrit (Hct), electrolytes (sodium-Na, potassium-K, chloride-Cl, carbon-dioxide-CO, glucose, creatinine-Cr) CPK isoenzymes (CPK-MB), PT, PTT, TT, platelet count, ABGs, CXR, ECG	Hct, electrolytes, CPK-MB, ABGs, CXR, ECG
TREATMENTS	Height, weight, enema, shave/prep, betadine shower	Foley catheter. intake/output (I & O), weight ————————▶ Oxygen by ventilator ——▶ face mask/cannula ——▶ Pulmonary artery with continous venous oxygen & arterial pressure monitoring ————————▶ Cardiac monitoring ————————▶ Epicardial pacing prn ————————▶ Chest tubes ———————▶ Discontinue (DC) 24-48 hours Intravenous (IV) access (2) ————————▶ Nasogastric tube prn ———▶ DC 24-48 hours	
MEDICATIONS	Continue patients own meds	IV antibiotic ————————————▶ Morphine sulfate ———————————▶ Vasoactive, antidysrhythmic ———————▶ and KCl drips prn Digoxin and diuretics prn ———————▶	
DIET	Regular ⟶ nothing by mouth after midnight	NPO —————————▶ Clear liquids ——————▶	
ACTIVITY	Up ad lib, self-care	Level I: Bedrest, passive range of motion (ROM) & turning. Total care	Level II: Dangle/stand at bedside, active assistive ROM. Partial self-care/feed
EDUCATION	Preoperative instruction by CNS, PT, RT, primary nurse; Visit to ICU or ICU video, Open-heart video		
DISCHARGE PLANNING	Assessments/plan of care initiated by healthcare team		

FIGURE 6-1. Coronary Artery Bypass Surgery Management Pathway *(Developed by Osguthorpe S, Tidwell S, Smith G, and Perkins T)*

Continued.

POSTOP DAY 2	**POSTOP DAY 3**	**POSTOP DAY 4**	**POSTOP DAY 5/6**
Transfer to acute care	Acute care	Acute care	Acute care
Cardiologist, CT surgeon, CNS, PT, RT	Cardiologist, CT surgeon, CNS, PT, RT	Cardiologist, CT surgeon, CNS, PT, RT	Cardiologist, CT surgeon, CNS, PT, RT
Hct, Electrolytes, CPK-MB, ABGs, CXR, after chest tubes DC'd	Hct ?, Electrolytes ? Pulse oximetry oxygen saturation	CXR after pacer wires DC'd. Pulse oximetry oxygen saturation	
DC foley catheter. ----------------→		DC I & O when preop wt	
nasal cannula ----------------→		DC when oxygen saturation > 90% on room air	
DC pulmonary artery and arterial lines			
Telemetry monitoring ----------------→		DC after 48 hours sinus rhythm or atrial fibrillation with rate < 100	
Pacer at bedside on standby if stable ----------------→		DC pacer wires if sinus rhythm or atrial fibrillation with rate < 100	
Heparin lock, 1 IV ----------------→		DC heparin lock	
DC antibiotic			
Analgesic, aspirin dipyridamole, ? digoxin docusate. Milk of magnesia (MOM) prn ----------------→		MOM if no bowel movement (BM)	Bisacodyl suppository and/or enema until BM
Low-fat, low cholesterol diet, ? sodium restriction in some individuals ----------------→			
Level III-IV: Out of bed/chair, ambulate in room 2-5 minutes Self-care	Level V: Ambulate in room prn and hall for 5-7 minutes Self-care	Level VI-VII: Ambulate in hall 7-10 minutes, 1/2 flight stairs. Self-care, shower if pacer wires are out	Level VII: Ambulate in hall 7-10 minutes, full flight stairs. Consider referral for Phase II cardiac rehabilitation program. Self-care
	Classes per cardiac rehabilitation program schedule for Heart Surgery, Up & About, You & Your Diet, and Coping with Heart Surgery		Medications, Review of Individualized Diet, Activity, Wound Management, Signs & Symptoms
			Follow-up appointment scheduled

Table 6-1. MANAGED-CARE ACCOUNTABILITIES

1. Admission history, physical, and medical treatment plan, including monitoring the therapeutic effectiveness of tests, treatments, and medications. Facilitate daily rounds on nursing units—maintain and update patient progress tool.	Cardiac fellow Surgical house staff
2. Admission history, physical, and nursing care plan, including monitoring patient progress in achieving goals related to education and independent activities of daily living. Coordination of class attendance and consultations with PT, OT, the cardiothoracic CNS, the dietician, and the social worker.	Telemetry and ICU primary nurses
3. Patient activity progression and conducting "Up and About" class.	Physical therapy Occupational therapy
4. Nutritional evaluation and assessment. Conducting individualized risk factor counseling and conducting "Diet" class.	Dietician
5. Assessment and intervention to increase effectiveness of patient/family coping, strengthening of formal and informal support systems, and facilitating continuity of care during transfers and following discharge. Conduct "Coping" class.	Social worker
6. General nursing management consultant and posthospital follow-up of all open-heart patients. Case management of patients with failure to progress. Facilitate weekly care conferences. Conduct "Heart Surgery" class.	Cardiothoracic clinical nurse specialist
7. Overall nursing direction and management of ICU. Facilitate hospital support and changes in the patient care delivery system to support collaborative practice. Facilitate quarterly collaborative practice meetings.	Nurse manager
8. Overall direction and management of cardiovascular program	Cardiothoracic surgery attending physicians
9. Overall medical direction and management of the ICU.	ICU medical director

SYSTEMS SUPPORT

The ICU medical director and the nurse manager meet with the director of nursing, the chief of staff, and a consultant from the finance department. The nurse manager proposes a trial of managed care for open-heart surgery patients to achieve more effective patient outcomes while minimizing cost. The finance consultant develops a computerized tracking system that requires minimal input from clinical personnel, and uses the managed care pathway and monitoring tool in conjunction with patient billing input and with medical record department input. She also

Collaborative practice 91

Patient Stamp								Attending Physician
								Primary Nurse
Date	2/10/91	2/11/91	2/12/91	2/13/91	2/14/91	2/15/91	2/16/91	2/17/91	2/18/91
Pathday	Preop	OR	Day 1	Day 2	Day 3	Day 4	Day 5	Day 6	Day 7

CORONARY ARTERY BYPASS SURGERY
MANAGEMENT PATHWAY PROGRESS TOOL

CONSULTS

TESTS

TREATMENTS

MEDICATIONS

DIET

ACTIVITY

EDUCATION

DISCHARGE PLANNING

Risk Factors (Circle all that apply)
Over 65 years old
Over 70 years old
Male/Female
Family History
Race
Decreased activity
Type A personality
New York Heart Association Class I, II, III, IV

Total cholesterol   > 200   > 240
              LDL > 130   > 160
Diabetic   Type   I   II
Weight   ideal   15%   20%
Hypertension systolic   > 140
              diastolic   > 100
Chronic Obstructive Pulmonary Disease

Ejection fraction < 50% < 30%
Reoperation
Failed coronary angioplasty
ICU/CCU patient
Preoperative intra-aortic ballon
Urgent Operation/Emergent Operation
Chronic Renal Failure/Dialysis
Impending Sense of Doom

FIGURE 6-2. Coronary Artery Bypass Surgery Management Pathway Progress Tool *(Developed by Osguthorpe S).*

presents summary data at the collaborative practice quarterly meetings for review. Many of the high-risk factors documented with the patient progress tool are identified as those that contribute to a prolonged length of stay and poor postoperative patient progress. Patient population subgroup care-planning is undertaken to manage the high-risk patients.

To enhance optimal unit management, the nurse manager and medical director incorporate the collaborative practice model of the American Association of Critical-Care Nurses[1] and the Council of the Society of Critical Care Medicine (see the following box).

The nurse manager compares the collaborative practice environment and managed care as it evolves in her unit with the recommendations of the National Joint Practice Commission (NJPC).[5] The five essential elements delineated by the NJPC

COLLABORATIVE PRACTICE MODEL PRINCIPLES

1. Responsibility and accountability for effective functioning of a critical care unit must be vested in physician and nurse directors who are on an equal decision-making level.

2. These directors must be appropriately prepared and educated. In addition to competence in patient management, they need knowledge and experience in the following areas: management principles, resources management, and skills in interpersonal relationships (including conflict resolution).

3. The organizational structure of a critical care unit must insure that physicians are autonomous when dealing with issues that affect medical practice.

4. The organizational structure of a critical care unit must ensure that nurses are autonomous when dealing with issues that affect nursing practice.

5. Some aspects of patient care require interdependence between physicians and nurses. These aspects must be identified and addressed jointly.

6. Every critically ill person requires medical and nursing care. The services of additional disciplines may also be required in specific situations. In order to provide a holistic approach, the care delivered by other health team members must be coordinated by the physician and nurse directors.

7. Unit support services must be organized to enable the directors to optimally carry out their primary responsibilities in the practice of their respective disciplines (that is, patient care).

8. The directors are accountable for the evaluation of the quality and efficiency of care and the financial provision of that care. They must develop a unit-specific system for the evaluation of care on a timely basis.

9. The directors are responsible for creating and maintaining an environment in which individuals have opportunities to realize their potentials.

10. Close collaboration between the directors is essential for successful management. This collaboration can be enhanced by daily rounds, weekly meetings, and other means that will ensure continuous, open communication.

American Association of Critical-Care Nurses: Collaborative practice model: the organization of human resources in critical care unit, AACN Position Statement, October, 1982.

are primary nursing, the integrated patient record, clinical decision-making by nursing, a joint practice committee, and joint care review.[8,13] Although the ICU has an all-RN staff (which enhances primary nursing and collaborative practice), the telemetry unit utilizes some non-RN support personnel. Despite this, the managed-care model worked very well on the telemetry unit and achieved the goals of managed care described by Bower.[5]

The nurse managers of ICU and the telemetry unit work closely with other ancillary and support services to minimize the need for nurses to perform non–nursing tasks, particularly during the evening and night shifts. Working with the other departments enables nursing to meet their accountabilities.

Formulating the integrated patient record involves developing a multidisciplinary charting document that includes progress notes by health care providers, documentation of patient education, and assessment information. The usual hospital progress note is used by all disciplines for specific patient problems, and the patient progress tool is used to track patients on a day-to-day basis, although it is not part of the permanent record. The managed-care plan is used to orient practitioners from all health care disciplines to the management and treatment of the open-heart patient population.

The decision-making by nurses and other health care providers is enhanced by establishing a written guideline (see Figure 6-1). Each health care provider is accountable for reporting and resolving patient care problems, which is easy during daily rounds and weekly care conferences. General changes and recommendations in the managed-care plan occur often at the quarterly collaborative practice meeting.

The quarterly collaborative practice meeting is used as a joint practice committee, although the ICU committee continues to deal with management and policy of the critical care unit. The quality assurance activities developed around the managed-care plan are regularly reviewed by the ICU committee, as well as by the collaborative practice group. Joint review is accomplished through daily unit rounds and weekly care conferences. It became clear after several months that six key issues (regarding the clarity of patient care goals and communication) should trigger a care conference within twenty-four hours:

1. Unclear perception of treatment goals by any member of the health care team
2. Unpredictable transfer or discharge date due to poor patient progress
3. Inadequately written care plan
4. Lack of consensus among health care providers on care plan
5. Patient and family concerns
6. Patients with major unresolved complications and prolonged lengths of stay

EVALUATING THE PROCESS

The managed-care process and collaborative practice environment are evaluated after six months. The evaluation outcomes appear in the next box.

CONCLUSION

Collaborative practice and managed care enhance each other, improve patient outcomes and maximize resource utilization. Like all planned change, the imple-

MANAGED CARE EVALUATION

1. Economic. Patient stay was decreased by one day in the high-risk group and by two days in the normal-risk group. All services were decreased, and some services were significantly decreased because they were stopped several days before discharge rather than on the day of discharge. These included IV therapy, oxygen therapy, and telemetry monitoring. Many lab tests were found to be redundant and not contributory to improving patient outcome.

2. Education. Nurses, physicians, and other healthcare providers were very familiar with services provided by each specialty and made more appropriate and timely requests for consultation for patients at high risk or patients that failed to progress. Fewer significant differences of opinion occurred regarding patient care and treatment goals. Differences of opinion were presented in light of patient outcomes rather than an ongoing power struggle or turfbattle.

3. Litigation. Although few actual litigious situations had occurred in this patient population before managed care, the health care providers reported that they perceived (a) better patient care and outcomes, (b) increased knowledge of patient/family problems, and (c) earlier resolution of problems, issues, and delays. Patients reported increased satisfaction with the care provided.

4. Administration. Increased communication between and among the health care providers increased the amount of decision making at lower levels and resulted in better decision-making for the entire cardiovascular program.

5. Patient Education. Patients were provided with group classes stressing important aspects of care and recovery on a consistent basis. Individualized education was completed earlier and more appropriately. Patient education materials were developed, and these contributed to more effective retention of important aspects of care and recovery. Physicians and the cardiothoracic CNS reported a decrease in telephone calls postdischarge, and an increase in patient compliance with the treatment plan.

6. Record Keeping. Integrated record keeping was developed as part of the managed-care trial. Some records were kept at the patient's bedside to minimize redundant charting by nursing and to facilitate rounds. Health care providers indicated that the multidisciplinary record and patient progress tool increased their knowledge of individual patient responses to the treatment plan.

7. Nursing Satisfaction. Nurses reported greater job satisfaction with their increased accountability and communication, which was borne out by a decease in turnover. The lower turnover resulted in increased familiarity with patient care management and decreased utilization of agency nurses.

8. Physician Satisfaction. Attending physicians indicated less need for supervision and improved coordination in patient care management. House staff indicated that nurse-physician communication was significantly improved, and much more collaborative in nature.

Adapted from Ritter HA: Collaborative practice: what's in it for medicine? Nursing Administration Quarterly 1983 7(4): 31-36.

mentation process is purposeful and time-consuming. Both collaborative practice and managed-care depend upon professional role clarification, professional accountability and assertiveness, as well as the cooperative efforts of all health care providers. It is clear that the goals of collaborative practice benefit the nurse, the physician, the institution, and the patient.[8] Collaborative practice

- gives the nurse increased job satisfaction through changes in role definition and decision-making processes
- gives the physician the need for less supervision and the development of better coordination with other health care providers
- gives the institution greater patient satisfaction with better use of professional staff and other resources
- gives the patient more personalized and individualized care that optimizes patient outcomes while assuring appropriate utilization of expensive resources

Finally, in the words of Jacob Javits, "In critical care, it strikes me that the issues are three: realism, dignity, and love."[9] For nurse managers and health care providers, it is not just the delivery of critical care that is important, but the optimization of the human process of caring.

REFERENCES

1. American Association of Critical Care Nurses: Collaborative practice model: the organization of human resources in critical care units, AACN Position Statement, Newport Beach, Calif, October 1982, The Association.
2. American Association of Critical Care Nurses: Role expectations for the critical care manager. AACN Position Statement, Newport Beach, Calif, June 1986, The Association.
3. American Association of Critical Care Nurses: Scope of critical care nursing practice, AACN Position Statement, Newport Beach, Calif, November 1986, The Association.
4. American Nurses' Association: Nursing: a social policy statement, ANA Position Statement. Kansas City, Mo, 1980, The Association.
5. Bower KA: Managed care: controlling costs, guaranteeing outcomes. Definition: The Center for Nursing Case Management 3(3):1-3, 1988.
6. Clemmer TP and Orme JF: An integrated approach to the patient with acute respiratory failure. In Clemmer, TP and Orme JF, editors, Critical Care Medicine, Salt Lake City, 1981, LDS Hospital.
7. Clochesy JM: Planning for various settings in critical care. In Cardin S and Ward CR, editors, Personnel Management in Critical Care Nursing, Baltimore, 1989, Williams and Wilkins.
8. Devereux PM: Essential elements of nurse-physician collaboration. Journal of Nursing Administration 11:19-23, 1981.
9. Javits J: 1986 Inspirational Award Honoree. Foundation for Critical Care. 1001 Connecticut Ave. NW, Suite 428, Washington, DC, 20036.
10. Kilmann RH and Thomas KW: Developing a forced-choice measure of conflict-handling behavior: The "MODE" instrument. Educational and Psychological Measurement 37:309-25, 1977.

11. Knaus WA, Draper EA, Wagner DP, and Zimmerman JE: An evaluation of outcome from intensive care in major medical centers, Annals of Internal Medicine 104:410-18, 1986.
12. Koerner BL, Cohen JR, and Armstrong DM: Professional behavior in collaborative practice, Journal of Nursing Administration 16(10):39-43, 1986.
13. National Joint Practice Commission: Guidelines for establishing joint or collaborative practice in hospitals, Chicago, 1981, Neely Printing Co, Inc.
14. Ritter HA: Collaborative practice: what's in it for medicine? Nursing Administration Quarterly (Summer):31-36, 1983.
15. Styles MM: Reflections on collaboration and unification, Image: The Journal of Nursing Scholarship 16:21-23, 1984.

Unit II

Developing Managerial Skills

Chapter 7

STANDARDS OF CARE

Sarah J. Sanford

CONCEPTUAL FRAMEWORK FOR STANDARDS IMPLEMENTATION

Standards of care provide a framework for delivery of optimal nursing care. If implemented effectively they help define, organize, deliver, and evaluate the care provided to patients. To implement standards of care, however, nursing must be envisioned as the problem-solving approach to individualizing and delivering nursing care.

The second edition of the AACN's *Standards for Nursing Care of the Critically Ill*[1] advises its readers to begin by individualizing and adapting its statements and concepts to fit the particular practice environment. AACN's standards statements are in two sections: process (clinical practice) standards and structure (environmental) standards. The comprehensive *process* standards are as follows:

    I. Data shall be collected continuously on all critically ill patients wherever they may be located.

   II. The identification of patient problems/needs and their priority shall be based upon collected data.

  III. An appropriate plan of nursing care shall be formulated.

  IV. The plan of nursing care shall be implemented according to the priority of identified problems/needs.

V. The results of nursing care shall be continuously evaluated.

The comprehensive *structure* standards include the following:[1]

I. The critical care unit shall be designed to ensure a safe and supportive environment for critically ill patients and for the personnel who care for them.
II. The critical care unit shall be constructed, equipped, and operated in a manner which protects patients, visitors, and personnel from electrical hazards.
III. The critical care unit shall be constructed, equipped, and operated in a manner which protects patients, visitors, and personnel from fire hazard.
IV. The critical care nurse shall have essential equipment, services, and supplies immediately available at all times.
V. The critical care unit shall have a comprehensive infection control program.
VI. The critical care unit shall be managed in a manner which ensures the delivery of safe and effective care to the critically ill.
VII. The critical care unit shall have appropriately qualified staff to provide care on a 24-hour basis.
VIII. The critical care nurse shall be competent and current in critical care nursing.
IX. The critical care nurse's performance appraisal shall be based upon the roles and responsibilities identified in the position description.
X. The critical care unit shall have an explicit, systematic, and ongoing program to evaluate care of the critically ill.
XI. Critical care nursing practice shall include both the conduct and utilization of clinical research.
XII. The critical care nurse shall ensure the delivery of safe nursing care to patients, being cognizant of the various "causes of action" for which the nurse may be liable.
XIII. The critical care unit shall be managed in a manner which assures the delivery of humane and ethical care.

The comprehensive standards are stated in general terms. The process standards describe the nursing process. Therefore, although they are targeted at critical care nursing practice, they are broadly applicable to all acute care settings. The structure standards, on the other hand, relate to the practice environment, and thus are more specific to critical care practice.

Because the comprehensive standards statements are so broad, supporting standards statements* have also been defined. Each supporting standard statement delineates a key concept implicit in the general comprehensive statement:

---

* Reprinted from: AACN Standards for Nursing Care of the Critically Ill (2nd edition). Used with permission.

STANDARDS OF CARE IN THE CRITICALLY ILL

Comprehensive Standard I.   Data shall be collected continuously on all critically ill patients wherever they may be located.
Supporting Standards.   The critical care nurse shall

a. determine the gravity of the patient's problems/needs.
b. collect subjective and objective data within a time period which reflects the gravity of the patient's problems/needs.
c. collect data in an organized, systematic fashion to ensure completeness of assessment.
d. utilize appropriate physical examination techniques.
e. demonstrate technical competency in gathering objective data.
f. demonstrate competency in communication skills.
g. gather pertinent social and psychological data from the patient, significant others, and other health team members.
h. collect pertinent data from previous patient records.
i. collaborate with other health team members to collect data.
j. facilitate the availability of pertinent data to all health team members.
k. revise the data base as new information is available.
l. document all pertinent data in the patient's record.

Comprehensive Standard II.   The identification of patient problems/needs and their priority shall be based upon collected data.
Supporting Standards: The critical care nurse shall

a. utilize collected data to establish a list of actual and potential patient problems/needs.
b. collaborate with the patient, significant others, and other health team members in identification of problems/needs.
c. utilize collected data to formulate hypotheses as to the etiologic bases for each identified actual or potential problem/need.
d. utilize nursing diagnoses for the actual or potential problems/needs which nurses, by virtue of education and experience, are able, responsible, and accountable to treat.
e. establish the priority of problems/needs according to the actual/potential threat to the patient.
f. reassess the list of actual or potential problems/needs and their priority as the data base changes.
g. record identified actual or potential problems/needs, indicating priority, in the patient's record.

Reprinted from AACN Standards for nursing care of the critically ill, ed 2, Sanford S and Disch J, editors, Norwalk, Conn, and San Mateo, Calif, 1989, Appleton & Lange Publishing Co. Used with permission.

Continued.

STANDARDS OF CARE IN THE CRITICALLY ILL — cont'd

Comprehensive Standard III. An appropriate plan of nursing care shall be formulated.
Supporting Standards: The critical care nurse shall

a. develop the plan of care in collaboration with the patient, significant others, and other health team members.
b. determine nursing interventions for each problem/need.
c. incorporate interventions for each problem/need.
d. identify areas for education of the patient and significant others.
e. develop appropriate goals for each problem/need in collaboration with the patient, significant others, and other health team members.
f. organize the plan to reflect the priority of identified probems/needs.
g. revise the plan of care to reflect the patient's current status.
h. identify activities through which care will be evaluated.
i. communicate the plan to those involved in the patient's care.
j. record the plan of nursing care in the patient record.

Comprehensive Standard IV. The plan of nursing care shall be implemented according to the priority of identified problems/needs.
Supporting Standards: The critical care nurse shall

a. implement the plan of nursing care in collaboration with the patient, significant others, and other health team members.
b. support and promote patient participation in care.
c. deliver care in an organized, humanistic manner.
d. integrate current scientific knowledge with technical and psychomotor competency.
e. provide care in such a way as to prevent complications and life-threatening situations.
f. coordinate care delivered by other health team members.
g. document interventions in the record.

Comprehensive Standard V. The results of nursing care shall be continuously evaluated.
Supporting Standards: The critical care nurse shall

a. assure the relevance of nursing interventions to identified patient problems/needs.
b. collect data for evaluation within an appropriate time interval after intervention.
c. compare the patient's response with expected results.
d. base the evaluation on data from pertinent sources.
e. collaborate with the patient, significant others, and other health team members in the evaluation process.
f. attempt to determine the cause of any significant differences between the patient's response and the expected response.
g. review the plan of care and revise it based on the evaluation results.
h. document evaluation findings in the patient record.

Table 7-1. THREE-COLUMN FORMAT
Comprehensive Standard _____

SUPPORTING STANDARDS	SKILLS/ ACTIVITIES	REFERENCES

Modified with permission from: AACN Standards for Nursing Care of the Critically Ill, ed 2, Norwalk, Conn, and San Mateo, Calif, 1989, Appleton & Lange.

AACN recommends using a three-column format like that in Table 7-1 to facilitate the adaptation of these standards to the specific practice setting. This format allows maximum creativity and flexibility, and simultaneously reinforces the link between the standard and the actual activities in the practice environment.

To use this format, write the comprehensive standard across the top. List supporting standards in the left-hand column. Complete the middle and right-hand columns during the individualization process. That is, for each supporting standard in the left-hand column, list in the middle column the specific skills or activities required to comply with it. List references, such as applicable policies and procedures, relevant articles or texts, and even specific individuals, in the right-hand column.

During implementation, it is often necessary to reflect institutional or unit idiosyncracies. Concepts reflected in several AACN supporting standards statements may be consolidated in one statement to fit the practice setting so that tasks typically linked together can continue to be linked. As long as the key concepts are preserved in the unit-based adaptations, supporting standards statements may be streamlined to increase their relevance.

The Joint Commission on Accreditation of Healthcare Organizations (JCAHO)[2] and state regulatory agencies require delivery of nursing care in accordance with individual patient needs. The comprehensive and supporting standards of AACN help determine the scope of practice, the related activities, and the measurement criteria for critical care nursing in any given practice setting. Thus, if adapted effectively, the AACN standards can facilitate JCAHO accreditation and regulatory compliance.

Case Study: Critical Care Manager

As an experienced critical care manager, you have decided to move across the country to be near your aging parents. While looking for the ideal position you attend a meeting of the local chapter of the American Association of Critical-Care Nurses (AACN). At the meeting, you overhear two nurses discussing the lack of quality care in a critical care unit of a hospital you had always thought of as "home." You had graduated from that hospital's diploma program sixteen years ago, and you are appalled with this derogatory talk about the unit. This unit had accepted you as a new graduate. The nurse manager and instructor had tailored an effective orientation specifically to your needs. Although you went on to complete your master's degree years ago, you still have fond memories of your first work experience in this hospital. Furthermore, you strongly believe that this initial, positive work experience played a major role in the rewarding and exciting career in critical care you have enjoyed since. After much thought, you decide to explore work opportunities in this unit.

During the interview with the director of medical-surgical practice, you discover a number of disquieting things. The former nurse manager had stayed only nine months. Out of 76 budgeted positions, there are 25 vacancies—a 33 percent vacancy rate. Annual turnover is 43 percent, and more than 90 percent of the staff has less than two years of experience in critical care. Three different agencies are used routinely to keep the unit staffed. Morale among the regular staff is at an all-time low, and nurses from the hospital's PRN pool refuse to work in the unit. As if that's not bad enough, two serious incidents associated with poor-quality care had occurred in the past six months. Physicians are complaining about the poor attitude; so are several of the hospital's ancillary departments. You are not surprised when you hear that there had been no qualified applicants for the nurse manager position.

Undaunted, you continue the interview process and request a meeting with the chief nurse executive. You plan for this meeting carefully, recognizing that you must discover her personal philosophy, as well as the departmental philosophy. You must also determine her willingness to support major change, and her commitment to improving the unacceptable situation in the unit.

The chief nurse executive is open and forthright. You are satisfied that you will have the full support of the chief nursing executive and director of medical-surgical practice. You accept the nurse manager position, fully understanding that the task ahead will be difficult.

You strongly believe that the unit needs leadership and participatory decision-making. Moreover, the chief nurse executive, the director of medical-surgical practice, and you have reached a consensus that care standards are necessary to provide a framework, first for stability, and eventually for growth. Having implemented standards of care based on AACN standards[1] twice before, you are sure you can work with the staff to do it again.

BEGINNING THE PROCESS

You begin the implementation of standards, recognizing that you and the staff will be undergoing a significant change. You hold staff meetings and solicit volunteers to develop a plan to make the unit more effective with patients and more satisfying for staff. You realize that many committees need to be established or reactivated to address issues with as much staff participation as possible.

Ideas for specific committees and committee membership guidelines are presented during a staff meeting. After staff review and input, the unit committee list is finalized:

- Standards committee
- Quality assurance committee
- Documentation committee
- Procedure and policy committee
- Journal club

Guidelines for membership* are also revised with staff input. Each Committee will have

- Representation from all shifts
- A chairperson elected by the third meeting
- At least five staff members
- Minutes taken; copies to be made and distributed by the unit clerk

Meetings will be

- Alternated weekly between A.M. and P.M. shifts
- Held at predictable, consistent times
- Held in the lounge after report

Other details about committee meetings are also discussed at staff meetings. It is agreed that staff would receive pay for one hour of overtime when they attend committee meetings during a shift they do not normally work. After the first three months, staff would work on committee projects during scheduled work time, and overtime for committee work would no longer be necessary. Committees would meet even if some members were not on duty, as long as there were at least two members present. Minutes would be taken by the unit clerk on duty and would be posted in the lounge for review at shift report. After four consecutive days, the minutes would be sent to the nursing office for typing and then filed in the unit committee meeting notebook for future reference.

You attend the first two meetings of each committee and plan to attend one to two meetings a month of each committee for the first three months. Initially, you direct each committee by asking them to work on topics that overlap with standards of practice. Below is a summary of the initial direction you provide to each committee:

---

*Modified with permission from: AACN Standards for Nursing Care of the Critically Ill, ed 2, Norwalk, Conn, and San Mateo, Calif, 1989, Appleton & Lange.

Table 7-2. TEMPLATE FOR UNIT-SPECIFIC STANDARDS
Comprehensive Standard I. A comprehensive and dynamic database will be maintained on all patients admitted to the critical care unit.

SUPPORTING STANDARDS	SKILLS, ABILITIES, COMPETENCIES	REFERENCES
I.c. The critical care nurse shall collect assessment data in an organized, systematic fashion to assure completeness	I.c-1. Assessment will be systems-based, including the following: Neurosensory Respiratory Cardiovascular Gastrointestinal Fluid and Electrolytes Endocrine	

Modified with permission from: AACN Standards for Nursing Care of the Critically Ill, ed 2, Norwalk, Conn, and San Mateo, Calif, 1989, Appleton & Lange.

Standards committee. You supply each member with a copy of the AACN standards and ask them to discuss ways to adapt the process standards statements to the unit. You encourage the committee to consider adopting the recommended three-column format.

Quality assurance committee. You ask members to read the past year's unit QA reports, and suggest that the committee consider modifying the audit tool by using a three-column approach. The modified audit tool could use the established unit-based standards directly, with a change only in the right-hand column. You remind them that in the adaptation/individualization process they are defining minimum levels of compliance for each of the unit-based standards. To assure compliance with accreditation and regulatory guidelines, the QA committee would also select high-volume, high-risk, and significant elements of care for auditing.

Documentation committee. You ask members to explore the reasons that care plans were not being written, and to develop a strategy to remedy this. You remind them that, based upon the work of the standards committee, they will also be asked to assess ways in which the flow sheet could be utilized or modified to assure documentation in accordance with unit-based standards.

Procedure and policy committee. You ask members to review the critical care unit manual and revise or remove those procedures and policies that no longer reflect actual practice. You also remind them that they will be asked to develop procedures and policies to reflect the work of other committees.

Journal club. You ask members to review the literature on standards of practice in critical care. Each member is to read one article a week and bring it to committee meetings for discussion. You ask the committee to select the five most relevant articles presented; each member will receive a copy, and a copy will be posted in the staff lounge. Finally, you ask journal club members to present a 3-minute overview of an article at weekly staff meetings.

As planned, you attend the first two meetings of each committee to provide clarification of expectations and moral support. At each meeting you reassure committee members that regardless of specific committee emphasis, the goal is to develop reasonable, workable solutions from their particular perspective.

Initially some staff members are resistant, but by the end of the first month, 27 staff members (53 percent of existing staff) had attended at least one committee meeting.

Response to the committee structure and the direction provided is overwhelming. Excitement clearly is generated by involvement in the specific activities that are part of the comprehensive plan to make the unit a more organized, cohesive place to practice. As committees continually focus on ways to enhance patient care, active discussions about standards of care become more and more common. Along with the flurry of activity and positive interactions, morale begins to improve. Staff are smiling more readily and interactions with patients, families, physicians and ancillary departments are improving.

PROGRESS REPORT

When committee meetings address difficult issues that generate strong feelings, you encourage members to take brief breaks as needed. By doing this, staff return not only with renewed energy, but also with fresh perspectives that often came from informal discussions among themselves.

The standards committee adopted the three-column format, and after six months is now adapting supporting standards statements. You give them the template in Table 7-2 and stress that they are free to modify the AACN Supporting Standards Statements, as long as the central concepts are preserved. You ask them to focus on identifying skills and competencies (the middle column) relevant to their unit. You provide a few references for the right-hand column and encourage committee members to do the same, focusing on the need for the readily available and easily applicable resource materials.

As their deliberations progress, the committee summarizes their progress at staff meetings about once a month. As a result of staff feedback, several issues are referred to other committees, groups, or individuals for their opinions about procedures or competencies. Staff meetings, discussions, and referrals to others result in ongoing dissemination of information and facilitate widespread unit staff involvement.

A small group that had chosen not to be involved in committees challenges the standards committee on issues of clarity and applicability at early staff meetings. As a result, specific referrals are made to these individuals, and quite unknowingly, they provide invaluable insight.

At staff meetings, the QA committee discusses the lack of compliance with documentation of intravenous fluids and intravenous site condition. They propose incorporating specific areas on the flow sheet for this documentation. After discussion, consensus is achieved and the documentation committee is asked to incorporate the change into the flow sheet.

As directed, the documentation committee discusses barriers to staff development and to using meaningful care plans. They quickly discover that there are many varied and intense feelings about care plans. Feelings about nursing diagnosis are even more intense and polarized, even among committee members. Thus, they also bring issues to staff meetings.

Several themes emerge in the subsequent discussions. Some staff believe that no one reads care plans. Others think that the interdependent responsibilities defined by physician orders are all that is needed to provide quality care. Some staff complain that the care plan fragments the record and increases the nurse's paperwork. Progress is at a standstill with little hope in sight when someone from the standards committee suggests that the documentation committee work collaboratively with the standards committee to adapt the AACN comprehensive and supporting standards that address care plans (see page 102, Standard III) and to develop a care plan format that addresses these concerns.

As this collaborative effort begins the joint committee group quickly realizes that by addressing the care planning issue, they can also address the staff's wide dissatisfaction with their proficiency in patient teaching activities. The discussion focuses on adapting and identifying resources for Supporting Standard III.d: *The critical care nurse shall identify areas for education of the patient and significant others.* Momentum is gained. The joint committee group identifies several immediate needs: an information sheet about the unit targeted to patients, families, and significant others; a list of commonly asked questions about transferring from the unit to less intense settings; and "what you can expect" information about each of the most common diagnoses or procedures of patients in the unit. The joint committee group becomes excited as they realize that identifying tools to actively assist staff in teaching activities could result in a turnaround of the negative attitudes about the care-planning issue into more positive attitudes directed toward improving patient care.

With some trepidation the joint committee raises these ideas at the next staff meeting. Staff agree they are dissatisfied with the current patient teaching activities, and they also agree that there is a need for the support materials identified by the joint committee. Many say patient and family teaching would clearly be enhanced if staff did not have to "re-invent the wheel" every time teaching is needed. The joint committee is gratified when several staff members—and individuals who had not yet been active in any committees—volunteered to develop materials for future staff review. Furthermore, heads nod in agreement when you point out the lesson to be learned from the previous, often heated discussions is that the standards-based approach to patient care is a focus for addressing staff concerns and areas of dissatisfaction. Although by a narrow margin, a staff vote confirms the need to establish care planning as a unit expectation. A major breakthrough has clearly occurred.

In the meantime, the policy and procedure committee has been actively revising several policies. The policy for hemodynamic monitoring, which stated that tubing must be changed every 24 hours, was revised to fit the current practice of changing the tubing every 48 hours. Similarly, the committee strengthened the arterial blood sample policy by adding the requirement that gloves be worn in accordance with the Center for Disease Control's guidelines and hospital policy. As these and other changes are discussed at staff meetings, staff members begin to realize that this committee and others are centered on the real world of bedside practice.

The journal club had identified and given staff specific articles addressing the implementation of standards. While not all staff members have read the posted articles, many have. Some staff asked to borrow copies of the AACN Standards from standards committee members, some posted articles they found relevant, and some volunteered to review and provide feedback to the standards committee as the adaptation process evolved.

As an outgrowth of the care planning issue, and specifically the role of nursing diagnosis, journal club members were asked to include specific articles focusing on the benefits and logistics of implementing nursing diagnosis in their literature review. Brief summary presentations are presented at staff meetings and result in increasingly more open discussion about the best ways to describe patient problems and needs. Although six months into the process, complete consensus has not yet been reached, staff are actively engaged in defining ways to describe and intervene optimally in patient care delivery.

Looking back to the beginning, you are very proud of the unit staff's initial efforts. You recognize that the money spent to pay overtime for initial committee meetings and to provide copying and secretarial support to committees were significant factors in establishing the current momentum. In fact, you had adapted the key steps to facilitate change suggested by the AACN (see the box on the next page). The high participation also contributed to success—further evidence that unit staff truly are the experts when what is realistic, appropriate, and relevant for bedside practice must be determined.

Throughout the process, you had regularly compared progress with the committee guidelines and steps to facilitate change; specifically you had checked to assure appropriate shift mix on committees and adequate support for ongoing deliberations. You made yourself available to provide clarification and encouragement, and reminded all of the need to have committee recommendations truly reflect unit needs and realities.

A YEAR LATER

As the first year of your tenure as nurse manager ends, a new picture emerges. The momentum generated as a result of the care plan/patient teaching discussions has led to formation of a task force of unit staff and hospital service

> **STEPS TO FACILITATE CHANGE**
>
> Ensure that committee members are representative of staff.
> Provide support for committee work.
> Ensure that the nursing process is central to practice.
> Develop a consistent format.
> Adapt and modify AACN's standards.
> Translate standards into activities and competencies.
> Identify and address constraints to success.
> Assure that final product is clear, relevant, realistic, and measurable.

Modified with permission from: AACN Standards for Nursing Care of the Critically Ill, ed 2, Norwalk, Conn, and San Mateo, Calif, 1989, Appleton & Lange.

managers to address amenities for patient families and significant others. Plans are progressing to make minor but significant changes within the critical care waiting area, such as beverages, new curtains, new furniture, and a phone. Similarly, unit staff are reviewing visiting guidelines and ways optimal mobilization of the hospital chaplain and social work staff could help support patient loved ones, and assist unit staff in facilitating effective learning and coping by families and significant others.

Another staff task force has decided that the standards prepared by the standards committee might be useful as an orientation guide for new staff. It is also investigating whether an abbreviated version that focuses on high-risk, high-volume activities could be used as a mini-orientation tool for agency nurses and nurses in the hospital's PRN pool.

The QA committee has adopted a columnar format for the unit audit tool. They retitled the right-hand column, as suggested in the AACN Standards, to read *Minimum Standard* and have started defining minimum compliance measurement criteria for the newly developed unit-based standards. Audit results have become routine agenda items for staff meetings and result in energetic discussions about the unit-based standards and the most relevant ways to measure compliance. In several instances these discussions resulted in clarification and revision of specific standards statements. To you it seems as if there are increasingly frequent instances when staff express ownership of the unit-based standards and cohesiveness around the need for clear articulation and consistent implementation of standards.

After a staff meeting discussion, you begin reviewing and revising job descriptions based upon the expectations expressed in the unit's standards. Two staff members volunteer to work with you in a task force studying the issue of job descriptions for the institution as a whole.

Tangible results of the unit's progress are visible. The attrition rate has dropped remarkably to slightly less than 10 percent. Twelve nurses have been hired, and despite the fact that thirteen positions remain to be filled, the unit's dependence on agencies has decreased to less than 25 percent of last year's agency usage.

Staff enthusiasm has never been higher, and you observe that individual staff members are vocal and anxious to share their ideas and progress with peers among the unit staff and external to it as well. No longer do PRN pool nurses avoid the unit; in fact, two are expressing interest in regular positions.

As you assess the progress of the unit you feel extremely proud of the staff. A unit potluck is held—it reinforces the fact that the highly participatory nature of the accomplishments, and the organizing framework provided by the AACN standards, were responsible for all the improvements. The process had been neither easy nor without conflicts, but as you remind them, they have come a long, long way. Everyone is encouraged to look back and to truly appreciate not only their own energy and investment, but that of their peers, as well.

You know that much remains to be done. You know that ahead lie disagreements and complex issues. You know there will be difficult times, but most of all, you know it is good to be "home."

CONCLUSION

This chapter has provided a practical approach to implementing standards of care. The nurse manager's commitment to the value of the standards fosters the development of a process dedicated to defining, organizing, delivering, and evaluating patient care. Using a three-column format and adapting the existing time-proven AACN standards for critical care results in individualized, unit-specific standards that allows one to identify the appropriate skills and competencies for that unit. The nurse manager involves staff in the process at the beginning, and provides direction, support, and encouragement along the way. This results in the emergence of staff who truly are experts in implementing realistic and relevant practice issues.

REFERENCES
1. AACN Standards for nursing care of the critically ill, ed 2, Sanford S and Disch J, editors, Norwalk, Conn, and San Meteo, Calif, 1989, Appleton & Lange Publishing Co.
2. Joint Commission on Accreditation of Healthcare Organizations: Accreditation manual for hospitals/88, Chicago, 1987, The Commission.

SUGGESTED READINGS
1. Alspach J et al, editors: AACN's core curriculum for critical care nursing, ed 3, St Louis, 1985, The CV Mosby Co.
2. Kinney M et al, editors: AACN's clinical reference for critical care nursing, ed 2, New York, 1988, McGraw-Hill Book Co.
3. Millar S et al, editors, AACN procedure manual for critical care, ed 2, Philadelphia, 1985, WB Saunders Co.

Chapter 8

QUALITY ASSURANCE AND RISK MANAGEMENT

Jeanne S. Latimer
Mary Jane Spuhler-Gaughan

What exactly are quality assurance (QA) and risk management (RM)? If terms like *rhetoric, paper chase,* and *watch dogs* come to mind, it may be because of insufficient education, limited support mechanisms, poorly planned systems, and less-than-positive experiences. QA and RM can be dynamic forces for change and growth if they are properly understood and applied in day-to-day patient-care settings.

This chapter examines the dynamics of QA and RM specifically for critical care nurse managers. The workings of QA and RM are the same regardless of the setting; however, because the pace of critical care nursing practice is swift and intense, these activities tend to be considered superfluous and burdensome. The critical care nurse manager is the key to effective promotion and conduction of unit QA and RM programs. The objective of this chapter is to provide nurse managers with a working knowledge of QA and RM by defining the terminology, describing the methodology, reviewing the examples, and examining the benefits and pitfalls of QA and RM activities.

Misconceptions of QA and RM result from overemphasizing the regulatory requirements and repercussions that surround these two activities. *Quality* is a

> **ATTRIBUTES OF INNOVATIVE AND EXCELLENT ORGANIZATIONS**
>
> 1. Action-oriented and creative project groups to solve problems and make decisions.
> 2. Customer-focused projects.
> 3. Entrepreneurial autonomy.
> 4. Recognizing staff promotes quality and productivity.
> 5. Hands-on experience by the top executives.
> 6. Focus on one product.
> 7. Decentralized simplicity.
> 8. Central direction and maximum individualism.

Excerpt from In Search of Excellence by Thomas J. Peters and Robert H. Waterman, Jr. Copyright © 1982 by Peters and Waterman. Reprinted with permission of Harper & Row Publishers, Inc.

very nebulous term; quality is strongly subjective and difficult to measure. Peters and Waterman,[7] the authors of *In Search of Excellence,* researched the ways that organizations maintain vitality and excellence. They identified eight interrelated attributes distinctive to innovative, excellent organizations, which can be applied by the nurse manager to the critical care setting. The box above highlights these. The motivators to achieve excellence, according to Peters and Waterman, are simplicity, creativity, experimentation, and involvement. Outstanding performance is related to people's values.

The objective of QA is to facilitate the provision of optimal, cost-effective care. Because regulatory agencies often dictate the framework used to measure QA components, nurses often focus on meeting the requirements, rather than on providing quality care. The goal of QA and RM programs is to achieve both.

Progress is gaining momentum. Programs are being developed not only to assure quality and reduce risks, but to build sound nursing practices in all settings. Nursing research programs are being linked directly with QA programs to accomplish this. In addition, nursing models that portray value systems are being tested and utilized with great success in a variety of settings. A basic understanding of the key elements that compose QA and RM assists the nurse manager in broadening her knowledge base.

The dynamics of QA and RM, and their effects on nursing practice, should be clearly understood. QA and RM now fit more effectively into patient care goals. QA has been defined by some as the result of mandates, and by others as a part of professional accountability. The Joint Commission on Accreditation of Hospital Organizations (JCAHO) defines QA in terms of process requirements that relate to basic professional practice. The American Nurses Association (ANA) defines QA as the continuous evaluation of nursing care against objective measurements of structure, process, and outcome. The ANA recognizes that RM is a major component of QA, because RM alerts everyone to those occurrences that have the greatest potential effect upon the patients' well-being.[8]

CONCEPTS AND TERMINOLOGY IN QUALITY ASSURANCE

Care givers depend on QA to measure patient outcomes. A good understanding of nursing quality assurance (NQA) concepts and terminology fosters positive response, commitment to practice, opportunity for accountability, and staff involvement; and is also the first step of effective implementation of an NQA program. The box below provides definitions to illustrate that QA and RM are components of daily nursing activities and professional values.

QUALITY ASSURANCE TERMINOLOGY AND CONCEPTS

Quality Assurance (QA). JCAHO defines QA as the process of monitoring, evaluating, and assuring the quality and the appropriateness of health care.[6]

Risk Management (RM). RM is a review of quality of care on an individual patient basis. RM is designed to minimize liability for an institution as well as to protect the patient.

Scope of Care. The scope of care is the range of services provided by a department or organization, including treatments provided, procedures used, patient populations served, locations where care is provided, time when care is provided, and the personnel providing care.[6]

Important Aspects of Care. Important aspects of care are the activities within the scope of patient care that are of greatest significance to the health and safety of the patient. Activities that are identified as important aspects of care because they are high-volume and/or high-risk to the patient, and/or problem-prone for patients or care givers are the focus of NQA monitoring and evaluation.[6]

Threshold for Evaluation. A threshold is a pre-established level of performance for a practitioner, department, or organization related to a specific indicator of the quality of an important aspect of care.

Indicator. An indicator can be described as a well-defined objective and measurable tool used to monitor the quality of an important aspect of care. The three types of indicators are *structure*, *process*, and *outcome* indicators.

Monitoring. Monitoring is the planned, systematic, and ongoing collection and organization of data about an indicator of an important aspect of care, and the comparison of data to a pre-established level of performance (threshold).

Criteria. Criteria are measurable variables that allow compliance with a standard to be determined. Criteria are the units of measurement that make up the indicator.

Standard. A standard is an agreed upon level of excellence.[1] There are three types of standards: *standards of care* address patient outcomes, *standards of practice* address nursing care activities, and *standards of performance* address quality of nursing practice.

NQA PROGRAM

JCAHO requires that hospitals conduct an ongoing QA program and mandates that nursing departments monitor and evaluate the quality and appropriateness of patient care, as well as resolve any identified problems. The box on page 119 illustrates the JCAHO Ten-Step model, a valuable tool for developing effective QA and RM programs.

CASE STUDY: NQA CONCEPTS AND THE TEN-STEP MODEL*

You are the nurse manager of a 14-bed cardiac intensive care unit (CCU) in a 320-bed teaching institution that provides acute and nonacute care. Other specialized units include ambulatory care, intermediate care, critical care, telemetry, emergency care, oncology, general medical-surgical, orthopedic, operating room, postanesthesia care, and eating disorders. The hospital employs an all–registered nurse (RN) staff, and follows a primary care philosophy.

The nursing department is decentralized, and it participates in hospitalwide programs and projects, which fosters a team approach and professional commitment. The vice president of patient care services is ultimately responsible for implementing the NQA program and for resolving problems and issues related to nursing care delivery. The NQA coordinator organizes, maintains, and evaluates the NQA program; facilitates the flow of QA information; and acts as an interdepartmental liaison for NQA issues.

This institution's NQA program operates through the departmental NQA council and the unit-based NQA committees. Figure 8-1 illustrates the institution's flow of NQA activities and compares it with B. Neuman's Health Care Systems model. B. Neuman's Nursing model is shown in Figure 8-2. It is germane to QA and RM endeavors because it extends beyond the "illness model and includes the concepts of problem identification and prevention."[5] Utilizing a nursing model to support NQA strengthens the commitment not only to nursing, but to a program that is based on a solid framework.

NURSING QUALITY ASSURANCE COUNCIL

The NQA council is composed of one staff nurse representative from every nursing unit, one member from the infection control division, nursing administration, and the continuing education office. The council is chaired by the NQA coordinator. Each member has an equal vote. Monthly meetings last approximately one hour. The council's charge is to oversee all NQA activities that are undertaken on a departmentwide level and to serve as an advisory body for unit-based monitoring. The NQA council assists its members and the units in focusing on potential areas to improve care and in directing the evaluation and resolution of identified problems. It also promotes collaboration between critical care units that share similar concerns. The box on page 120 delineates NQA council responsibilities.

---

*Adapted from JCAHO: Update on nursing services monitoring and evaluation, Chicago, 1989, JCAHO.

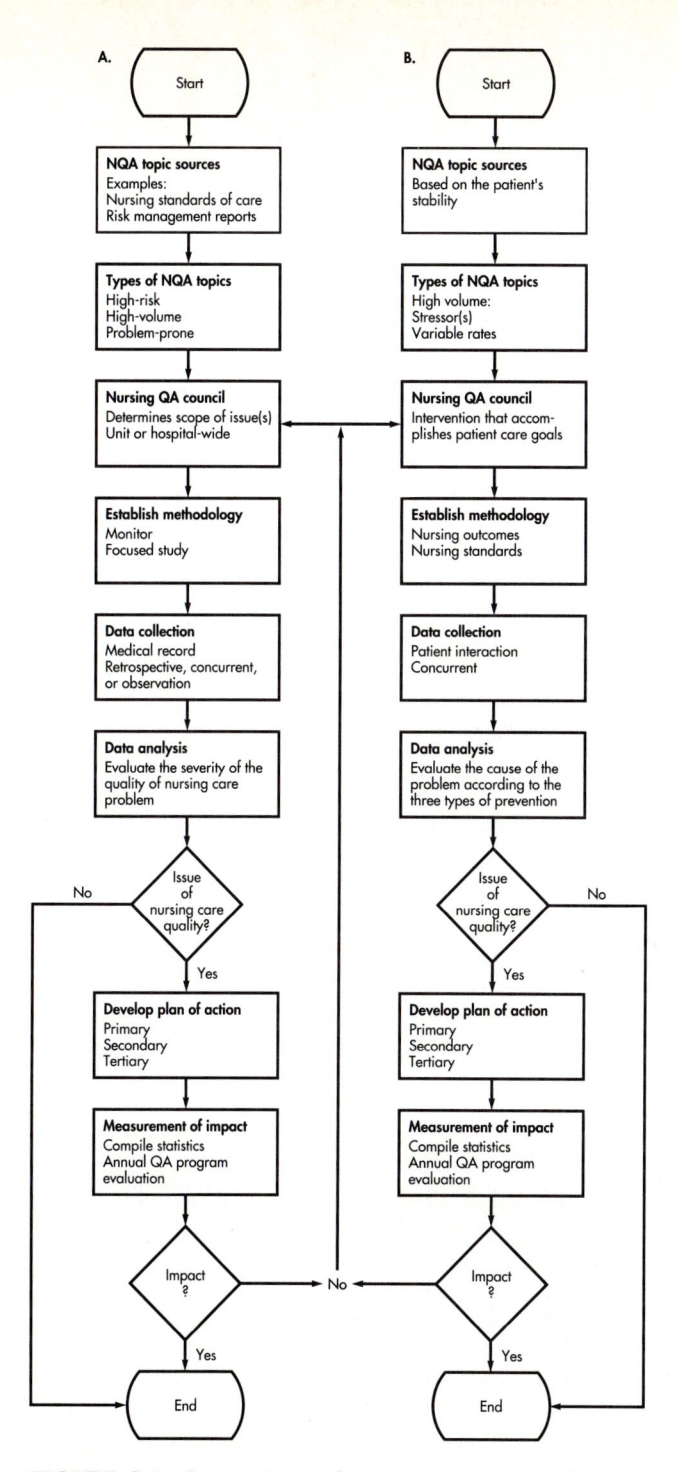

FIGURE 8-1. Comparison of an Institution's Application of the Newman Model (A) with the Newman Model (B). (Redrawn with permission from Graduate Hospital, Philadelphia, Pa.)

118 *Chapter 8*

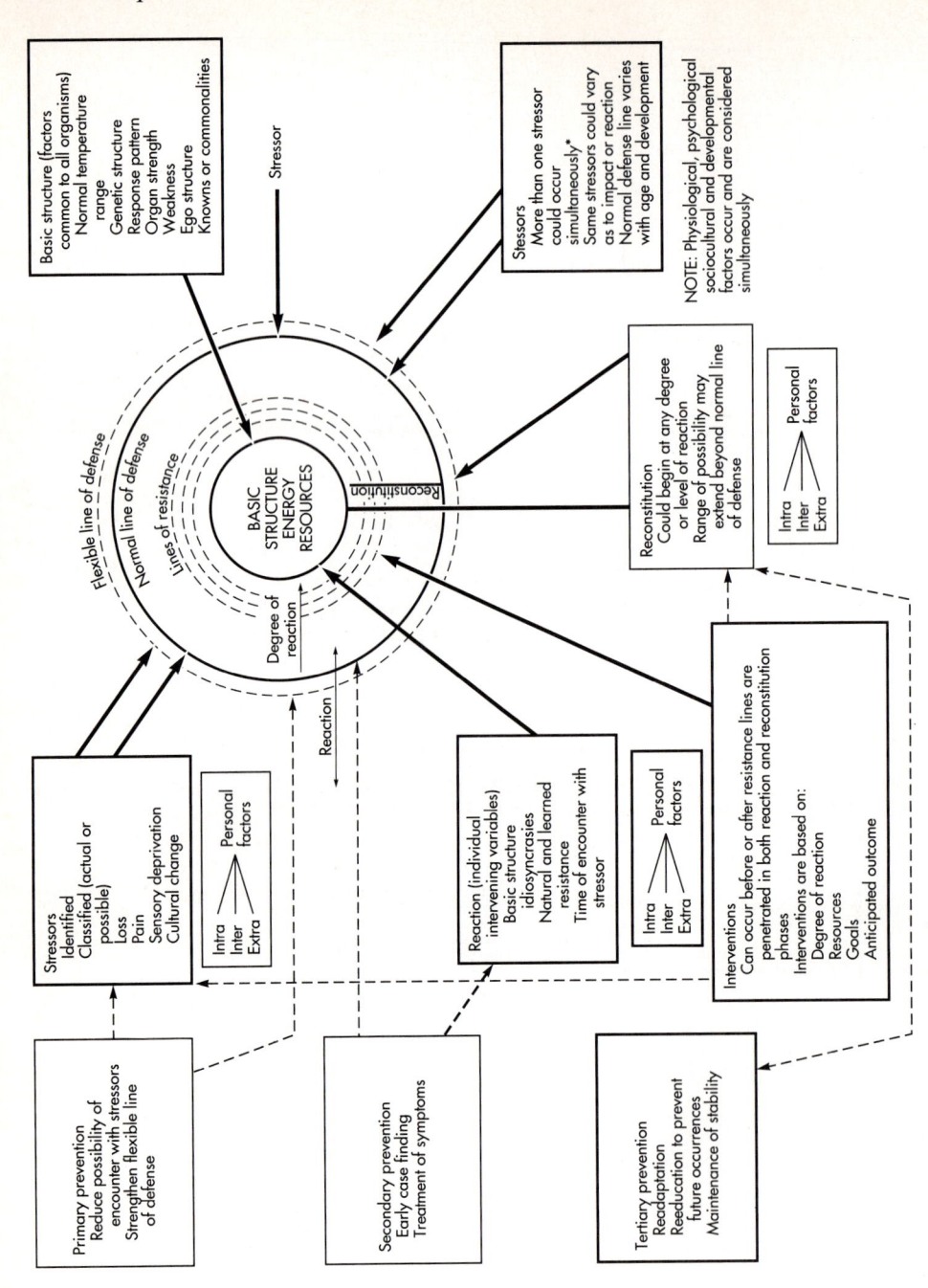

FIGURE 8-2. The Neuman System Model. (Used with permission from B. Neuman, Beverly, Oh. From The Neuman Systems Model Application to Nursing Education and for Nursing Practice, ed 2, 1989, Appleton & Lange, Norwalk, Conn.)

> **THE TEN-STEP MODEL FOR MONITORING AND EVALUATION**
>
> 1. Assign responsibility.
> 2. Describe scope of patient care.
> 3. Identify important aspects of care.
> 4. Identify indicators.
> 5. Establish thresholds for evaluation.
> 6. Collect and organize data.
> 7. Evaluate.
> 8. Take actions to resolve identified problems.
> 9. Assess the actions and document improvement.
> 10. Communicate information to the organizationwide QA program.[6]

UNIT-BASED NQA COMMITTEES

Each nursing unit has a unit-based NQA committee, which consists of representatives from all shifts and the nurse manager. Membership is voluntary and no one is denied participation. Continuing education instructors are available as expert clinical resources and often attend committee meetings. The unit representative to the NQA council acts as the committee facilitator. Each committee meets at least monthly.

NQA PROGRAM GOALS

The unit-based NQA committee is responsible for monitoring, evaluating, and resolving the specific "quality of nursing care" issues that arise on the unit. The box on page 121 highlights the responsibilities of the unit-based NQA committee.

These program goals outlined are achieved through a unit-based NQA system. Nursing QA and RM authorities support the need for unit-based NQA programs. For example, *Nursing Management*[4] reported,

> A recent study of staff nurses revealed that they believe involvement in QA activities is an important role for the professional nurse. Activities directly linked to patient care were valued most highly. A unit-based NQA program provides a forum for staff nurses to enhance their professional practice while solving patient care problems.

The box on p. 121 lists additional advantages of unit-based NQA programs.

Ideally involvement at the staff level facilitates a practical approach to promoting high-quality care. Staff observe and understand the relationship between the care given and the outcomes obtained. Furthermore, if risk management (RM) events are identified in a timely fashion, meaningful indicators can be developed to evaluate ways to reduce future occurrences.

The nursing department's philosophy promotes the nurses' accountability, advocacy, education, research, and collaboration. Nursing personnel believe that by utilizing the Ten-Step model, their philosophy is fully supported. The program

NQA COUNCIL RESPONSIBILITIES

1. Departmentwide annual review of important aspects of care and generic indicators.
2. Determine the scope of identified quality-of-care issues.
3. Identify and prioritize departmentwide quality-of-care issues.
4. Approve all departmentwide monitors and thresholds for evaluation.
5. Monitor departmentwide problems or potential problems as requested by the NQA Coordinator.
6. Review and analyze data from departmentwide NQA activities, make recommendations for action, and evaluate plan implementation.
7. Support continued growth of the unit-based NQA program by providing guidance to unit-based committees.
8. Incorporate educational workshops for council members.
9. Support and utilize the nursing process.
10. Facilitate and promote all nursing research activities.
11. Comply with JCAHO, state, and other regulatory agencies' requirements for NQA.
12. Increase divisionwide awareness of the importance of quality review activities for accreditation and third-party payment.

UNIT-BASED NQA COMMITTEE RESPONSIBILITIES

1. Identify unit scope and important aspects of care.
2. Formulate unit-specific standards of care and practice.
3. Utilize current standards of practice to monitor the quality and utilization of nursing care.
4. Set thresholds for evaluation of care practices.
5. Monitor departmentwide problems or potential problems as requested by the NQA council.
6. Implement effective actions to improve the quality of care.
7. Support excellence in nursing care to assure patient satisfaction.
8. Inform the NQA council and unit staff of NQA activities.
9. Review the unit-based program annually.

encourages all professional nurses to strive for clinical excellence in the ever-changing technical and economic environment of health care.

CRITICAL CARE NQA PLAN

As the nurse manager of a 14-bed CCU, you must develop and implement a unit-based NQA program on your unit. As the nurse manager, you have front-line responsibility for monitoring and evaluating NQA issues, and for implementing effective

NQA PROGRAM GOALS

1. Monitor clinical practice and determine compliance with nursing standards.
2. Initiate new standards relative to findings.
3. Evaluate identified problems.
4. Implement change to assure high-quality nursing care.
5. Provide a mechanism for unit-specific NQA.
6. Encourage staff involvement in all NQA activities.
7. Coordinate NQA activities in order to ensure efficiency.
8. Provide documentation and information concerning the results of NQA activities.
9. Foster participation with nursing research.
10. Promote collaboration among nursing units.

ADVANTAGES TO UNIT-BASED NQA

1. Decision making is decentralized.
2. Problem resolution is realistic and practical.
3. Patient care issues are routinely addressed.
4. Commitment to problem solving is heightened.
5. Staff assume leadership roles in NQA activities.
6. RM issues are addressed before they become problematic.
7. Staff exposure to the process fosters appreciation of NQA benefits to the patient.

actions to improve quality of care. Your role as nurse manager is explained further in the box on page 122.

The nurse manager must be willing to delegate and share the NQA responsibility with the nursing staff. Participating can be a new experience for some nurse managers who customarily direct. Placing a high value on staff involvement will increase their commitment to problem solving and their acceptance of accountability, and will heighten their morale; this results in a strong nursing staff who feel empowered. Only in a unified group whose members have equal power can shared responsibility for the unit's quality of care be attained. A recent study[9] examined

> whether nurses involved in QA programs perceived the nursing care they delivered differently from nurses not involved in QA programs. A significant difference was identified, indicating that nurses involved in QA activities perceived the care they delivered at a higher level than their uninvolved colleagues.

It is essential that the nurse manager obtain the assistance of the unit-based NQA committee in drafting a NQA plan. The JCAHO Ten-Step model is utilized for the CCU's NQA monitoring and evaluation plan. Before defining each step, the staff must

> **NQA: ROLE OF THE NURSE MANAGER**
>
> 1. Assist staff in the QA process by:
>   - Fostering effective approaches to monitoring and evalution that do not overburden the staff
>   - Arranging and attending unit-based committee meetings, but not setting the agenda
>   - Coordinating and facilitating staff involvement
>   - Supporting and encouraging staff involvement with unit-based and departmentwide activities
>   - Identifying problems and prioritizing unit-based NQA issues
>   - Ensuring the implementation of corrective action and evaluation of its effectiveness at the unit level
> 2. Assess and respond to specific RM occurrences by reviewing incident reports completed by the staff.
> 3. Insure implementation of corrective actions at the unit level and evaluate the effectiveness of the problem resolution through continued monitoring.
> 4. Foster collegiality and peer respect among staff members.
> 5. Incorporate the results of quality assessment activities into management decisions and performance evaluations.
> 6. Inform the Nursing Department of all unit-based activities.

understand all of the terminology, and must be involved in this defining. After each step is completed, it is reviewed by the entire staff for approval. The nursing department's NQA coordinator helps design the NQA unit-based program and confirms that the approach to important NQA issues is consistent across the nursing department.

The individual steps involved in implementing the CCU's unit-based NQA plan are as follows:

STEP 1. ASSIGN RESPONSIBILITY

Together you, as the nurse manager, and your staff must *assign responsibility* for monitoring and evaluation activities through the unit-based NQA committee, which is responsible for planning and delegating the monitoring activities. This committee assigns data collection activities to other staff members, who are accountable for completion of their assigned monitoring. Professional commitment to the unit's NQA program will be reflected on each staff member's yearly evaluation and merit pay increase.

Upon completion, the unit's NQA plan will be approved by the entire unit nursing staff, the NQA coordinator, and the vice president of patient care services. The plan will be assessed annually and modified accordingly.

STEP 2. DELINEATE SCOPE OF CARE

The *scope of care* is the range of services provided on the unit (treatments provided, procedures used, patient populations served, types of nursing staff who provide care). Delineating the scope of care ensures that all nursing activities are considered in the monitoring and evaluation.

The CCU staff members delineate their scope as follows: The CCU is a 14-bed intensive care unit that is staffed by RNs who have successfully completed the hospital's ICU course. The majority of the patient population consists of middle-aged patients with coronary artery disease. Mainly, post–myocardial infarction, pre– and post–cardiac catheterization, and angioplasty care are rendered. Frequent treatments and procedures include administration of intravenous antiarrythmics, invasive hemodynamic evaluation, and dysrhythmia detection.

STEP 3. IDENTIFY IMPORTANT ASPECTS OF CARE

Important aspects of care are identified using the scope of care as the basis. The nursing staff must take a careful look at care activities. Important aspects of care are activities that are high volume, high risk, or problem prone for the patient or nursing staff; they provide the focus of NQA monitoring and evaluation. Important aspects of care do not represent care problems. They are nursing activities that can be monitored and evaluated periodically to determine whether or not care can be improved.

The CCU staff chooses the following important aspects of care: nursing process, patient education, unit-specific standards of care, medication administration, patient safety, and psychosocial support. These aspects will be monitored and evaluated quarterly by the CCU nursing staff.

STEP 4. FORMULATE INDICATORS

Indicators are paramount to the NQA monitoring process. An *indicator* is an objective and measurable tool used to collect data regarding important aspects of care and the quality of care. The data collected for each indicator facilitate potential opportunities for improving care. There are three types of indicators: *structure* indicators are methods used to review resources, such as utilization of staff or equipment; *process* indicators are techniques that focus on nursing care activities, such as medication administration; and *outcome* indicators are measures of the effect of nursing care, such as patient participation. All three types of indicators can be used to measure the effect of care. Each important aspect of care selected must be evaluated by at least one type of indicator.

Indicators should be derived from exemplary patterns or standards of nursing care. Nursing standards of care should not be the sole source of indicators, because exclusive reliance on them may allow error and misidentification of NQA issues. It is especially important to avoid obsolete or incomplete standards of care. Current nursing literature, when used in conjunction with established standards of care, increases the likelihood of high quality care promotion.

The CCU staff formulates and approves unit-based indicators. The data collection format includes the data-collection time period, sources for the data collection (medical record, patient interview, observation), the designated data abstractor, and the acceptable level of compliance (threshold). Simple indicators enhance the ease of data collection, especially on a busy unit. It is important that the staff consider the indicators practical and reliable. An example of the indicator developed by the CCU staff to measure their important aspects of care is the NQA problem identification tool.

The NQA problem identification tool was developed to further increase staff involvement with QA activities. The form is available on all nursing units, and is completed when isolated problems become apparent. The tool is devised to assist

NQA PROBLEM IDENTIFICATION TOOL

Instructions: Staff member who identifies a potential or actual NQA issue should complete this form.

I. Staff member identifying issue:

Name: _____ Date: _____
(Person may remain anonymous if desired.)

II. Issue Description:

III. Source of Issue:
    A. Individual   B. Group   C. Department
    D. Institution   E. Other (specify)

IV. When should this issue be resolved (e.g. immediately or routinely)?

V. How could this issue be solved?

Modified and used with permission of The Graduate Hospital's Department of Nursing, Philadelphia, PA.

staff in applying problem-solving techniques. The completed report is forwarded to the NQA coordinator for review. For example, through spontaneous staff discussion, the CCU staff discovers that there is a lack of familiarity with the use of a particular pacemaker. To solve the problem, in-services are conducted by the nurse manager. The staff follow-up is a quiz to ensure adequate knowledge. The NQA problem identification form allows the CCU nursing staff to document discovery of the problem, formulation of the action plan, and follow-up of the plan's effectiveness in a easy standardized manner.

As part of the annual evaluation of the NQA plan, the unit-based committee shall reevaluate all indicators and vote on prior and prospective indicators for the upcoming year. Active staff participation in this ensures an effective program.

STEP 5. ESTABLISH THRESHOLDS FOR EVALUATION

The *threshold for evaluation* is the level of performance of an indicator that represents the point below which an intensive evaluation should be initiated. Setting this boundary facilitates better use of the staff's time, because if time were spent investigating every instance in which the indicator is not met (specifically, random occurrences), the progress and benefits of the program would be impeded.

Sources used to establish thresholds include standards, current literature, professional organizations, and professional expertise and consensus. Nursing staff may choose to set a threshold at a point where they consider an opportunity to improve nursing care to be present. Some indicators pertain to such significant events that every instance in which the indicator is not met should be evaluated. For example, the CCU nursing staff completes a code evaluation at the end of each event. Any noncompliance with the evaluation tool is reviewed and follow-up action taken. Thus, the threshold for this indicator is 100 percent. An approved threshold may be applied to the entire nursing department or to the entire nursing unit. For the standards of care indicator on cardiac monitoring, the CCU staff sets the threshold at the departmentwide standard of 85 percent.

STEP 6. COLLECT AND ORGANIZE DATA

The CCU nursing staff organizes a schedule for data collection by establishing the calendar of monitoring events shown in the next box. Each indicator to be scheduled is approved by the unit-based NQA committee and added to the monitoring calendar. Data sources vary with the indicator; however, those that are easily accessible (for example, medical records and incident reports) are selected. In compliance with the JCAHO sample size requirements, the nursing department already collects data on 5 percent of the population or 20 cases per indicator per review.[2] The method of data collection is standardized throughout the department (see the box on page 126) on the standardized indicator form, which makes it easy to understand the indicator topics. In addition, as the staff becomes familiar with the tool, the speed of data collection increases.

The nursing staff are instructed how to retrieve indicator data. After the data are collected, the results are sent for compilation and analysis by the NQA coordinator,

UNIT-BASED NQA MONITORING CALENDAR

Indicator	Jan	Feb	Mar	Apr	May	Jun	Jul	Aug	Sep	Oct	Nov	Dec
Patient safety survey	X			X			X			X		
Care plan review		X			X			X			X	
IV medication administration			X			X			X			X
Cardiac monitoring	X			X			X			X		
Documentation of psychosocial interventions		X			X			X			X	
Documentation of patient education			X			X			X			X

Modified and used with permission of the Graduate Hospital's Department of Nursing, Philadelphia, PA.

NQA PROGRAM INDICATOR FORM

Important Aspect of Care: <u>Cardiac Monitoring</u>   Nursing Unit: <u>CCU</u>

Date of Review: _____ Data collected by: _____

Criteria:

1. On admission, all patients are connected to the cardiac monitor.
2. All monitor alarms are on at all times.
3. Rhythm strips are taken and placed in the chart at least every 8 hours.
4. QRS-complex measurements are documented at least every 8 hours.
5. Rhythm strip and QRS-complex measurements are taken with any change in patient status.
6. The physician is notified of any new dysrhythmias that are symptomatic.
7. The patient is observed at all times.
8. The patient understands and demonstrates knowledge of the reason for and process of monitoring.
9. The patient understands the importance of necessary electrical safety measures taken during cardiac monitoring.

Threshold: <u>85%</u>   Data Source: <u>X</u>   Medical Record: <u>X</u>   Patient <u>X</u>
Environment _____   Other _____

Subject_____ Criteria_____
Number_____

Name or #	1	2	3	4	5	6	7	Comments

% Compliance

Data Collection Key
+ subject meets criterion
− subject does not meet criterion
e subject meets identified exception

Overall indicator compliance:_____

Modified and used with permission of the Graduate Hospital's Department of Nursing, Philadelphia, PA.

who applies the following questions to evaluate patterns of care: What is actually occurring? Was the threshold for evaluation met? Is there an issue that can be resolved? The NQA coordinator returns a monthly summary report of the subthreshold practices to the unit-based NQA committee for follow-up.

STEP 7. EVALUATE CARE

If the threshold of a particular indicator has been achieved, the data collection continues on the quarterly schedule until the annual review. If the threshold of an indicator has not been achieved, an evaluation must be initiated. The unit-based NQA committee will determine if care can be improved. The analysis process should be designed to objectively examine the causes for the substandard level of performance and to recommend action to improve care based on these causes.

A complete examination of the monitoring results will reveal the source to be either a system, knowledge, or behavior problem. For instance, the CCU QA committee finds that the QRS-complex measurements are inadequately documented. Likely causes for the problem are identified as lack of readily accessible calipers (system problem), insufficient familiarity with the measurement procedure (knowledge problem), and reluctance to comply with standards of care (behavior problem).

Assessment of risk management issues is an essential duty of the nurse manager. A risk management issue is identified by the nursing staff and discussed in a staff meeting. For example, a CCU staff nurse discovered a defect in a certain brand of arterial line tubing. Fortunately, the problem was identified promptly and no adverse outcomes occurred. The staff regarded this as a high-risk occurrence that necessitated immediate action. Upon staff approval, the unit-based NQA committee recommended that the manufacturer be notified and be requested to perform an investigation of the manufacturing procedures. The nurse manager implemented this recommendation by contacting the manufacturer and completing an incident report for the hospital's risk management department.

STEP 8. TAKE ACTION TO SOLVE IDENTIFIED PROBLEM

If the unit-based NQA committee's data identifies a problem, the committee will then determine the appropriate action and make recommendations for follow-up. The following series of considerations support the unit-based NQA committee with identification of a relevant plan for improvement: How many patients are affected by this problem? How many departments have identified this problem? How often does this problem occur? How does the problem affect cost to the patient and to the hospital? How long has the problem existed? What is the likelihood of recurrence? What effect will resolving this problem have on other problems? What is the likelihood of a successful solution? How severe are the consequences of this problem to the patient.[3]

All plans of action should address the following: Who is expected to change? What corrective actions are to be taken? Who is responsible for implementing the plan? When is the change anticipated to take place? The plan of action plan is approved by the unit staff and the nurse manager before it is implemented.

The CCU unit-based committee meets with the nursing staff to review the documentation problem discussed earlier. Staff members agree that the problem is twofold. A set of calipers is not readily available for use, and the nurses had become uneasy with their understanding of the QRS-complex measurements. The unit-based NQA committee recommends that educational programs be provided for the entire nursing staff, and that several sets of calipers be purchased and kept near the cardiac monitors.

STEP 9. ASSESS EFFECTIVENESS OF ACTION

NQA assessments do not end when actions are taken. The nursing staff continues to monitor the important aspects of care to ascertain whether actions taken were effective in improving care. One month after the action plan is implemented, the relevant indicator is monitored. If the threshold is still not met and the problem has not been resolved, the plan of action is modified, reimplemented and reevaluated. Quarterly monitoring by the unit-based NQA committee and staff will resume for indicators whose thresholds were attained with adequate problem resolution.

STEP 10. COMMUNICATION OF NQA ACTIVITIES

Communication within the nursing department and with other departments is essential to the success of NQA activities. Information sharing minimizes duplication of efforts and enhances the dissemination of innovative ideas. Initial contact originates at the unit level. The unit-based NQA committee is responsible for providing relevant information at unit staff meetings. Sharing information demonstrates to staff that participation and commitment are an integral part of the NQA program. Results of monitoring, recommendations, and actions of monitoring and evaluation are reported monthly to the departmentwide NQA council. Council members convey information from these meetings to the unit staff.

The NQA coordinator distributes information about the ongoing monitoring process. All information presented in the NQA council should be recorded in the minutes. In addition, unit-specific summary reports outlining unit compliance with both departmentwide and unit-specific indicators are shared with nurse managers, staff members, and nurse administrators. Unit-specific reports can be drafted in the form of staff meeting minutes. Reports should contain conclusions, recommendations, and actions.

The NQA program should be directly linked to the hospitalwide QA program. Thus, the NQA coordinator communicates relevant departmentwide information at the quarterly hospitalwide QA forum. This affiliation provides for the exchange of information, concerns, and ideas, which encourages a collaborative approach to patient care issues. In addition, it assures that problems affecting nursing care, but beyond the domain of the nursing department (for example, delays in receiving laboratory results), are addressed and resolved. Figure 8-3 highlights the institution's information paths.

DEPARTMENTWIDE NQA MONITORING

Many care activities remain constant throughout a department, and therefore, centralized quality review is appropriate. For example, administration of medication is typically standardized. In this case, only one generic indicator is needed to ensure consistent monitoring. Identification of these departmentwide activities allows individual nursing units to focus on developing indicators that address unit-specific issues instead of "reinventing the wheel" for generic issues.

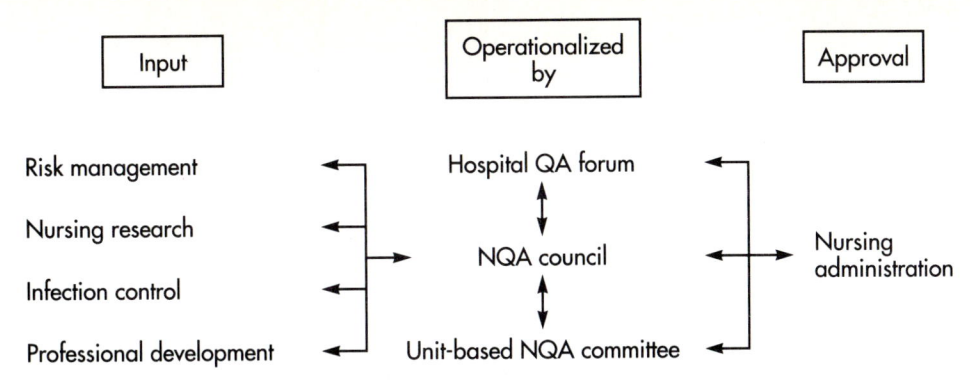

FIGURE 8-3. Nursing Quality Assurance Information Paths. (Used with permission from Graduate Hospital, Philadelphia, Pa.)

The overall departmentwide NQA plan identifies common areas of concern. Important aspects of care for the general program include patient safety, nursing process, patient satisfaction, staffing resources, medication administration, and standards of care. These important aspects of care are reviewed and approved annually by the NQA council.

Departmentwide indicators are also monitored on a quarterly basis. These indicators are selected in accordance with the current important aspects of care. Like the important aspects of care, these indicators are annually reviewed and approved by the NQA council. Actual data collection takes place on the nursing units and is performed by the nursing staff. Generic indicators include the following: nursing care plan review, patient satisfaction survey, incident reporting review, patient classification review, and the infection control report.

With unit-based NQA monitoring results, the general indicator monitoring results are forwarded to the NQA coordinator for analysis and report. The NQA council reviews these results and, if the thresholds are not met, makes recommendations for action. All NQA council recommendations are approved by the vice president of patient care services before they are implemented. The nurse manager assumes a key role in ensuring that NQA council recommendations are implemented at the unit level.

These assessments do not always indicate the need for improvement. Some demonstrate excellence of care, and are just as valuable. The council may acknowledge a particular unit or staff member for an outstanding performance. Names of the recipients or units are published in the hospital newsletter and are submitted for the hospital's annual Excellence in Practice award.

ADDITIONAL SOURCES OF NQA INFORMATION

Patient quality of care issues usually arise from routine unit-based monitoring. Other sources include departmentwide generic indicators, the NQA Problem Identification Tool as shown on p. 124 (staff concerns), hospitalwide committees (nursing research or code review committee), continuing education staff findings, utilization review reports, and direct patient contact.

The nursing research committee identifies current trends and national issues, while the code review committee recognizes issues involving emergent situations. Many issues of particular interest to critical care nursing staff arise in the code review committee.

CONCLUSION

This chapter assembled all the essential components of a NQA and RM program for a critical care nurse manager. Developing a unit-based program facilitates a simple and practical approach to nursing quality assurance that readily gains staff support, particularly in acute care settings. Autonomy, creativity, and self-esteem are maintained with a unit-specific program. By focusing on these fundamental values, professional excellence is realized. This excellence fosters quality.

REFERENCES

1. Beckman J: What is a standard of practice? Journal of Nursing Quality Assurance 1(2):19, 1987.
2. Coons M and others: Unit or service standard, Nursing Clinics of North America 23(3):639, 1988.
3. Haskin J and Marx L: Nursing QA: step V, the problem-focused study, Journal of Quality and Participation. 29, 1988.
4. New NA and New JR: Quality assurance that works, Nurse Management 20(6):21, 1989.
5. Neuman B: The Neuman systems model Application to nursing education and practice, Norwalk, Conn, 1989, Appleton & Lange.
6. Peters TJ and Waterman RH: In search of excellence, New York, 1982, Warner Books.
7. Professional nurses' role in quality assurance, Northridge, Calif, 1980, ANA and Sutherland Learning Associates Inc.
8. Schroeder P: Directions and dilemmas in nursing quality assurance, Nursing Clinics of North America 23(3):657, 1988.
9. Update on nursing services monitoring and evaluation, Chicago, 1989, JCAHO.

SUGGESTED READINGS

1. Bertalanffy L: General systems theory, New York, 1968, George Brazeller.
2. Birdsall C: Risk management and quality assurance strategies in critical care. In Fein IA and Strosberg MA, editors: Managing the critical care unit, Rockville, Md, 1987, Aspen Publishers.
3. Chinn R: Conceptual models for nursing practice. In Riehl JP and Roy C, editors: Conceptual models for nursing practice, New York, 1980, Appleton-Century-Crofts.
4. Marx L and Haskin J: Nursing QA: Step VI, determining thresholds for evaluation, Journal of Quality and Participation. 15 and 21, 1989.
5. McGee KB: Quality assurance can be more than just an exercise on paper, Focus on Critical Care 15 (20):27, 1988.
6. Neuman B: The Betty Neuman health-care systems model: a total person approach to patient problems. In Riehl JP and Roy C, editors: Conceptual models for nursing practice, Norwalk, Conn, 1974, Appleton & Lange.
7. Patterson CH: Standards of pateint care: the Joint Commission focus on nursing quality assurance, Nursing Clinics of North America 23(3):625, 1988.

Chapter 9

PATIENT CLASSIFICATION

Carole Birdsall

Patient classification is a tool used by most hospitals to quantify nursing resource use. A patient classification system that relates patient mix to budget, productivity, patient outcomes, and quality care would be ideal for nurse managers. However, most systems are not used in this way; in fact, they are usually used to predict staffing. Nurse managers responsible for increasing productivity by changing unit organization or practice can learn to use these systems for several purposes.

Knowledge about the various classification systems increases the nurse manager's options. If the interpretation of the data from each is maximized, resource consumption can be better understood. This chapter discusses the common patient classification systems and the components of effective nursing classification systems, and provides information about hospital reimbursement, diagnosis related groups (DRGs), and systems used in critical care practice. A case study demonstrates how the nurse manager uses classification data advantageously.

In the current economic environment, understanding the methods of reimbursement is imperative. The *prospective payment system* (PPS) is used to reimburse hospitals for Medicare. An average fee for services based on national standards is provided. PPS promotes strong incentives to discharge patients as soon as possible; the intent is to ensure that hospitals are efficient.

The historical types of patients and volume of those types comprise the hospital's *case mix profile,* which is used to calculate the money the institution *prospectively* receives for the component of the hospital budget associated with Medicare reimbursement. Other third party payors use similar approaches in which payment is based on the patient classification system that uses *diagnosis related groups* (DRGs).

DIAGNOSIS RELATED GROUPS (DRGS)

There are a total of 475 mutually exclusive medical and surgical DRG categories. Each patient can be placed in only one correct DRG. The DRG is determined by the *principal diagnosis,* or the reason the patient was admitted to the hospital. The principal diagnosis must be accurately determined for reimbursement; and therefore, the chart is carefully reviewed to determine the chief condition responsible for hospital admission. Once this is done, the dimensions associated with treatment and complications can be properly evaluated.

For elective surgical patients, the DRG decision is relatively clear; for emergency and medical patients, it is less so. Those who are older than 69 and those who have complications and co-morbidities belong in different DRGs. *Co-morbidity* is the presence of a preexisting secondary disease; for instance, the co-morbidity of a diabetic patient admitted for heart surgery would be diabetes mellitus.

Although DRG coding for third-party payment purposes is *retrospective* (completed after discharge by the medical records clerk), most hospitals use *concurrent* DRG coding in an effort to prevent excessive lengths of patient stays. Usually concurrent and retrospective DRG codings are accurate—coding is used to renegotiate reimbursement at predetermined times when the hospital submits its case mix to state and third-party payors to appeal for a higher level of reimbursement. This is a rather simplified explanation of the role of case mix in reimbursement.

Each DRG is assigned by Medicare a predetermined weight that is associated with the amount of money reimbursed to all institutions for that DRG, regardless of the specific institution's actual cost. It is important to recognize the difference between costs and charges. *Costs* reflect the actual money needed to provide care; *charges* reflect the price tag put on the service by the provider. Under PPS (Medicare and many third-party payors), the hospital can charge whatever it wants, but can only be reimbursed according to the predetermined *costs per DRG.* Therefore, charging steep prices has little effect unless the institution has many self-pay patients.[3]

Each DRG has a preassigned *length of stay (LOS)* used to calculate the amount of reimbursement. A patient who is admitted, cared for, and discharged within the applicable DRG time-frame is called an *inlier.* A patient who, for any reason, stays more than 1.5 standard deviations beyond the DRG-assigned LOS, or incurs care costs that exceed the norm, is called an *outlier.* Notice that an inlier does not become an outlier immediately at the end of the inlier time-frame. The *trim point* is the number of days or the amount of money above which a patient is considered an outlier. The patient must remain in the hospital 1.5 standard deviations beyond the inlier time before becoming an outlier.

The method of reimbursement during the outlier time frame is calculated differently, and research has demonstrated that financial reimbursement for outliers never fully covers the actual cost of the care provided.[5]

Costs versus charges

Many hospitals divide costs into two cost centers, ancillary and patient care, to determine the average total cost of one patient stay. The *ancillary* cost center includes costs for operating a service and the charges associated for each particular service. To arrive at the charge, the cost of keeping the service within the institution, and the cost of providing the specific service are added together.

For example, the radiology department uses a certain amount of money annually to operate. This cost includes the department's portion of the hospital's overhead (heat, light, etc.). Radiology's portion of overhead is divided and prorated according to annual volume and type of radiologic procedures to reach an overhead cost per procedure. In addition, each specific procedure is associated with a cost that is based on the amount of time the procedure takes, the number of personnel needed to perform the procedure, the complexity of the procedure, and the amount of equipment and supplies used in the procedure. This cost plus the overhead cost will give a unique charge for each procedure. This figure is the typical patient charge for the specific radiology service. All ancillary departments handle charges similarly.

Conversely, the *patient care* cost center is usually divided into *room* and *board* charges. Nursing is usually subsumed under these. There is a major difference between these costs and charges and the previous ones: The ancillary charge is a *per item* charge while room and board are *per diem* charges. The per diem cost (the cost per day) is calculated according to whether the patient is receiving *special* care (critical care) or *routine* care. The special care per diem rate for nursing, dietary, and room is higher than the routine care per diem rate for the same services. Routine per diem cost is the average daily cost for all patients receiving routine care. Special care per diem cost is the average daily cost for all patients receiving special care. To arrive at the total cost of hospitalization, the average cost of routine and special care is multiplied by the average LOS for routine and special care respectively, and the products added. The calculation of cost varies somewhat from state to state, but per diem methodology was used for all reimbursement until the advent of PPS. Because the per diem rate does not truly reflect costs, institutions are developing new ways to calculate them.

The DRG nursing cost component is based on average costs, not on specific patient care requirements. The result of recent cutbacks to large teaching hospitals that service inner-city populations has been increased attention to nursing costs and specific patient care needs in an attempt to find a way to enhance DRG specificity. Research has shown that nursing intensity varies considerably across different DRGs and within a single DRG. Many nursing departments are prorating and billing for nursing services. By separating nursing services from room and board, nursing itself is becoming a cost center that generates charges as do the ancillary services.[11,12] Although it has not increased the actual PPS disbursements, this data can be used by nursing departments to support and maintain the staff needed to care for the case mix.

Compressed Acuity

One major disadvantage of the DRG system is the shortened LOS, which has resulted in the compressed acuity seen in health care facilities—particularly in critical care units. Figure 9-1 identifies the elements that contribute to compressed acuity and hence to the current health care crisis.

Many health care facilities are in a crisis because of inadequate financial resources as a result of PPS. In the past, hospitals could remain solvent by relying on cross-subsidization, in which funds from money-makers (such as elective plastic surgery) were used to offset the costs of providing care to money-losers (such as complicated medical care to patients with multisystem failure). But rules have changed, and with PPS cross-subsidization no longer exists. Thus, there is no longer any extra money available as there was before the DRG system was instituted, when hospitals were reimbursed on the per diem basis. Furthermore, as the number of PPS-mandated outpatient services increases, the inpatient mix becomes more acute.

Other rules have also changed. The purchase of equipment is now carefully scrutinized; only equipment that is absolutely necessary to operate is purchased and supplied. The critical care unit no longer has the influence it enjoyed in the past. Now the services that are highlighted and encouraged are those that bring in DRG money. For example, obstetrical patients are lured by offers of rooming-in, homelike deliveries, and amenities for mother and father. To maximize reimbursement by filling beds to capacity, hospital emergency departments have stopped transferring patients to other institutions, instead keeping them in the E.D. in a holding pattern for sometimes days on end. Patients who should be admitted to the medical critical care unit for monitoring are sometimes sent to a telemetry bed on a routine floor, because the critical care unit is full of patients with far more demanding needs.

Ambulatory centers have opened, shifting the in-house operating room (OR) caseload. The expanded OR hours have resulted in changes in postanesthesia units. Shortened length of stays increase the number of admissions and change the utilization of critical care beds. Medical-surgical units have seen an increase of patients who used to be in critical care beds. Questions are being posed about the place in critical care for patients who are frail and elderly, patients with terminal cancer, and patients with acquired immune deficiency syndrome (AIDS).

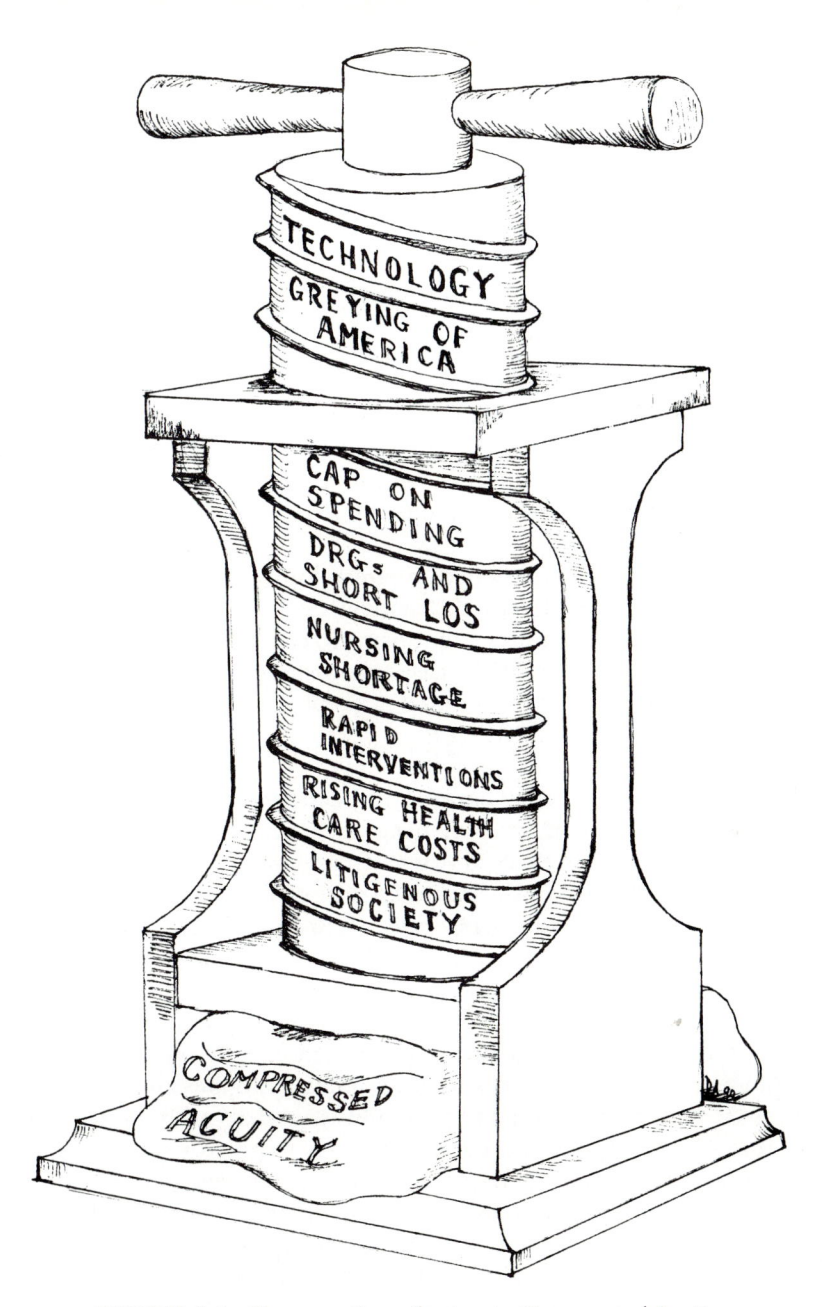

FIGURE 9-1. Elements Contributing to Compressed Acuity.

Rationing care and dealing with the "Do not resuscitate" (DNR) patient in the critical care unit are being discussed.[2]

The indigent, especially those in urban areas, have limited access to health care—which fosters a population of patients who only seek health care in crisis because the cost is so prohibitive. Therefore, by the time these patients are admitted, they are often sicker than those in more affluent patient populations, and require longer to recover. However, PPS mandates that the lengths of their stays fit into a prescribed DRG LOS. And to make matters even worse, most states promulgate patients' rights that encourage patients to challenge early discharge. The two paradoxically opposite poles frustrate health care providers.

Third-party payors assume that within each DRG, homogenous groups of patients consume resources in similar patterns. However, all patients are not exactly alike; within a DRG, care for some patients costs more than care for others. When the hospital is reimbursed more money than the actual cost of the service provided, the hospital keeps the difference. The designers of this system expected that institutions would receive over time an equitable reimbursement for the care of all patients in the case mix. Equitable reimbursement depends on the institution's case mix.

As institutions gained experience in streamlining hospitalizations, compression within DRGs resulted. Research has demonstrated that PPS is causing near financial ruin for those institutions that provide care to the poor and the chronically ill; this is especially true if the case mix includes many outliers.

Impact of DRGs on Practice

The impact of DRGs on practice has not yet been fully realized. Most health care workers, patients, and families reel from the speed with which patients are admitted, treated, and discharged. Health care providers are aware that the system feels like an out-of-control roller coaster careening down a hill; and how steep the track is and how long the ride is has not yet been determined. The federal government is content with the cutbacks in revenue spending to date, and, in fact, may end up legislating additional cutbacks.

Critical care practitioners are very aware of compressed acuity, because they experience the nursing shortage, inadequate staffing, tight budgets, short lengths of stay, older and sicker patients, and often limited supplies and equipment. The nurse manager must interpret and enforce institutional policy, support her staff, and see that the necessary resources are available to provide quality patient care. Identifying problems is not enough. Nurse managers need substantive information to explain, to justify, and to plan for change in this era of economic cutbacks. The effects of shortened LOS and compressed acuity on nursing practice must be accurately documented. Concrete methods based on hours of nursing care are necessary to justify needed changes in staffing. With a basic understanding of DRGs, of how the institution is reimbursed, and of how nursing charges (and room and board charges) are calculated, the nurse manager can assess and use patient classification data—specifically, DRG accounting data. The progressive nurse manager seeks out the case mix, average LOS, cost and LOS of outliers, patient age data, and the number of critical care days. Many hospitals also have data on the average LOS by MD or medical group practice, specific ancillary services per case type and the standard deviation associated with the service, and the remaining deficit after reimbursement for that DRG.

The nurse manager's first step is to determine the DRG case mix in the unit. Determine which 20 percent of the unit's DRGs accounts for 80 percent of the work load. This DRG profile is then used to analyze and forecast the budget and to examine current practice.

The nurse manager documents the kind of care needed by the patient mix. Nursing intensity is related to the specific care required for patients in each DRG. By justifying costs on the basis of required care, and by keeping track of trends that emerge with particular DRGs, data can be gathered and used when DRG refinement occurs. (DRGs are probably here to stay; once federal controls are established they are unlikely to be removed. The classification system used to identify case mix is more likely to change.) Thus, it behooves the nurse manager to develop systems that facilitate data collection, and that accurately measure the nursing intensity required for each DRG.

PATIENT CLASSIFICATION SYSTEMS IN NURSING

Patient classification systems are used in nursing to project staffing needs, to ensure equitable patient care assignments, to justify the budget, and to provide a basis for nursing charges. In addition, some are used in quality assurance audits. A patient classification system is mandated by the Joint Commission of Accreditation for Healthcare Organizations and some state health departments. Knowledge of the way these systems were developed enables a better understanding of what the data represent.

In nursing, a patient classification system is either a prototype or factor system. A *prototype* system is based on broad descriptions of the typical characteristics of patient categories (see the following box). Each category represents relative need for nursing care, which is usually quantified in hours of care per day. To use this type of system, the rater reads the category *descriptors* and then chooses the category that best fits the patient. Usually there are one to four categories; some systems may have as many as seven. This example has five and begins with Category II because Category I patients are in step-down units.

For the most part, the category descriptor is written to ensure that the patient fits into only one category, and thus the categories are mutually exclusive. Although not based on discrete tasks, the categories are quantified by time-motion studies to determine the average nursing time per category. Note that the descriptors can easily be interpreted by a practitioner, which makes the system easy to use. Because of the system's simplicity, a patient can be rapidly classified once the practitioner is familiar with the descriptors.

PROTOTYPE SYSTEM

Care Needs	CATEGORY II (4.5 hours)	CATEGORY III (8 hours)	CATEGORY IV (12 hours)	CATEGORY V (18 hours)
ACTIVITIES OF DAILY LIVING	Assistance: bath, meals, turning, etc.	Total care: bath, meals, turning, etc.	Totally dependent, can be comatose	ADL not a priority, cannot be unattended
GENERAL HEALTH	Satisfactory	Moderately ill	Acutely ill	Acute crisis
THERAPEUTIC NEEDS	VS q4h, probable transfer in 24 h	VS q2h, stable on pressors, monitoring, IVs, meds, tubes, etc	VS q1h, fluctuating status, arrest within past 24 h	Multi-system-failure, deteriorating status, grave outlook
TEACHING AND EMOTIONAL SUPPORT	Routine	Reinforcement of plan; mood variation	Anxious, confused or disoriented	Resistive to teaching; patient or family severe emotional response

Factor systems classify patients by determining the discrete nursing tasks required by the patient (see the following box). A standard number of points based on time is associated with each task. (The minutes of care are converted into standard units or points, for convenience.) The time values are based upon time-motion studies, published standards, group consensus, or a combination of these. The rater reads each discrete task and selects those that are applicable. The points are added and the total usually determines the patient category, which will have a number from II to V. The category expresses the care hours, or nursing intensity, required by the patient. GRASP, Medicus, and the military workload management system are widely used factor evaluative systems.

Factor Systems versus Prototype Systems

Factor evaluative systems are very objective, easy to use, task oriented, and point driven. Because factor systems are objective, results can be easily replicated. Unfortunately, factor systems often capture only the selected nursing activities. Because they are task driven, factor systems have no related sense of professional activity; thus staff often object to using factor systems.

Prototype systems are difficult to monitor. Subjective manipulation can occur subconsciously on busy days. In other words, when stressed, the rater may

FACTOR SYSTEM

Select highest applicable in each field and total the points below.

DIET		CLEANLINESS		TURNING		VITAL SIGNS	
Tube feeding	24	Special needs	7	Multiple staff	24	>q1h	20
Total feed	11	Bed bath	5	Bedfast	13	q1h	16
Some help	7	Some help	3	Some help	6	q2h	8
Independent	1	Independent	2	Independent	0	q4h	4

OUTPUT		SPECIAL		ASSESSMENTS		SUCTION	
Incontinent w/diarrhea	12	Isolation	10	Hypothermia	12	No tube	10
Incontinent urine	8	Draining wound	9	Cardiac monitor	5	q1h	8
I & O q1h	4	Ostomy/skin	5	Halo vest, pacemaker	5	q2h	6
		Dressings	2			q4h	3

RESPIRATORY		MEDICATIONS		FLUIDS	
Assisted ventilation	12	IV, NG q1h	24	> 3 drips	15
IMV/CPAP	8	IV, NG g2h	12	> 3 lines	10
Oxygen	4	IV, NG q4h	6	> changes per shift	5
		IV, NG q6h	4		
Subtotal	___		___		___
Total	___				

Circle point category

Points	Category	Hours of Care
136–170	IV	18.0
104–136	III	12.0
70–103	II	8.0
36–69	I	4.5

perceive patient acuity to be higher than it actually is. Thus, when nurses rate patients on hectic days, many patients jump to a higher category. Interrater reliability is much more difficult to replicate with prototype systems.

Problems with Systems

Before assuming that the nursing classification system used in the critical care area is effective, the nurse manager must be able to answer the questions listed in the box below. Each question helps the nurse manager understand the system so that the data collected is more meaningful when applied to patient mix.

Definitions of direct, indirect, and non-nursing time are needed to determine what the classification system includes. *Direct* care time is the time spent at the patient's bedside providing patient care, and talking, teaching, or interacting

> **QUESTIONS ABOUT PATIENT CLASSIFICATION SYSTEMS**
>
> What indirect and non-nursing time is built into the system?
> How does the system handle time for patient and family teaching and emotional support?
> Were time-motion studies completed to check the time value assigned to some of the specialized tasks?
> Were reliability and validity studies ever done?
> How was the system adapted to the individual hospital and critical care unit and by whom?
> If used for staffing, is the workload realistic, and are productivity measures evaluated?
> Was the system designed to charge for nursing services?

either with the patient or with the family. *Indirect* time includes all the time spent on the patient's behalf away from the bedside. Indirect care activities are associated with the way care is delivered, the geography of the unit, and the responsibilities of staff to equipment and supplies. Activities like patient care conferences and physician communications are considered indirect time. Indirect care time is expressed in minutes per patient per day. Each specialty area requires a different indirect care factor, because these activities vary from service to service and from unit to unit.

Non-nursing time is that spent cleaning up spills, gathering equipment, or looking up laboratory values. Much of non-nursing time is wasted nursing time, but until health care facilities hire adequate nonprofessional help, most systems must count this as indirect time.[4]

Each system allocates time for teaching and for being with patients differently. Some incorporate this time into the total; others allow the rater to select a specific amount for an item if it is supported by written documentation; still others build teaching time and time with the patient into the tool, as do most prototype systems.

The time standards developed for each task must reflect the actual time it takes to perform the task in that particular unit. The data from the original time studies of the late 1960s and early 1970s still reflect the actual time it takes to complete most basic nursing tasks, such as bathing patients. However, since that time, critical care practice has emerged as a highly complex and technical specialty. Changes in critical care practice demand a reevaluation of time-to-task ratings.

Both the reliability and the validity of patient classification systems are important if the data collected are used to justify staffing or costs. *Reliability* measures how consistent or homogeneous an individual's responses are with the tool; how equal or consistent the results are across investigators (interrater reliability) or tools (instrument reliability); and finally, how stable the tool is with repeated applications. *Interrater reliability* measures the consistency of the results when the classification instrument is used by different raters. The system's most important aspect is *instrument reliability*.[3]

Validity is the degree to which an instrument actually measures what it is supposed to measure. Ensuring validity is complex and difficult. *Content validity* means the classification instrument truly represents the domain it measures. *Predictive validity* is the ability of the instrument to predict nursing requirements accurately.

Unfortunately, the literature does not always provide adequate information about the reliability and validity of classification instruments.[3] In addition, no single nursing classification system is widely accepted, is generalizable across services, and is applicable to all institutions. Each system must be modified for the particular nursing service and unit.

Patient classification systems that are good indicators of patient care needs are often used for scheduling and staffing. However, an old classification system may be unrealistic for use in staffing, because old numbers do not address current staffing needs. The system must take today's case mix and DRGs into consideration. If the system is old and the number of required staff no longer reflects reality, consider the potential legal ramifications. For example, if a system deems that eight nurses per shift are adequate, but because of budget cuts or availability constraints, the unit is routinely staffed with six, what could happen during litigation over a patient incident? Could an aggressive attorney use the required staffing determined by the patient classification instrument to demonstrate the institution's failure to provide safe staffing ratios? The aware nurse manager can ensure that the records reflect reality.

Often classification systems are used to establish workload standards and to measure productivity, based on the predicted number of staff necessary and the variance. The nurse manager then evaluates the quality of care and the workload to determine whether actual practice meets the productivity standard. Consider what happens when the expected staffing cannot be supplied and how this influences the staff's workload and productivity.

If the classification system is used to determine nursing costs, the astute nurse manager asks, "Do the amounts reflect the change when the unit does not comply with the staffing standard?" and, "How are records kept in these instances?" Some systems require that data be collected on every shift. However, Nauert and colleagues[10] reported that additional data obtained this way is not relevant. Some of the newer cardiac monitor terminals can automatically adjust the classification by using special software that tracks the monitored parameters. In other words, each time a calculation of cardiac output occurs, its assigned time is automatically added to the classification value. The usefulness of a real-time patient classification factor remains unknown.

ADDITIONAL SYSTEMS

In addition to hospital reimbursement methods, DRGs, and general nursing classification systems, the nurse manager should understand another category of classification systems: those that were designed to measure specific aspects of care. This category includes the Severity of Illness index,[7] APACHE II,[9] and TISS scoring.[8]

Severity of Illness

The severity of illness index developed by Susan Horn is a patient classification system used by many hospitals.[7] This is a retrospective system (the scoring is completed by the medical records clerk after the patient's discharge). The severity of illness index is composed of seven dimensions, each of which has four different choices of severity, Level I (minimal) to Level IV (highest) severity. Within each dimension and under each level there are several descriptors that are used by the medical records clerk to determine the severity rating for each (see Table 9-1).

The *stage of the principal diagnosis* rating is based on the existing manifestations of this illness at admission. *Complications of the principal condition* result from the hospitalization, whether from the diagnosed illness, the treatment given, or a mistake. The *concurrent interacting conditions* rating is based on the existence of problems unrelated to the principal diagnosis. Interacting conditions also include complications that have no physiological relationship to the principal diagnosis but still require treatment. Pathology that contributed to or caused the illness are also included in this dimension.[7]

Dependency on hospital staff reflects how dependent the patient is, especially for activities of daily living. *Non–operating room procedures* include noninvasive therapeutic procedures. For example, mechanical ventilation is given a severity rating of III; cardiopulmonary resuscitation, Level IV. The *rate of response to therapy* is scored similarly. The *resolution of acute signs or symptoms,* or residual effect, is the degree of signs or symptoms of the illness that prompted the principal diagnosis, remaining on discharge.[6] Note that the first three dimensions relate to the severity of illness that existed before hospitalization, the next two relate to treatment within the hospital, and the last two relate to the way the patient recovered from the hospitalization.[7] Therefore, this tool identifies how sick the patient is on admission, as well as the burden of illness that exists on discharge.

For example, patients who are severely ill on admission with complex previous multisystem problems are often discharged with no change in level of severity. Patients with spinal cord injuries and limb amputations have higher severity scores than patients who do not have these problems. The burden of illness of a patient who walks into the hospital for a carotid endarterectomy, but leaves with a hemiparesis from a cerebral vascular accident (CVA), is much higher than it

Table 9-1. HORN'S SEVERITY OF ILLNESS

	LEVEL I	LEVEL II	LEVEL III	LEVEL IV
Stage of the principal diagnosis	Asymptomatic	Moderate	Major	Catastrophic
Complications of the principle condition	None or minor	Moderate	Major	Catastrophic
Concurrent interacting conditions that affect the hospital course	None or minor	Moderate	Major	Catastrophic
Dependency on hospital staff	Low	Moderate	Major	Extreme
Extent of non-operating room life-support procedures	Non-invasive minor diagnostic	Invasive diagnostic therapeutic	Non-emergent life support	Emergency life support
Rate of response to therapy or rate of recovery	Prompt	Moderate	Serious	No response
Resolution of acute signs/symptoms	Minor	Moderate residual	Major	Catastrophic

Compiled from Horn SD, Sharkey PD, Chambers AF, and Horn RA: Severity of illness within DRGs. Impact on prospective payment, American Journal of Public Health 75(10): 1195-99, 1985.

would have been if the CVA had not happened. If the unit patient population has a high severity of illness index, the case mix reflects high acuity, and thus the critical care unit costs more to operate because more resources are needed to provide care.

To use Horn's Severity of Illness index, the rater reads the descriptors associated with each level. All seven dimensions are rated, and then the final severity level is determined either by taking the overall level of four or more dimensions or by averaging the seven dimensions. Death is rated as Level IV.[7]

The nurse manager must ask that severity of illness data, like DRG data, be made available. The major problem with using DRGs for patient classification is

Table 9-2. SAMPLE APACHE II SCORE

PARAMETER	WORSE VALUE PAST 24 HOURS	SCORE
Temperature	38.5	1
Mean arterial pressure	49	4
Heart rate	118	2
Respiratory rate	35	3
Arterial blood gas oxygen level	68	1
Arterial blood gas pH	7.32	2
Serum sodium	150	1
Serum potassium	3.4	1
Serum creatinine	1.8	2
Hematocrit	46	1
White blood count	7	0
Neurologic points	5	5
Total		23

that DRGs are based on a *medical* model. In nursing we look at *nursing* resources. As severity increases, nursing care hours increase. But what is the relationship between *hours* of care and severity? And how can the DRG code, the severity of illness, and the hours of care be related? The best way to find out is by using the existing systems and recording the hours of care, the DRG, and the severity of illness. Over time the data will show trends and provide an average range of nursing care hours per DRG at the associated severity of illness.

APACHE II

APACHE II is a classification system designed for and specifically used in critical care. APACHE is an acronym for Acute Physiologic And Chronic Health Evaluation, and most recent is the second or abbreviated version that was developed by Knaus and associates[9] at George Washington University Medical Center. APACHE II reflects the patient's severity of disease by rating the degree of abnormality of the tool's parameters. APACHE II is relatively easy to use and requires that the admission score or the worst score for each parameter in 24 hours be used to produce the total score. The instrument is designed to rate the degree of abnormal values—low or high—for vital signs, neurologic function, and laboratory values; in addition, factors for age and chronic health problems are included.[9] Table 9-2 lists these parameters and shows sample values.

A value for each of the twelve parameters is preassigned. These twelve parameters are weighted for degrees of abnormality and then assigned ratings of 0 (normal), 1, 2, 3, or 4 (very abnormal). The rater reviews the medical record, chooses the worst value in 24 hours, compares that value with the values chart, selects the appropriate point score, and adds points for age and chronic

Table 9-3. TISS SCORING

POINTS SCORED	PATIENT CLASSIFICATION
< 10	I
10-19	II
20-39	III
>40	IV

From Keene R and Cullen D: Therapeutic intervention scoring system, update 1983, Critical Care Medicine 11(1): 1-3, 1983.

health. This is the total APACHE II score. The highest obtainable score is 71. The majority of critically ill patients fall in the 20–30 point range. Scores of 40 suggest a poor prognosis and scores of 50 are rarely if ever seen.[9] For example, a 54-year-old CCU patient who was admitted in cardiogenic shock had an APACHE II score of 23. This patient had no previous history of chronic health problems. The values and scores of this patient might be similar to those in our sample, Table 9-2.

Experience has demonstrated that APACHE II is extremely useful for medical patients and for emergent surgical patients. It has proven to be less useful for routine postoperative assessment. Although the developers have used the instrument to predict survival, it is not always used in this way. In addition, the instrument may or may not help the clinician decide if the prescribed therapy is effective. When therapy is begun to treat a problem, the score should decrease. The major advantage of APACHE II is that it is widely accepted by physicians. Because it is based on easily discernible numbers, it is an objective measure of acuity.

TISS Scoring

Another classification tool used specifically for critical care is the Therapeutic Intervention Scoring System (TISS) developed by Cullen and associates at Massachusetts General Hospital. This is the critical care version of the factor-evaluative patient classification system. TISS measures the intensity of nursing care required during a 24-hour period. A fixed number of points ranging from 1 (low) to 4 (high) is assigned to each specific activity that is commonly done in critical care; in all, TISS scores 57 medical and surgical interventions. The total TISS points are added up, and then each patient is placed in a category that reflects nursing intensity. Table 9-3 depicts TISS.

Each patient should be classified at the same time each day. An item is counted if the task has been done anytime in the past twenty-four hours. However, only the highest possible score is counted for related interventions (such as different kinds of ventilation). The total TISS score decreases as the patient gets better.[8]

Table 9-4. PATIENT CLASSIFICATION COMPARISON CHART

SYSTEM	NUMBER OF CHOICES	ITEM MEASURED OR CLASSIFIED	RANGE OF SCORE	SCORE REPORTED
DRGs	475	Medical Diagnoses	Not applicable	Not applicable
Prototype	1-5	Descriptors of patient types	I–V	I–V
Factor	39	Tasks-to-time, or factors	36–170	I–IV
APACHE II	14	Abnormal physiologic factors	0–71	0–71
TISS	57	Therapeutic interventions (tasks)	9–70	I–IV
Severity	28	Burden of illness on discharge	I–IV	I–IV

OVERVIEW

This chapter has described DRGs as a medical model, severity of illness as the burden of illness at discharge, nursing prototype as a descriptor, nursing factor as time-to-task score, APACHE II as abnormal physiological parameters, and TISS as the number of critical care interventions done. Table 9-4 summarizes these systems.

Thus, patient classification can be based on medical, nursing, or patient needs. Each system provides a different view of the patient. Each measures a different factor related to the hospitalization, and each has a different purpose. The American Association of Critical Care Nurses[1] stated:

> A careful account of patient care needs is needed for scarce resources to be applied most effectively to meet those needs. Priorities for care can be determined and changes in individual patients can be monitored through use of a PCS [patient classification system]. In addition, analysis of patient classification data can be helpful in identifying trends in patient care needs so proactive, rather than reactive, steps can be taken to meet those challenges.

Table 9-5 is a score comparison chart of critical care patients with a sample range of scores for recovering, moderately ill, and severely ill patients. In practice the relationship between systems is not as clear as it is portrayed in the table.

Relationship of Data

Generally speaking, each classification system measures a different thing. Comparisons are useful only when knowledge matches application. The next box identifies some suggested relationships among patient classification systems. As expected, high intensity and acuity often yield high APACHE II scores. High severity can mean high acuity if the unit is a regional trauma center that admits transferred accident victims managed elsewhere. High severity means poor outcomes, which may also be associated with substandard care in a poorly staffed unit.

Table 9-5. SCORE COMPARISON CHART FOR CRITICAL CARE PATIENTS

	RECOVERING PATIENT SCORE	MODERATELY ILL PATIENT SCORE	SEVERELY ILL PATIENT SCORE
APACHE II	10-15	20-30	> 30
TISS	I (< 10)	III (20-39)	IV (> 40)
Prototype	I or II	III or IV	V
Factor	I or II	III	IV
Severity	I or II	II or III	III or IV

RELATIONSHIPS OF PATIENT CLASSIFICATION SYSTEMS

High DRG intensity = High acuity = High APACHE II scores
High severity = High acuity *or* Substandard care
High prototype + Low APACHE II = ? Admitting criteria
High TISS + High severity = Negative patient outcomes
High APACHE II + Severity < III = Good quality care

If the pattern of scores includes a high prototype category with low APACHE II scores, explore admitting patterns to see if non–critical care candidates are being admitted to the unit over the weekend because the staffing on the regular floors is not sufficient.

If the pattern reveals a high TISS with a Level IV severity score (meaning death), this should be discussed with the medical director. The time, energy, and resources that are put into negative outcomes need to be addressed. If the TISS score is high but the severity score is low, the nurse manager might want to keep track of physician ordering patterns for treatments such as pulmonary artery lines. Perhaps all patients are treated with pulmonary artery catheters without thought as to need.

High APACHE II scores with severities less than III indicate that the care given was superior because the outcome of that care was positive, considering the acuity present on admission. This information should be shared with staff so they can take pride in the excellent job they did in caring for these patients.

Case Study: Patient Classification

> The nurse manager in an 8-bed medical-surgical critical care unit wants to document the need for more staff. Although this manager has worked in the unit for three years, she has been the manager for only eight months. Several new changes have affected the unit, including the addition of a vascular surgeon and an oncologist who specializes in adult leukemia. Prior to this time, the unit comfortably served this 200-bed community hospital in this medium-size midwestern city. The previous nurse manager had established a comprehensive data base for collecting patient information, but had resigned before using the information in any way.

148 Chapter 9

Table 9-6. SCORE COMPARISON CHART

DIAGNOSIS	APACHE	TISS	PROTOTYPE	FACTOR	SEVERITY	DRG
CVA	19	19	IV	II	III	16
AAA	9	21	III	I	I	111
SHOCK	29	43	V	IV	IV	123
LUNG LACERATION	14	17	III	II	I	84
LEUKEMIC	33	36	V	III	III	401
PTCA	5	19	II	I	II	5
CAROTID	8	16	II	I	II	112
BOWEL	20	20	III	II	IV	148

The diagnosis of the patient is listed along the y axis and the score, level or number for each of the identified patient classification systems is listed under the appropriate heading.

The nurse manager receives a monthly medical records report that includes the DRG coding and severity of illness score for each patient who had been cared for in the unit. This data includes LOS compared with DRG-allowable LOS, hospital costs, hospital reimbursement for that DRG, and the variance. The unit secretary enters this retrospective information, plus admissions, transfers, deaths, census, APACHE II scores, TISS scores, nursing prototype category and nursing factor level of all patients cared for in the unit in the past twenty-four hours, into a data base management program daily. Patient data can be retrieved by matching the patient ID number; unit data can be retrieved as a day of the week unit total.

USING PATIENT CLASSIFICATION DATA

Because the data base is extensive and ongoing, there is minimal difficulty in finding out information. If a nurse manager must begin with establishing a data base, it is paramount that she secure help from medical records, and (if available) from computer support personnel. The chief nurse executive can be helpful in gaining access to data from other departments. The nurse manager, whose role is to interpret data, must find a way to get the data with minimal personal daily involvement.

The nurse manager begins by picking one day that represents the unit's case mix and workload, and has this day's data printed for all patients. Table 9-6 gives the classification scores of all eight patients. This table is difficult to understand in its entirety because of the amount of information it contains. Therefore, a basic picture of each patient will be discussed separately so the scores can be better understood. When viewing the scores, the nurse manager is aware that severity and DRG coding are completed after discharge and thus represent retrospective data.

Patient 1 was an 86-year-old male admitted over the weekend by the first medical director (who is no longer active) of the critical care unit. Although CVAs rarely come to the unit, this patient was a town councilman actively campaigning when he sustained the stroke. He had suffered a respiratory arrest in the ambulance on the way to the hospital and was successfully resuscitated. He survived the hospitalization but sustained a total right-sided paralysis and a speech loss. The classification scores are for the day of admission.

	APACHE	TISS	Prototype	Factor	Severity	DRG
CVA	19	19	IV	II	III	16

The APACHE II score falls in the normal critical care range, and reflects mostly the poor neurologic function. The TISS score is only a medium value because of the postarrest status, assorted treatment modalities, monitoring, and few necessary therapeutic interventions. Note that the prototype score is higher than the factor score. The prototype descriptors are based on the patient's ability to be independent in activities of daily living. Since the patient had a CVA, the category that best described his acuity was IV. Because the factor system uses tasks, the category was II. This example demonstrates the inconsistency of the relationship between prototype and factor systems. At discharge this patient had a total paralysis with a burden of illness or severity score of III.

Patient 2 was a 63-year-old female admitted to the unit postoperatively after an abdominal aortic aneurysm repair. This patient did well. This data was obtained on the second postoperative day.

	APACHE	TISS	Prototype	Factor	Severity	DRG
AAA	9	21	III	I	I	111

The low APACHE II score affirms that physiological parameters remain normal in stable postoperative patients. The TISS score is also relatively low, despite the fact that a pulmonary artery catheter was inserted. The prototype score is higher because of the immediacy of assessment and teaching needed after surgery as rated with the tool. The factor system reflects low time-to-task activities. Because the patient did well and went home symptom-free, the Severity score of I is normal.

Patient 3 was a 69-year-old female admitted to the unit in cardiogenic shock. She had advanced coronary artery disease and died despite balloon support and investigational drug therapy. These values were taken on her second day of hospitalization, when she died.

	APACHE	TISS	Prototype	Factor	Severity	DRG
SHOCK	29	43	V	IV	IV	123

This APACHE II score clearly reflects the acute nature of this patient's illness. The high TISS score identifies the complexity of the patient care. The prototype and factor system scores are in the highest category. Since the patient died, the severity score was IV. In this instance all five measurement scales clearly indicate a high degree of nursing intensity needed to care for this patient.

Patient 4 was a 19-year-old male who was stabbed in the chest during a barroom brawl. He was admitted to the unit after surgical repair of the wound. He was intoxicated at the time of the incident and was not readily responsive for the first twenty-four hours. These values reflect his status within the first twenty-four hours of injury.

	APACHE	TISS	Prototype	Factor	Severity	DRG
LUNG LACERATION	14	17	III	II	I	84

This patient is both young and healthy. The APACHE II score demonstrates the residual effect of anesthesia and probably intoxication. The low TISS score shows that very few therapeutic interventions were required once the initial surgery was completed. Both the prototype and factor systems rate the patient as moderately ill. However, this demonstrates why specific critical care tools are better than generic nursing classification systems for measuring critical care activities. Note that this patient went home with no burden of illness.

Patient 5 was a 56-year-old female admitted in leukemic crisis. She had been in the unit two weeks ago, and was transferred from the medical floor two days ago in renal and respiratory failure after another episode of frank GI bleeding.

	APACHE	TISS	Prototype	Factor	Severity	DRG
LEUKEMIC	33	36	V	III	III	401

The APACHE II score identifies the patient acuity. The TISS score reflects the relatively frequent therapeutic interventions needed. The prototype system recognizes the seriousness of this individual's condition, while the factor system results in a moderate score since critical care tasks were not evaluated. This woman chose to go home to die, despite the fact that she was totally incapacitated; she was assigned a severity rating of III on discharge.

Patient 6 was a 51-year-old male with proximal single vessel disease of the right coronary artery, admitted for percutaneous transluminal coronary angioplasty (PTCA). During this successful procedure the patient had two recurrent episodes of ventricular tachycardia. He was admitted to the unit because the attending physician chose to keep the arterial line in place and to insert a pulmonary artery catheter to monitor the patient. The physician was concerned about a potential small vessel tear from the procedure and wanted the patient observed closely. This data represents postprocedure day 1.

	APACHE	TISS	Prototype	Factor	Severity	DRG
PTCA	5	19	II	I	II	5

Note the low APACHE II score. There are no abnormal physiological parameters. The patient is in the unit primarily for monitoring rather than therapeutic interventions. The prototype system reflects a satisfactory category assignment while the factor system rates the patient as requiring very few tasks. However, upon discharge the chart reflected that the patient had some degree of burden of illness (severity score of II), which might have been an infection or some other problem.

Patient 7 was a 58-year-old diabetic male admitted for an elective carotid endarterectomy. During the surgical procedure he sustained a mild CVA and remained in the unit for three days on pressors for blood pressure instability. These values represent day 3.

	APACHE	TISS	Prototype	Factor	Severity	DRG
CAROTID	8	16	II	I	II	112

For the most part these values in all four classification systems reflect low-level critical care needs, which demonstrates the inconsistency seen when patients simply require monitoring. Had this patient not needed pressor support, he would not have been in the unit. In addition, since the cardiovascular surgeon was relatively new, staff inexperience with this type of patient might have contributed to a longer stay. Note that on discharge the burden of illness was rated at a level II secondary to the mild CVA.

> **INTENSITY FACTOR**
>
> *DRG 111: Abdominal Aortic Aneurysm*
>
> | Day | Hours of care |
> |-----|---------------|
> | 1 | 15 |
> | 2 | 12 |
> | 3 | 10 |
> | 4* | 6 |
> | Total | 43 |
>
> Intensity per stay = 43 ÷ 4 = 10.75 hours of nursing care

*Transferred to floor

Patient 8 was a 72-year-old female admitted with a perforated bowel secondary to advanced ovarian cancer. Palliative surgery was performed and she expired on the tenth postoperative day. These values represent day 10.

	APACHE	TISS	Prototype	Factor	Severity	DRG
BOWEL	20	20	III	II	IV	148

The APACHE II and TISS score reflect normal critical care values. The high moderate prototype score is related to the patient's total dependence for activities of daily living and the low factor score is related to the limited non-ICU tasks required. The severity score of IV reflects the patient's death.

Since this only represents one day, the nurse manager would look at several months' data before drawing inferences about the overall unit nursing intensity. For demonstration purposes, the nurse manager for this unit evaluated daily data for three months; she gained an understanding of the relationship of patient classification to nursing intensity by analyzing the trends.

In addition to the patient classification values, the nurse manager examines the other puzzle pieces for insight into intensity: the hours of care per patient per day (actual versus the overall average); admitting patterns (weekend versus weekday); ordering patterns of the physicians by DRG; staffing and productivity evaluation (number needed versus number available); and finally, supply and equipment costs per patient per day.

It is necessary to decide whether to examine patient intensity for each patient per day or the overall average intensity per unit stay. For example, if the DRG case mix for the unit includes the abdominal aortic aneurysm (AAA) patient discussed earlier, averaging the nursing intensity over the 4-day critical care stay develops an overall intensity factor for that DRG type. Based on trended data, an abdominal aortic aneurism required the hours of care depicted in the box. Note that a 4-day average of 10.75 hours of nursing provides an overall DRG intensity.

The manager alternatively can use the exact daily intensity of all patients in the unit to develop a daily intensity pattern. When analyzing data, consider the total hours of care provided on a routine day (24 hours). For example, data can be calculated into hours of care per DRG type by classification system. There are

152 Chapter 9

Table 9-7. 24-HOUR NURSING INTENSITY

	DRG	APACHE SCORE	TISS HOURS	PROTOTYPE HOURS	FACTOR HOURS	OVERALL AVERAGE
CVA	16	19	10	12.0	8.0	10.0
AAA	111	9	10	8.0	4.5*	7.5
SHOCK	123	29	20	18.0	18.0	18.6
LUNG LACERATION	84	14	5	12.0	8.0	7.0
LEUKEMIC	401	33	20	18.0	12.0	16.6
PTCA	5	5	10	4.5	4.5	6.3
CAROTID	112	8	5	4.5	4.5	4.6
BOWEL	148	20	10	8.0	8.0	8.6
TOTAL						79.2

*This value skews the average.

several additional bits of information that are helpful. One nurse can care for approximately 40 TISS points. In a unit with 12-hour staffing, one nurse has 10 productive hours per 12-hour shift. Thus a 40-point TISS score would require 20 hours of nursing care, or two nurses per 24 hours. The hours for the prototype and factor systems are predetermined and listed with the sample of each in the boxes on p. 138 and p. 139.

Table 9-7 reflects the care hours for the unit (80.5) based on the patient classification data given. This number indicates that the unit requires a minimum of four nurses per 12-hour shift to care for these eight patients based on the 10-hour per nurse productivity factor. There are several pitfalls in looking at required nursing intensity data as opposed to the actual staffing patterns. It remains illogical to use intensity values that are not reality based. For example, if the unit had only three nurses on the night shift of a particular day, the nurse manager would note that 30 hours of care, not 40, were given. This lower factor is then used when calculating the overall unit trends.

The nurse manager can relate the hours of care per nurse to the cost of supplies and equipment used in the unit to provide this care. Over time a cost per patient and eventually a cost per patient type can be determined. This cost can be evaluated periodically to assess the potential for inefficiency or waste. Skill at using this data is enhanced through computerization. Access to data and the ability to manipulate and cross match findings is easier and more manageable when the data are computerized. Once computerized, variations for unit specific parameters can be evaluated and changed if needed to enhance effectiveness and efficiency.

CONCLUSION

Patient classification systems attempt to quantify patient needs by measuring nursing intensity and matching the available resources to reimbursement. No existing patient classification system does everything. The ideal patient classification system of the future will reveal the individual patient's true nursing costs. Until it is developed, interpretation rests with the astute manager who can use the data to plan and predict future directions. Regardless of the systems currently used, the nurse manager should be able to extract enough information to develop a sense of patient intensity. The classification systems measure the discrepancy between the needs, the resources, and the financial status of the unit.

Patient classification is a management tool used along with task performance and analysis, financial management, and the interpretation of the economic status of the unit. The results of patient classification are used to look at the variance in resource use. The ability of the nurse manager to describe nursing intensity and use patient classification data is imperative to facilitate meaningful future change.

REFERENCES

1. American Association of Critical Care Nurses: Statement on patient classification in critical care nursing, Newport Beach, Ca, 1986, The Association.
2. Baker R: Ethics and the management of critical care units. In Fein IA and Strosberg M, editors: Managing the critical care unit, pp. 247-73, Rockville, Md, 1987, Aspen Publishers, Inc.
3. Cromwell J and Harrow B: An evaluation of Medicare's current method of allocating nursing costs and an examination of alternative approaches: summary and critique of patient classification systems, Health Economics Research Contract No. T-31415512 RFP: 01-85-PROPAC For Mary Kay Willian, PhD, Washington, DC, 1985, Prospective Payment Assessment Commission.
4. Freitas CA, Helmer FT, and Cousins N: The development and management uses of a patient classification system for a high-risk perinatal center, Journal Obstetrics Gynecological Neonatal Nursing 16(5):330-339, 1987.
5. Green J, McClure M, Wintfeld N, Birdsall C, and Reider K: Severity of illness and nursing intensity: going beyond DRGs. In Patients and Purse Strings II, p. 207-30, New York, 1988, National League for Nursing Press, Pub # 20-2191.
6. Horn SD: Severity of illness: case mix beyond DRGs. In Franklin A. Shaffer, editor: Costing out nursing, pricing our product, NLN Publication 20-1982, p. 225-35, New York, 1984.
7. Horn SD, Sharkey PD, Chambers AF, and Horn RA: Severity of illness within DRGs: impact on prospective payment, American Journal of Public Health 75(10):1195-99, 1985.
8. Keene R and Cullen D: Therapeutic intervention scoring system: update 1983, Critical Care Medicine 11(1):1-3, 1983.
9. Knaus WA, Draper EA, Wagner DP, and Zimmerman JE: APACHE II: a severity of disease classification system, Critical Care Medicine 13(10):818-27, 1985.
10. Nauert LB, Leach KM, and Watson PM: Finding the productivity standard in your acuity system, Journal of Nursing Administration 18(1):25-30, 1988.
11. Panniers TL: Severity of illness, quality of care and physician practice as determinants of hospital resource consumption, Quarterly Review Bulletin 13(5):158-65, 1987.
12. Trofino J: A reality-based system for pricing nursing service, Nursing Management 17(1):19-24, 1986.

SUGGESTED READINGS

1. Ambutas S: Evaluating a patient classification system, Dimensions in Critical Care Nursing 6(6):364-67, 1987.
2. Berman RA, Green J, Kwo D, Safian K, and Botnick L: Severity of illness and the teaching hospital, Journal of Medical Education 61(1):1-9, 1986.
3. Dijker M, Paradise T, and Maxwell M: Pitfalls of using patient classification systems for costing nursing care. In Franklin A. Shaffer, editor: Patients and purse strings, NLN Publication, [03Z] p. 3-20, (20-2155), 1986.
4. Fosbinder D: Nursing costs/DRG: a patient classification system and comparative study, Journal Nursing Administration 16(11):18-23, 1986.
5. Harrell JS: Predicting nursing care costs with a patient classification system. In Franklin A Shaffer, editor: Patients and purse strings NLN Publication [03Z] p. 149-63, (20-2155), 1986.
6. Horn SD, Sharkey PD, and Bertram D: Measuring severity of illness: homogeneous case mix groups, Medical Care 21:14-31, 1985.
7. Kinley J and Cronenwett LR: Multiple shift patient classification: is it necessary? Journal Nursing Administration 17(2):22-25, 1987.
8. Meyer D: GRASP: making the most of nursing budgets, Healthcare Financial Management, 34:32-36, 1980.
9. Nagaprasanna B: Patient classification systems: strategies for the 1990s, Nursing Management 19(3):105-6, 108, 113, 1988.
10. Thompson JD and Diers D: Management of nursing intensity, (Yale Nursing Intensity Project) Nursing Clinics of North America 23(3):473-92, 1988.
11. Sherrod SM: Patient classification system: a link between diagnosis-related groupings and acuity fators, Military Medicine 149(9):506-11, 1984.
12. Williams MD: When you don't develop your own: validation methods for patient classification systems, Nursing Management 19(3):90-2, 94, 96, 1988.

Chapter 10

TWENTY-FOUR HOUR STAFFING

Susan Craig Schulmerich

Volumes have been written about the nursing shortage, which continues despite national recognition and despite the many strategies suggested to reverse the trend. Meanwhile, health care consumption continues to escalate, and even though there are more nurses than ever before, the demand for even more continues to grow. In 1988, according to the Georgia Nurses Association, 91 nurses were needed to care for every 100 patients.[2] This is an increase from 50 nurses per 100 patients in 1973. The shortage has resulted in a need for more efficient and effective ways to staff critical care areas. The nurse manager bases staffing plans on the hours of care needed, the funds allocated, the available staff, the institution's past practices, and the manager's skill at interpreting data that support the need for staffing changes. This chapter provides an overview of 24-hour staffing. The material is based on data collected and stored by computer using the LOTUS 1-2-3 electronic spreadsheet.

STAFFING POLICIES OF THE PAST

In the 1970s and early 1980s, many hospitals assumed a rigid position on staffing. A nurse had to work a full shift, had to commit to working a set number of days per week, and had to have experience for a specialty assignment in critical care. Foreign recruitment was uncommon, although foreign graduates were always welcome after they had immigrated and passed state boards. The average staff nurse had little say in which days, shifts, or weekends were assigned to her. Attitude and practice changes accompanied increased opportunities for nurses with the advent of the nursing shortage. Hospitals have adjusted shift hours, introduced job sharing, started weekend plans (the Baylor model), begun recruiting in foreign countries; and they now offer a variety of creative work schedules and benefits.

The nursing shortage has resulted in the emergence of staff retention as a major goal of most institutions.[3] Job satisfaction from the feeling of autonomy in practice is the main factor in staff retention; however, institutional parameters, individual unit organization, and staffing also contribute. Today the nurse manager must be flexible and creative to retain staff.

IDENTIFYING NEEDED STAFF

Many institutions use patient classification to determine the hours of care needed and thus the number of staff needed. The Joint Commission on Accreditation of Healthcare Organizations (JCAHO)[4] mandates in Standard NR 4.4:

> The nursing department/service defines, implements, and maintains a system for determining patient requirements for nursing care on the basis of demonstrated patient needs, appropriate nursing intervention, and priority of care.

The traditional nurse-to-patient ratio of one nurse to two patients was used extensively in the late 1970s and early 1980s; however, it does not meet current JCAHO requirements, and may fall short of actual patient requirements. A patient classification system is the most accurate and valid predictor of nursing care hours.

Technologic and pharmacologic advances have not lessened the required nursing care hours in critical care units, but instead have escalated them. It is not unusual that 1.5 or 2.0 nurses are required to provide nursing care to a critically ill, unstable patient. A patient classification system captures and reflects nursing intensity.

Adams and Johnson[1] used the Spectra Medical Information System to identify the appropriateness of using paraprofessional staff, specifically licensed practical nurses or licensed vocational nurses (LPNs or LVNs), as adjuncts to professional staff. The computerized classification system had qualifiers that identified percentages of required registered nurse (RN) activity and LPN activity. For example, the qualifiers classified ventilator monitoring, and hemodynamic measurements and monitoring as 100 percent RN activities; forcing fluids as 50 percent RN and 50 percent LPN activity; and special mouth care as 30 percent RN and 70 percent LPN activity. Based on these data, an appropriate RN-to-LPN skill mix of 2.5 to 1 was established for that specific unit.

With the growing demand for and shrinking supply of RNs, LPNs can supplement the staff of critical care areas. When paraprofessional staff are available, the nurse manager can explore specific tasks such as those identified by using a similar system.

Nursing Care Hours and Full-Time Equivalents

A *full-time equivalent (FTE)* represents a hypothetical staff person who has an annual full-time commitment of 1950 hours (37.5-hour work week) or 2080 hours (40-hour work week). If an FTE is defined by 1950 annual hours, 875 annual hours designates 0.5 FTE (part-time), and so on. The key word here is *equivalent*. An FTE does not refer to an actual employee—an FTE reflects the amount of *hours needed to staff the unit*. FTEs can be converted into actual employees by taking into consideration vacation, holiday, sick time, and education days that are paid–time-off for actual employees. When planning staffing for a unit, however, the nurse manager must consistently use FTEs instead of real employees. If actual staff positions are used, the staffing will not meet patient care needs because the paid–time off each employee has for vacation, holiday, sick, and education leave would be included. FTEs are converted into actual employees only after all other calculations are finished. Table 10-1 illustrates the way actual staff hours are calculated from FTEs for a 37.5-hour work week and a 40-hour work week. The FTE hours less the benefit package translates into actual hours worked. Benefit time should be adjusted by the nurse manager to apply to the institution and the individual critical care unit.

Over a period of time, the trends in patient classification data are used to project the number of FTEs required to meet average patient care needs. One year's retrospective, accurate data allow the nurse manager to project staffing requirements if care needs remain constant. The more data available, the more accurate the projection.

Table 10-2 is used to project staffing needs for upcoming years based on retrospective data (census and NCH) for a 12-bed critical care unit. The FTEs budgeted for 1984, the baseline year, were calculated using the ratio 1 nurse/2 patients: If the average census is 10 patients/day, 5 RNs per 8-hour shift would be

Table 10-1. FTE HOURS VERSUS ACTUAL HOURS

	ANNUAL HOURS	
	37.5-HOUR WORK WEEK	40-HOUR WORK WEEK
1 FTE (260 shifts)*	1950.0	2080
less 20 vacation days	150.0	160
less 10 holidays	75.0	80
less 7 sick days	52.5	56
less 5 education days	37.5	40
ACTUAL HOURS WORKED	1635.0 (218 days)	1744 (218 days)

*For a 37.5-hour work week, use 7.5 hours per shift. For a 40-hour work week, use 8 hours per shift.

158 Chapter 10

Table 10-2. PROJECTING STAFF REQUIREMENTS

A YEAR	B AVERAGE CENSUS (PTS/DAY)	C FTES* BUDGETED	D AVERAGE NCH (HRS/PT/DAY)	E PROJECTED FTES
1984	10	21.06†	10.5	19.65
1985	10	19.65	10.0	18.72
1986	11	18.72	13.0	26.77
1987	12	26.77	15.0	33.69
1988	12	33.69	15.6	35.04
1989	12	35.04	15.8	35.49
1990‡		35.49		

*One FTE equals 1950 hours.
†1984 budgeted FTEs based on 1:2 ratio instead of classification system.
‡To project FTEs for 1991,
   a. multiply the 1990 average census by the NCH for 1990 determined from the patient classification system,
   b. multiply that number by 365,
   c. divide that number by 1,950.

needed, or 15 RNs per 24-hour day. Multiplying 15 RNs/day by 365 days/yr gives a total of 5,475 tours/yr of RNs:

$$10 \text{ pts/day} \times 1 \text{ RN/2pts/shift} \times 3 \text{ shifts/day} = 15 \text{ RNs/day};$$

$$15 \text{ RNs/day} \times 365 \text{ days/yr} = 5475 \text{ RN tours/yr}.$$

By definition, 1 FTE equals 260 shifts (tours). Thus if we divide 5475 tours/yr by 260 tours/FTE, we will obtain the total FTEs needed for the year:

$$5475 \text{ tours/yr} \div 260 \text{ tours/FTE} = 21.06 \text{ FTEs}.$$

At the end of 1984 when the patient classification system had been in place for a year, the average nursing care hours was found to be 10.5 h/day/patient. To project the FTEs needed for 1985 (assuming census and nursing intensity remain constant), use the 1984 data in Table 10-2: multiply the census by the NCH, then multiply by 365 days/yr, and then divide by the defined hours of an FTE (see Table 10-1). In other words:

$$\begin{aligned} \text{FTEs needed} &= \text{Census} \times \text{NCH} \times 365 \div \text{FTE hours} \\ &= 10 \times 10.5 \times 365 \div 1950 \\ &= 19.65. \end{aligned}$$

Thus, 19.65 FTEs are budgeted for 1985, and this number can be seen in column E (1984) and column C (1985).

At the end of 1986, retrospective data indicated an increase in census and in nursing care hours per patient. Thus the actual need for FTEs was much higher than the 18.72 FTEs budgeted:

$$\text{FTEs needed} = \text{Census} \times \text{NCH} \times 365 \div \text{FTE hours}$$
$$= 11 \times 13 \times 365 \div 1950$$
$$= 26.77.$$

The increase in staff that the unit needed in 1986 is thus easily justified by the numbers. Nursing care hours were determined by the patient classification system, and the higher intensity made it necessary for the unit to pay overtime, use agency nurses, and add float nurses to supplement the underbudgeted FTEs.

Historical Data

Three historical trends are determined to complete the request and justification for the staffing budget. These annual trends include sick time utilization, education and conference days, and overtime. The total number of sick days used by all staff is divided by the number of FTEs. (Remember to be consistent about the use of FTEs instead of staff!) For example, in 1988 if a total of 200 sick days was consumed by 30 FTEs in the unit, the historical sick days per FTE is 6.67, which is rounded up to 7 days.

Education time is based on the in-house and out-of-house education and conference paid–time off for all staff. Mandatory programs include one day for CPR, two days for ACLS, and one day for fire, safety, and infection control: total, 4 days per RN. Calculate the additional number of paid staff conference days and divide it by the number of FTEs. If 30 conference days were used and there are 30 FTEs, then an average of 1 additional day per FTE was used, which brings the total education time to 5 days per FTE.

Overtime (time-and-a-half) must be converted back into actual hours worked to determine the real FTE requirement of the unit. Separate the time-and-a-half hours from the regular hours paid, then determine the actual hours worked (that were paid at the higher rate) and convert them into FTEs. For example, if the budget reflects that 2925 hours were time-and-a-half hours the nurse manager divides this by 1.5 to get the actual hours worked.

$$2925 \div 1.5 = 1950 \text{ actual hours}$$

The nurse manager can now calculate the actual cost in hours of care for 1988 by converting these numbers to FTEs, and then converting FTEs into actual employees. Using the data from Table 10-2 for 1988,

$$\text{Annual hours} = \text{Census} \times \text{NCH} \times 365$$
$$= 12 \times 15.6 \times 365$$
$$= 68,328.$$

In Table 10-1 it can be seen that an employee on a 37.5-hour work week actually works 1635 hours after paid-time off is subtracted from the FTE-defined 1950 hours. Thus:

$$\text{Employees needed} = 68{,}328 \text{ annual hours} \div 1635 \text{ hours/FTE}$$
$$= 41.75.$$

The difference between this number and the 35.04 FTEs listed in Table 10-2 for 1988 is the total hours paid, but not actually worked. More detailed information on budget development can be found in other chapters of this book.

Developing Staffing Patterns

Once the required FTEs have been determined, a staffing pattern for the 24-hour period is developed. The primary objective of the staffing pattern is to have the appropriate number of staff present to meet the usual activities of the unit. Depending on the type of patient and the type of critical care unit, some times of the day may be more active than others. For instance, a surgical critical care unit may be busier in the afternoon and evening as a result of patient movement from the operating room and post-anesthesia care unit.

Admission, transfer, and discharge (ADT) activity can be used to determine a unit trend. Logs reflecting the ADT activity are universally kept in critical care areas; this log is the first information source for investigating peak activity times and interpreting their effect on NCH consumption.

Visiting hours also should be reflected in the staffing pattern. If the unit is in a teaching hospital, the day tour will be hectic because of physician activity. ADT activity, visiting hours, physician rounds, and institutional idiosyncracies should be considered in developing the most appropriate utilization of staff.

Tour Hours

Critical care units where tour hours are set at 8 or 12 hours/shift have conformity in tour hours. For this kind of unit, creating the staffing sheets may be time-consuming, but not particularly difficult. To determine the required staff per tour for each day, a simple calculation is necessary. Using the 1986 data from Table 10-2, we see that

$$11 \text{ [census]} \times 13 \text{ [NCH]} = 143 \text{ daily nursing hours.}$$

For 8-hour tours, 7.5 hours are worked:

$$143 \text{ hours} \div 7.5 \text{ hours} = 19.07 \text{ RNs needed.}$$

For 12-hour tours, 11.5 hours are worked;

$$143 \text{ hours} \div 11.5 \text{ hours} = 12.43 \text{ RNs needed.}$$

These numbers are rounded off to 19 RNs for the 8-hour tour and 12 RNs for the 12-hour tour.

Further consideration of the staffing pattern is dependent upon whether or not the individual unit activities warrant the addition of a flexible (flex) shift to provide additional coverage during specific times. Through analysis of the ADT, visiting hours, and physician activity, the nurse manager can create flex shifts to meet these needs.

Figure 10-1 represents a 3-week staffing pattern for 12-hour tours. In the middle of Figure 10-1, note that the nurse manager has scheduled a flex tour from 12 noon to 12 midnight. This staffing plan has a total of 31.5 FTEs. The pattern is designed to have 6 nurses working 7 AM to 7 PM, 1 nurse working 12 noon to 12 midnight, and 5 nurses working 7 PM to 7 AM.

Figure 10-2 represents a 3-week staffing pattern for a fully flexible unit. Note that the FTEs with flex staffing increase to 31.8 to deliver the same hours of care. To analyze the efficiency of Figure 10-1, the nurse manager looks at several things including the number of FTEs by tour and the contribution each tour and FTE makes to the average hours worked. Rather than totaling the various shifts, since so many overlap, simply determine the aggregate number of staff present during a 12-hour period. The staff working 11 AM to 9 PM are counted with the 7 AM to 7 PM staff because most of their hours are during the 7 AM to 7 PM time period. Conversely the 9 PM to 7 AM staff are counted with the 7 PM to 7 AM staff because their hours are within this time period.

Table 10-3 provides the breakdown of the data from Figure 10-2. Note that each FTE per tour is added up, converted to a percentage, and multiplied by the

Table 10-3. FLEX HOUR CONTRIBUTION TO AVERAGE HOURS WORKED

A TOUR	B NUMBER OF FTES	C PROPORTION OF TOTAL HOURS	D ACTUAL HOURS WORKED	E HOURS CONTRIBUTED TO AVERAGE HOURS WORKED‡
12-hour	10	0.32	11.5	3.68
10-hour	8	0.26	9.5	2.47
8-hour	13	0.42	7.5	3.15
Total	31	1.00	28.5	9.30

CALCULATION:
1. Determine how many FTEs work 12-, 10- and 8-hour shifts, and total them (31 FTEs in this example).
2. Divide the number of FTEs per tour by the total FTEs to obtain the proportion of the total contributed by each tour.
3. Multiply the actual hours worked by the proportion to determine the number of hours each tour contributes to the average hours worked.

*Column B ÷ total of column B.
‡Column C × column D.

FIGURE 10-1. 12-HOUR STAFFING

FTE	MONTH / DATE / ---NAME---	APR 16 SU	17 MO	18 TU	19 WE	20 TH	21 FR	22 SA	23 SU	24 MO	25 TU	26 WE	27 TH	28 FR	29 SA	30 SU	MAY 1 MO	2 TU	3 WE	4 TH	5 FR	6 SA
	SHIFT 7AM–7PM																					
1	SMITH		7	H				7	7		7	7							7	7	12	
1	BROWN	7		7	7							7	7	7			7	7				7
1	JONES		7			7	7			7	7				7	7		7	7			
1	HILL	7				7	7			7	7	H							7	7		7
1	GREEN				7	7		7	7				7	7			V	V	V			
1	JOHNSON		V	V	V						7	7			7	7				7	7	
1	KEENAN	7		7	7							E	7	7			7	7				7
1	CRAIG			7			7	7	7			7	7				7	7	7			
1	BOYD		7	R	7	R	7			7	R		R	7	7	7		R	7	R	7	
1	NOONAN	7		7	7							7	7	7				7			7	7
1	DROWNE			7	7			7	7										7	7	7	
1	WILLIAMS		7	7		7				7		R		7	7	7			R	7	7	
0.5	BLAKE	7				7					7						7					7
0.5	ROSEN		7					7	7				7					7				
0.5	WRIGHT		7							7					7	7				7		
0.5	GOODE	7					7					7					7					7
0.5	KNIGHT						7	7	7								12				7	
0.5	WASHINGTON					7				7					7	7	7					
	TOTAL 7AM–7PM	**6**	**6**	**6**	**6**	**6**	**6**	**6**	**6**	**6**	**5**	**6**	**6**	**6**	**6**	**6**	**6**	**6**	**6**	**6**	**6**	**6**
	SHIFT 12N–12M																					
1	MURPHY				12	12		12	12				12	12			V	V	V			
1	RODGERS	12				12	12			12	12	12							12	12		12
0.5	HOFFER		12	12							12				12	12		12				
	TOTAL 12N–12M	**1**	**1**	**1**	**1**	**2**	**1**	**1**	**1**	**1**	**2**	**1**	**1**	**1**	**1**	**1**	**1**	**1**	**1**	**1**	**1**	**1**
	SHIFT 7PM–7AM																					
1	BLACK	V	V				V				H	7	7				7	7				7
1	MALONE		7	7				7	7	7		E							7	7	7	
1	JACKSON		7	7	7							7	7		7	7			H	7		
1	DAY	7				7	7			H	7	7							7	7		7
1	ROBERTS				H	7		7	7	7		E					7	7	7			
1	WILSON		7	7	7							7	7		7	7		7	R	R	7	
1	MC ADAMS	7				7	7			7	7		7				V	V				V
1	STRONG			7	7			7	7		7	7							H	7	7	
1	JAMES				7	7	7				7			7	7	7		7	7			
1	HARRIS	7		7	7							E	7	7			7	7				7
1	WARD			V	V			V	V		V	V						7		7	7	
0.5	JENSON		V	V						7					7	7						
0.5	HOLBROOK	7								7	7										7	7
0.5	WINSLOW		7					7	7			E							7			
0.5	SMALL					7	7							7	7	7						
0.5	BARNES	7	7											7			7					7
0.5	MANLEY						7	7	7					7			7					
	TOTAL 7PM–7AM	**5**	**5**	**5**	**5**	**5**	**5**	**5**	**5**	**5**	**5**	**5**	**5**	**5**	**5**	**5**	**5**	**6**	**5**	**5**	**5**	**5**
31.5	TOTAL FTEs																					
	TOTAL 24 HOURS	12	12	12	12	13	12	12	12	12	12	12	12	12	12	12	12	13	12	12	12	12
0	SICK (S)	0	0	0	0	0	0	0	0	0	0	0	0	0	0	0	0	0	0	0	0	0
7	HOLIDAY (H)	0	0	1	1	0	0	0	0	1	1	1	0	0	0	0	0	0	2	0	0	0
23	VACATION (V)	1	3	3	2	0	1	1	1	0	1	1	0	0	0	0	3	3	2	0	0	1
5	EDUCATION (E)	0	0	0	0	0	0	0	0	0	0	5	0	0	0	0	0	0	0	0	0	0
0	ABS. W/O PAY (A)	0	0	0	0	0	0	0	0	0	0	0	0	0	0	0	0	0	0	0	0	0
0	LOA (L)	0	0	0	0	0	0	0	0	0	0	0	0	0	0	0	0	0	0	0	0	0

FIGURE 10-1. Example of a 12-Hour Staffing Schedule. H = holiday; V = vacation; R = requested; E = education day.

actual hours worked for the day to provide the total number of hours each tour contributes to patient care. With this information, the nurse manager can determine how many nurses are required in a 24-hour period to meet patient care needs. For example, if the patient classification system indicates that 143 nursing care hours are required, the nurse manager would divide 143 by 9.3 average hours worked (calculated in Table 10-3) to identify that 15 RNs are needed every 24 hours to meet patient care needs.

$$\text{RNs required} = 143 \text{ [NCH]} \div 9.3 \text{ [average hours worked]}$$
$$= 15.05 \text{ (round to 15)}$$

As mentioned earlier, a true flex schedule requires more staff than does a schedule comprised of conforming tours. Using this model, Figure 10-1 shows that 12.5 RNs are needed while Figure 10-2 with flex time shows that 15 RNs are needed.

Staffing plans with flexible work hours are more cumbersome for the nurse manager and more difficult to design. An automated staffing system is ideal when flexible work hours are used but not all units can afford them. However, if the nurse manager must do the staffing by hand she must be adept in matching one nurse to another to complement the hours worked by both.

The staffing sheets shown in Figures 10-1 and 10-2 can be created on a commercially available electronic spreadsheet. The spreadsheet will count staff and benefit time once a template has been written; more sophisticated functions can be written into the template if desired. There are a variety of software packages available, but a commercially available electronic spreadsheet is much less expensive than a staffing software package. Use of a spreadsheet requires a certain level of computer expertise.

Parameters the nurse manager uses in the preparation of the time sheet are listed in the box on page 165.

Job Sharing

The concept of job sharing has existed for decades, but nurses who shared jobs were referred to as split-shifters. Any two staff members who work equal parts of a tour can be considered job sharing. The nurse manager must assure that staff who are job sharing understand their commitment to the unit and each other. The staffing sheet should reflect that the two job-sharing staff members are equivalent to one person in the total staff available for a particular tour of duty.

Agency Nurses

Price and Southerland[6] explain that the increase in use of agency nurses results from the decrease in availability of hospital-employed nurses. The cost of agency nurses is significant. In the classified section of the Sunday *New York Times*, (January 21, 1990) the highest annual salary offered by major metropolitan

FIGURE 10-2. FLEX STAFFING

FTE	MONTH / DATE / ---NAME---		APR 16 SU	17 MO	18 TU	19 WE	20 TH	21 FR	22 SA	23 SU	24 MO	25 TU	26 WE	27 TH	28 FR	29 SA	30 SU	MAY 1 MO	2 TU	3 WE	4 TH	5 FR	6 SA
	SHIFT 7AM–7PM																						
1	MARSH	R	7	7			7				7	7	R	7						7	H		7
1	LAWRENCE	R				7	7		7	7	7				7			7	7	H			
1	LOCKE	R		7	7	E						H^3	H	H		7	7	7			7		
1	ABEL	R			7			7				7	7		7				7			7	7
1	MORRIS	R	7			7		7	7	7			7	7						7	7	7	
PD	HENSON	R							7	7													7
	TOTAL 7AM–7PM		2	2	2	2	2	2	3	3	2	2	2	2	2	1	1	2	2	2	2	2	3
	SHIFT 7PM–7AM																						
1	WALSH	R		7	7	7								7	7	7	7				7	7	
1	REYES	R	7	7	R^5	H	R	R					7	7	7			7	7				7
1	SHERMAN	R				7	7		7	7	7		E^7					7	7	7			
1	WONG	R		7	7			7			7	7				7	7				7	7	7
1	GALBRAITH	R	7				7	7				7	7							7	H		
	TOTAL 7PM–7AM		2	3	2	2	2	2	1	1	2	2	2	2	2	2	1	2	2	2	2	2	2
	SHIFT 7AM–3PM																						
1	KING	R	7		7	7	7	H			7	7	7		7	7	7		7	7	7	7	
1	SIMON	R		7	7	7	7		7	7	7		H	7	7			7	7	7	7		7
1	BRANDON	R	7	7		7	7	7			7	7	7	7		7	7	7		7	7	7	
0.5	WALLACE	R			7			7	7	7		7						7				7	7
0.5	FISCHER	R	7	7										7	7	7	7		7				
	TOTAL 7AM–3PM		3	3	3	3	2	2	2	2	3	3	2	3	3	3	3	3	3	3	3	3	2
	SHIFT 3PM–11PM																						
1	SAMUELS	R	3		3	3	3	3			3	3	3		3	3	3		3	3	3	H	
1	MCNAMARA	R		3	3	3	3		3	3	3		3	3	3			3	3	3	3		3
0.5	MARGOLIS	R	3	3										3	3	3	3				3		
0.5	DANIELS	R			3			3	3	3		3							3			3	3
0.5	RICHARDS	R	3	3				3						3		3	3	3				3	
0.5	ROWLAND	R					3		3	3	3	3						3					3
	TOTAL 3PM–11PM		3	3	3	2	3	3	3	3	3	3	2	3	3	3	3	3	3	2	3	2	3
	SHIFT 11PM–7AM																						
1	KRAUSS	R	11		11	11	11	11			11	11	11	11		11	11		11	11	11	11	
1	HINES	R		11	11	11		11	11	11		11	11	11	H			11	11	11		11	11
1	RIOS	R	11	11		11	11	11			11	11	11		11	11	11	11		11	11	11	
0.5	WATSON	R			11				11	11	11				11						11		11
0.5	MANN	R	11	11										11		11	11	11	11				
0.5	JAMESON	R		11			11	11	11	11		11								11			
	TOTAL 11PM–7AM		3	4	3	3	3	4	3	3	3	4	3	3	2	3	3	3	4	4	3	3	3
	SHIFT 11AM–9PM																						
1	DELO	R		11	11			11	11	11	11		11	H					11	11	11		11
1	BENNIN	R	11		11	11	11					11	11	11		11	11	11	11			11	
1	FLETCHER	R		R	R	11	11	11	11	11	R	R	11	11	11			R	R	11	11	11	11
1	HIGGINS	R	V^4	V	V	V					11	11			11	11	11	H		H	H		
0.5	WOODS	R	11	11				11								11	11	11					
	TOTAL 11AM–9PM		2	2	2	2	2	3	2	2	2	2	3	2	2	3	3	2	2	2	2	2	2
	SHIFT 9PM–7AM																						
1	DEMPSEY	R		H	9	9			9	9	9		9	9					9	9	9		9
1	HARTMAN	R	9		9	9	9					9	9	9		9	9	9		E	9		
0.5	JOSEPH	R			E				9	9					9							9	9
0.5	RICKMAN	R	9					9							9	9	9					9	
0.5	WAKEFIELD	R					9		9	9	9											V	V
	TOTAL 9PM–7AM		2	0	2	2	2	1	3	3	2	1	2	2	2	2	2	1	1	1	2	2	2
	TOTAL 7AM–7PM		7	7	7	7	7	7	7	7	7	7	7	7	7	7	7	7	7	7	7	7	7
	TOTAL 7PM–7AM		7	7	7	7	7	7	7	7	7	7	7	7	6	7	7	6	7	7	7	7	6
	0=CHARGE																						
	30.5 TOTAL FTEs																						

FIGURE 10-2. Example of a Flex Staffing Schedule. H = holiday; V = vacation; R = requested; E = education day.

> **PARAMETERS FOR TIME SHEET PREPARATION**
>
> Staff actually work less than they are paid for since each staff member is entitled to paid break time.
> - Twelve-hour staff are paid for 34.5 hours three out of four weeks and work a fourth shift every four weeks in order to meet annual full-time commitment of 1950 hours.
> - Ten-hour staff are paid for 38 hours and will exceed annual 1950 hour commitment.
> - Eight-hour staff are paid for and work 37.5 hours.
> - No staff are paid overtime until they work beyond 40 hours in one week.
>
> Part-time staff work
> - Seven 12-hour tours in a 4-week period.
> - Eight 10-hour tours in a 4-week period.
> - Ten 8-hour tours in a 4-week period.
>
> Holiday, vacation, and education are part of scheduled work time.
> Since this is a 3-week projection, not all full time staff will have holiday time in the schedule.
> Part-time staff receive prorated holiday time on the day the hospital celebrates the holiday. If part-time staff work on a holiday, they bank the time for future use.
> Rotation is planned on an equitable basis.
> Weekend commitment is similar for full and part-time staff:
> - 12-hour staff work 1 in 3 weekends.
> - 10- and 8-hour staff work every other weekend.
> - Per diem staff work 3 weekend days in a 6-week period.
>
> (Weekend commitment is reduced in exclusive 12-hour tours. If the staff were to work every other weekend, there would be far too many staff on the weekends, and insufficient staff on the during the week.)
> An attempt is made to give every full-time
> - 12-hour staff member a 5- to 6-day weekend every 6 weeks;
> - 10-hour staff member a 4-day weekend every six weeks;
> - 8-hour staff member a 3-day weekend whenever holiday time is available to be placed before or after a weekend off.
>
> On weekends charge will be assigned to a 12-hour staff member.
> If a tour is short, the staff will be supplemented with staff in the following order of cost:
> 1. Floats or per diems
> 2. Overtime
> 3. Agency

hospitals was $53,425.[5] This is for a 1950-hour year and includes educational, experience, certification, and shift differentials. Also appearing in the same section is an ad for agency nurses at $37 per hour; annualized for a 1950-hour year the salary is $72,150. The agency nurse is paid $37 per hour, the hospital must pay the agency an even higher rate to cover agency expenses.

Although agency nurses can be very expensive for hospitals, costs for agency nurses can be reduced or offset. Agency nurses can be used strictly on an as-needed basis. The functions and responsibilities the agency must bear at their own expense can be written into the contract, including yearly physicals, reference verifications, workman's compensation, and personnel record keeping. Mandatory education, CPR, infection control, and fire and safety can be the responsibility of the agency or the individual agency nurse.

Given the current environment's increased need and short supply of nurses, agency services may be necessary for many facilities. Over the years, this author has witnessed the change in the attitude of the hospital employed registered nurse toward the agency nurse. Unfortunately the change has not been a positive one. Friction arises because the hospital nurses resent the agency nurses' high hourly wages. The high hourly rates paid to outsiders is demeaning to the hospital nurses, who feel undervalued and underpaid. In addition, agency nurses work the best shifts—the Monday through Friday day tour—while staff work weekends and rotate to cover the off shifts. Hospital nurses do not perceive that agency nurses are committed to patients, unit, and co-workers. Agencies do not pay vacation, holiday, sick and insurance benefits; these are generally the responsibility of the independent practitioner. To reduce staff dissatisfaction when agency nurses are necessary, the nurse manager should assign a particular agency nurse to the same unit to foster a sense of belonging and commitment.

Orientation costs can be shared by the facility and the agency by implementing a sliding scale in which the agency absorbs the salary cost of the agency nurse's orientation. In return, for every tour the agency nurse works, 10 percent of this is then reimbursed to the agency. When the agency nurse has worked ten tours, the agency will have recovered the entire orientation cost. In addition, the hospital has not paid to orient a nurse who will only work a few tours.

The cost of orientation can be further reduced for both the agency and the hospital by developing self-learning modules for orientation. The self-learning module should include a written exam as evidence that key elements have been learned. The test also permanently documents that the agency nurse is aware of important facility policies and procedures. The self-learning module could be completed on the agency nurse's own time.

The nurse manager routinely identifies the benefits and the cost of these benefits to staff. Vacation, holiday, sick time, education days, paid health and welfare benefits, and pension plans are all part of the staff nurse's salary.

Stress that quality patient care mandates experienced full-time staff on off shifts and weekends because medical and other department support is less. Thus, some of the prime weekday shifts are often filled by supplemental staff when support from these departments and nursing exists. Every effort is made by nursing management to utilize agency nurses for the shifts most difficult to cover when a safe balance of agency and experienced staff exists.

Quarterly performance appraisal of agency nurses (if required for risk management and quality assurance programs) can be problematic for the nurse manager. Frequent performance evaluations help maintain the integrity of unit standards.

Case Study: Converting to a 12-Hour Shift

You are the nurse manager of a 12-bed critical care unit. Your staff is currently scheduled on the traditional 8-hour shift with every other weekend off. The majority have expressed a desire to change to a 12-hour shift, but a few of the older staff with families want to stay with the traditional shift. The assistant director of nursing for critical care has requested that you develop a plan and cost it out. What will you do?

THE PLAN

It would simplify matters if all the staff were on the same shift; the benefits of 12-hour staffing should be explained to the staff. Benefits include:

1. less weekend time scheduled
2. less holiday time (staff would be scheduled to work two holidays instead of three of the six major holidays)
3. more time-off (one 6-day weekend once every six weeks, when possible)
4. less travel expense, because they come to work three days per week instead of five
5. less laundry expense

After a 3-month trial, staff may return to traditional staffing if they wish. If some cannot be persuaded to try the 12-hour shifts, then proceed with a flex schedule for the sake of the staff who are requesting the trial.

COSTING THE PLAN

1. Determine the number of FTEs to work 12-hour shifts, the number of FTEs to work 8-hour shifts and the percentages each contribute to staff.
2. According to patient classification data, calculate the nursing care hours per patient per day (NCH).
3. Multiply the NCH by the average census to determine the daily NCHs.
4. Determine the average number of hours worked by a staff nurse per shift when there is more than one length of tour.
5. Divide the average number of hours worked into the daily NCH to determine the number of FTEs per day necessary to deliver the required patient care.
6. Determine the number of hours per year that a staff nurse actually works after vacation, holiday, sick and educational days have been deducted.
7. To determine the annual nursing care hours, multiply the daily NCH by the average daily census, then multiply by 365 days per year.
8. Divide the annual nursing care hours by the number of hours actually worked by a staff nurse (7 ÷ 6) to determine the number of employees needed annually.
9. Multiply the employees needed annually by the unit's average of nurses' salary and compare it to the present salary cost. If the new model is more expensive, are there any benefits that offset the cost?

CONCLUSION

In many respects, the 1990s will be filled with exciting changes and advances for all health care professionals; staffing issues, however, will be a constant source of frustration. Methods to attract young people into the profession and to retain nurses currently practicing at the bedside are the challenges placed before the contemporary nurse manager.

REFERENCES
1. Adams R and Johnson B: Acuity and staffing under prospective payment, Journal of Nursing Administration 16(10):21-5, 1986.
2. Georgia Nurses Association: As a nurse, will you tolerate . . ., Atlanta, Ga, 1988, The Association.
3. Hospitals cast new baits and lures for nurses: recruiters ranks swelling as staffing thins [news], American Journal of Nursing 87(10):1366, 1372-84, 1987.
4. JCAHO accreditation manual for hospitals/88, p. 145, Chicago, 1987, The Commission.
5. New York Times: Classified Section, Sunday, January 21, 1990, W21-22.
6. Price C and Southerland A: Rethinking staffing patterns in Critical Care Nursing, Nursing Management 20(3): 80Q, T, V, 1989.

SUGGESTED READINGS
1. Alexander J: The effects of patient care unit organization on nursing turnover. Healthcare Management Review 13(2):61-72, 1988.
2. Friss L: Simultaneous strategies for solving the nursing shortage, Healthcare Management Review 13(4): 71-80, 1988.

Chapter 11

COMPETENCY BASED ORIENTATION

Janet Mackin
Donna Scully Watts
Carole Birdsall

Competency-based orientation (CBO) is an instructional program based on established performance standards. The emphasis of CBO is on mastery of clearly stated competencies that are measurable and observable. All instructional strategies are focused on this end. Although CBO is not a new model for nursing education, its prominence has increased recently because of the endorsement and support of del Bueno and other nursing leaders.[2-7]

The application of CBO to critical care merits further exploration. The demand for highly trained critical care practitioners has increased because of the rising level of patient acuity. As a result of the nursing shortage, the requirements to be a critical care nurse have also changed: New graduates, foreign-trained nurses, and nurses with limited clinical experience now accompany experienced medical-surgical nurses into critical care. The challenge of orienting this mixed group involves meeting the substantially different needs of these nurses, and achieving a guaranteed level of competency.

The purpose of this chapter is to provide the nurse manager with an overview of competency-based orientation. Nurse managers are generally not expected to design and implement orientation programs on their own. However, the nurse manager is expected to ensure that the orientation method adequately meets the needs of the orientee and the critical care unit. With an understanding of the educational foundation of CBO, the nurse manager will be better able to evaluate the effectiveness of the orientation program. The following case study illustrates some of the orientation issues frequently faced by critical care nurse managers. The remainder of the chapter will use examples from the case study to illustrate important concepts.

Case Study: Choosing Staff

Staff vacancies are high and soon to be higher on your critical care unit. Your goal is to fill the available positions with competent practitioners as soon as possible. The ideal would be to hire only experienced critical care nurses. The reality is that none of the candidates you have interviewed have a critical care background. Your pool of candidates includes an RN with less than one year's experience on a medical-surgical unit in another institution, an experienced psychiatric nurse from an affiliated psychiatric hospital, and a potential transfer from the pediatric emergency department. You are also being pressured by recruitment to hire several new graduates. There's still some hope that a newspaper advertisement will bring in at least a few experienced critical care nurses.

Can you hire this mixed group of practitioners and successfully orient them to your unit? What help do you need from the nursing education department? How can you prepare your experienced staff to assist in this orientation process?

Assessment is the first step in answering these questions. Although all nurses that work in critical care have graduated from a school of nursing and have completed a complex course of study, not all nurses are ready to assume the responsibilities of caring for a critically ill patient. Even an experienced medical-surgical nurse needs to learn the technology and scope of practice of critical care nursing. The nurse manager and the nurse educator share the responsibility of ensuring that incoming staff are adequately prepared to assume independent critical care practice. A solid orientation strengthens the foundation upon which advanced practice and skills are built.

The nurse manager is aware of the pressure associated with budgetary constraints, unfilled positions, increasing census, and need for an appropriate orientation. The goal of orientation is to produce competent practitioners quickly and cost-effectively. All three of these factors (competency, minimum cost, minimum time) are required for a successful orientation program. Six-month orientations that require intensive instructor lecturing with direct supervision are no longer acceptable. A lengthy program prevents the expedient filling of a vacant position.

A VIEW OF COMPETENCY

The nurse manager must first define *minimum competency*. Nurse educators from the hospital's nursing education department or from an affiliated academic institution can be of assistance to the nurse manager in this area. Once a minimum competency is determined, an orientation program can be structured to produce the desired level of competency. CBO efficiently and effectively produces competent practitioners; the cost and time depends on the needs of each practitioner. No nurse receives more or less orientation than is required, and all nurses attain the same minimal level of competency.

For example, one required competency of all critical care nurses is the ability to interpret an ECG and respond to aberrant ECGs with the appropriate intervention. The length of time it will take each of the new employees in the case study to meet this standard may vary considerably. The medical-surgical nurse was nervous about working in critical care and began studying dysrhythmias independently, which enhances her grasp of ECGs. The psychiatric nurse is intimidated by technology and finds electrophysiology difficult to grasp; thus, it is expected that it will take more time for her to learn this new material. The pediatric nurse has worked in the pediatric special care unit and can already recognize life-threatening dysrhythmias. She will need help with advanced dysrhythmia interpretation for the adult population.

By using CBO, each orientee is given the information needed to achieve competency and the time needed to master the information appropriate to the level of need. The pediatric nurse does not need to review basic ECG interpretation, but can start with more complex dysrhythmias. The medical-surgical nurse might catch up with the pediatric nurse quickly because of her independent study. The psychiatric nurse may need remediation on basic cardiac anatomy and physiology before even starting ECG interpretation.

DEFINING CBO

In a traditional orientation program, knowledge is the possession of the teacher, and it is presented to the learners in portions known as *lectures.* The same lecture is delivered to all participants—those with no knowledge, those who just need a review and those who are proficient. The lecture is delivered at the same speed to all learners, whether English is their primary or secondary language. Because the instructor is the source of the knowledge, content review requires instructor involvement.

On the other hand, CBO is a nontraditional approach to the teaching and learning process. Since the desired competencies are clearly defined, the learner knows what is expected from the beginning. The program starts with a self-assessment of existing skills, which may be combined with a pretest to validate knowledge and identify areas of weakness. From this point on, the orientation varies greatly from learner to learner.

Using the new hires identified in the case study, the following CBO strategy develops: All new graduates and the psychiatric nurse (who rated low on the self-assessment) are required to review learning packages on cardiac anatomy, cardiac physiology, and basic ECG interpretation, and to attend a workshop, in which the instructor assists and directs the orientees in interpreting rhythm strips of patients who are currently in CCU. Thus, knowledge acquired from CBO is immediately applied to patient care, which reinforces the learning process. After completing this workshop the orientees study the learning packages on life-threatening dysrhythmias. In three weeks, the orientees complete all aspects of basic ECG-interpretation and take the ECG posttest to demonstrate their competency. Clinical evidence of competency is also sought. While caring for a monitored patient, they interpret the cardiac rhythms; these interpretations are validated by the instructor or preceptor.

In contrast, the medical-surgical nurse and the pediatric nurse begin studying the advanced dysrhythmia learning packages immediately. The pediatric nurse "tests out" and passes the clinical and classroom competency components in one week, and the medical-surgical nurse successfully passes the posttest in two weeks.

Consider the following scenario. You have recruited two experienced practitioners who immediately take the posttest; the first passes it, validating an adequate level of knowledge; but the second does not pass. The testing process has therefore identified a lack of competency in an experienced practitioner, and has indicated a need for remediation and follow-through. This is a simple example because it only considers *one* competency. But CBO applies to *twenty-five or more* competencies. Each orientee's situation is evaluated individually, educational materials are provided, and time requirements are adjusted to the learner's pace. In addition, a specific method of evaluation is used to validate each competency.

BENEFITS OF CBO

The finish date of orientation varies significantly from learner to learner. An experienced practitioner who successfully completes all posttests and clinical validation is available for staffing. The psychiatric nurse may take six to eight weeks to complete the program. The other orientees may complete the CBO in one to four weeks. Although the motto "from each according to his ability, to each according to his need" initially applies in a CBO, the result is better described as "equality for all," because when orientation has been completed, all participants must equally prove a minimum level of competency.

Thus CBO allows for variable start dates for new nursing staff. In contrast, a traditional orientation program requires a significant amount of anticipatory planning and relatively fixed scheduling. This preplanning is necessary to accommodate instructors who have other clinical obligations and to contain the cost of presenting a program with sophisticated content that is needed in critical care.

In a highly competitive recruitment market, the nurse who must delay a work start-date to coincide with the orientation schedule is likely to seek employment elsewhere because of personal economic pressures. The possibility of losing the candidate for employment and the pressure of the nursing shortage may persuade the nurse manager to hire the applicant without delay, and provide interim clinical support until formal orientation begins. Although this meets the nurse's economic needs, it fails to promote the most nurturing environment for orientation—and it places an extra burden on experienced staff to monitor the actions of the new employee, whose level of knowledge and skill is unproved.

Greater flexibility with the variable start dates offered by CBO allows the critical care unit to gradually absorb replacement staff. This eliminates the stress that occurs with the sudden increase in staffing when a traditional critical care orientation course is offered. Often these new practitioners are still gaining confidence and developing a sense of job mastery, but are labeled "independent" because of the nature of the system.

The emphasis of traditional orientation is placed primarily on the *acquisition* of knowledge. The *application* of this knowledge in the critical care setting could be either overlooked, neglected, or poorly timed. Completion of the traditional orientation program occurs on completion of the didactic lectures. Acquisition of knowledge is tested with a final exam. Passing the exam could be incorrectly interpreted to mean the new nurse was competent and ready to function as an independent staff member.

CBO utilizes the principles of adult learning, and acknowledges the professional experience and the previous learning the nurse brings to the new job. All new employees have some degree of prior nursing knowledge, skills, and experience. Unfortunately, traditional orientation programs subject all new nursing staff to the very same material, forfeiting a resource upon which to capitalize.

CBO utilizes behaviorally stated competencies that have measurable, observable assessment parameters. The orientee can review the required proficiencies, identify those already mastered, and proceed independently to the assessment stage of the program. The nursing educator provides instruction and skill lab practice for those competencies the orientee is unable to meet. This practice reduces the nonproductive time of orientation and is a cost-effective strategy.

__Learner Benefits__

CBO avoids the boredom and anomie of the uniformly attended orientation, and demands that the new employee participate actively. The orientee identifies learning needs, participates, and assumes responsibility for personal learning. Thus, from the beginning, CBO fosters in the orientee a sense of responsibility and good judgment—traits prized in critical care nurses.

Because of the individual attention received by the orientee, CBO facilitates collaboration and shared professional responsibility between the orientee, the nurse educator, and the nurse manager. In fact, the orientee actually spends less time with the instructor in a CBO program than in a traditional orientation program, but the time spent is more valuable. For example, in a traditional orientation, the orientee spends hours in a classroom with an instructor—in a four-week didactic critical care orientation, a total of twenty days. In a competency-based orientation, the orientee will be with an instructor on clinical days (the number varies) and in workshops part of some days, but the total might be less than four days of this twenty-day period. The orientee spends the rest of the time reading learning packages, viewing video programs, and working with a preceptor.

In a traditional orientation program, the demands of lecturing are great, and the instructor may not speak individually with an orientee until the clinical experience begins. Shy or easily intimidated orientees may fail to learn. This is not identified until a posttest is given or until clinical deficiencies are noted. Unfortunately, the posttest of the traditional program is usually a single grand test given after weeks of lecturing. CBO provides clear markers for each competency.

CBO requires a continuous dialog between the orientee and the instructor. The competent orientee spends much less time with the instructor. Most orientees appreciate being recognized for the knowledge they already have and do not feel cheated by this. The instructor gives the less-competent practitioner more time and support without the pressure of group competition. The instructor's time is also used for answering questions and supervising practice. A CBO design tends to decrease resentment between learners; without the traditional classroom setting, no one can show off by asking advanced questions, and no one feels like a dullard by asking that material be repeated. The learning needs of one orientee do not impinge on the rate of learning of another. This does not prevent the informal coaching system that occurs between orientees. However, the coaching is purely voluntary; it is not necessary to move the class forward.

IMPLEMENTATION AND ADMINISTRATIVE SUPPORT

Although CBO offers straightforward solutions to several problems of traditional programs, administration must be committed to supporting the program, beginning with the planning and implementation phases. To gain the support of administrative personnel, the recruitment, scheduling time, and outcome benefits of a CBO must be clearly identified. This takes time and strategic planning. Frequent orientations that utilize innovative, individualized teaching techniques are excellent marketing tools for recruiters. The nurse recruiter can really be an ally, because the recruiter's advice is taken seriously by the other hospital administrators in this era of nursing shortages.

There are significant direct and indirect costs involved in the initial funding of a CBO program.[4,5,6] Items to be funded include office, classroom, and laboratory space; salaries for qualified educators and support staff; office and audiovisual equipment; personnel to develop educational programs and assessment protocols; and possibly, consultant fees.

Because most hospitals have already budgeted for orientation and education of critical care nursing staff, the cost of underwriting the CBO program may be offset in part by shifting these funds. Furthermore, some costs could be recovered later by contracting educational services to other facilities. When experienced practitioners are hired, a direct cost savings can be counted because nonproductive time is decreased when orientation time is decreased. In addition, the resource materials developed for CBO can also be used by incumbent staff who require remediation. The burden of remediation is shifted from the instructor to the learner—another cost-effective benefit of CBO.

Once CBO is formally adopted as an educational standard, the planning process begins.[11] Administrative policy decisions, such as establishing orientation time frames, must be made. Because successful orientation is completed when all competencies are met, the orientation time frames must be flexible. This flexibility allows the experienced nurse to finish in a shorter time than the novice practitioner. For example, policy may state that orientation will range between two and ten weeks for newly hired critical care staff nurses. A proviso can be added to the policy stating that extensions or abridgments must be recommended by the nurse manager and instructor.

Consultation with human resource experts is essential to comply with all federal and state equal opportunity regulations. A copy of the finalized CBO policy is provided to all new employees when orientation begins. This can be presented in a learning contract or a blueprint.[10] The box on the following page is an example of a learning contract. The process for opportunities to review and discuss mutual expectations and concerns are identified in writing.

COMPETENCIES IN CRITICAL CARE

There are no formally established critical care entry-level clinical competencies, although the need for them has been identified by the American Association of Critical Care Nurses and recommendations for actions made.[1] Identification of the required competencies of a new critical care nurse is therefore the responsibility of the nurse manager and the clinical instructor. To form this competency list—the crux of CBO—the nurse manager and the instructor investigate mandated topics, position descriptions, hospital policies and procedures, the unit case mix, Quality Assurance and Risk Management considerations, and staff input.

Mandated Topics

Mandated topics designated for state and JCAHO accreditation of professional staff have been clearly identified. JCAHO requires documented evidence of staff participation in an initial orientation and in annual updates on the following topics: fire/safety, infection control, electrical safety, and basic cardiac life support.[8] In addition, state requirements must be met, including professional conduct, incident reporting, role in disaster plan, HIV confidentiality, and organ donation (understanding the request law). Internal and local requirements may

> **LEARNING CONTRACT FOR CBO**
>
> Dear Professional Colleague,
>
> The orientation program is based upon adult learning principles. We call this program *competency-based orientation* (*CBO*). To derive the greatest benefit from the CBO, you need to be self-motivated and self-directed.
>
> The critical care orientation blueprint identifies the learning competencies you are expected to achieve by the end of orientation. In addition, the blueprint provides a working list of resources that will help you meet those goals. You are not expected to view or read all of the resources. However, there are several strategies that can be helpful to you so that learning "your way" is easier.
>
> Make sure you fully understand the competency for each topic. You may or may not have had critical care experience. If you believe you can demonstrate the required skills or that you know the procedure, it is not necessary for you to read or view the resources.
>
> The clinical instructor and nurse manager responsible for your unit will work with you to reinforce the learning that has occurred. This reinforcement will be in the form of questions about what you have learned and how you are relating your new knowledge to clinical practice.
>
> After you have completed the orientation, you are expected to pass a final exam with a score of 80 percent or better. If you require additional help in any area, please speak to your instructor or nurse manager.
>
> If you cannot meet the required level of competencies, you will be invited to a conference to plan how competency will be accomplished.
>
> We hope this letter has identified our expectations of you. We view this letter as a learning contract that holds you accountable for achieving the goals outlined. For clarification, please talk with the clinical instructor or nurse manager. Once your questions are answered, please sign and date two copies of this letter. Keep one copy for your personal records and give the other to the nurse manager, who will place it in your employee file.
>
> If at any time in the program you have questions or experience difficulties, please discuss them with either the instructor or the nurse manager. We hope this program will enable you to meet the hospital's requirements for practice in the critical care area and your own expectations of yourself as a critical care nurse.
>
> (signature) _____ RN
>
> (date) _____

also exist. For example, if the hospital is a trauma center, advanced cardiac life-support and advanced trauma life-support certification may be necessary. These mandated topics provide the core competencies around which the CBO is built.

Position Descriptions

A review of the position description of the critical care nurse reveals additional competencies required. For example, if the position description states that the nurse will document all aspects of the nursing process, competencies related to documentation of the nursing process must be included in the CBO.

If the position description is poorly written or not criterion-based, little competency information will be gleaned from it. It is recommended that inadequate position descriptions be revised before designing the CBO.

Hospital Policies and Procedures

Additional competencies can be found by reviewing the hospital's policies and procedures. Policies and procedures contain specific responsibilities that are not usually included in generic position descriptions. For example, if policy states that critical care nurses are permitted to draw blood for arterial blood gases, the design of the CBO must include a competency in arterial phlebotomy.

Unit-Specific DRG Statistics

Computers now give access to a quantity and type of data previously unavailable, such as the critical care unit's case mix by DRG, and average length of stay. This information can help identify the types and numbers of patients, the most frequent patient diagnoses, and the length of stay per DRG. These frequency and chronicity figures can be used in CBO development since competency selection and prioritization are determined by performance and associated risk frequency.[9]

For example, a review of a surgical critical care unit's statistics reveals that 65 percent of all patients admitted had thoracic or abdominal surgery, 10 percent had orthopedic surgery, 15 percent had head-and-neck surgery, 5 percent had trauma surgery and 5 percent had other admitting diagnoses. To begin identifying competencies, list the skills that are most frequently used. In this example, the general surgical nursing skills and those skills associated with the care of patients undergoing thoracic or abdominal surgery are priorities.

Further analysis of unit statistics may reveal that the length of stay of patients undergoing head-and-neck surgery is longer than the DRG average. The nurse manager investigates and explores the potential causes of this. For example, returning to the case study, the nurse manager finds that the medical-surgical nurse and the psychiatric nurse have been caring for many of the radical neck surgical patients. They both work 12-hour shifts and have alternate days off. Neither has taught the patient how to self-suction, which delays the patient's transfer from the unit and potentially the patient's discharge from the hospital.

Upon investigation, the nurse manager and instructor realize that the educational needs of patients undergoing radical neck surgery were not covered in orientation. A revision of the CBO and inclusion of a competency in patient education for self-suctioning techniques may help shorten the length of stay, improve the patient's independence and benefit the hospital financially.

Quality Assurance/Risk Management Data

Quality Assurance (QA) programs have been established to identify and monitor high-volume, high-risk, and problem-prone aspects of patient care. The nurse manager reviews QA audits with staff and institutes corrective actions. QA deficiencies are identified as compliance, practice, or knowledge problems. Deficiencies related to a lack of knowledge require the implementation of expanded and or improved educational programs.

For example, consider what happens when a QA audit reveals poor documentation of central-line dressing changes. The nurse manager identifies the problem as lack of knowledge because the staff were not taught the new guidelines. A two-pronged approach to this problem is needed. Not only should a review be provided for the incumbent staff, but a competency is included in orientation to ensure that all orientees are taught the procedure and policy. Once this procedure is incorporated in the orientation, the nurse manager is relatively sure that new employees will be able to perform a central-line dressing change and will know what documentation is required. A review of incident reports will pinpoint clinical errors that may have resulted from a deficit in nursing knowledge, judgment, or skill. To decrease the likelihood of future errors, strong consideration is given to incorporating specific learning experiences in the CBO. Inclusion should depend on the frequency of a particular incident or the gravity of the associated sequelae.

QA and Risk Management (RM) trends are monitored continuously. New findings may necessitate a revision of the CBO. Therefore, the CBO needs to be flexible and responsive to the changing needs of the institution.

Staff Input

The input and opinions of the incumbent staff, the critical care clinical specialists, and the direct line administrators are needed when designing the CBO program. Nurses from all levels can add valuable suggestions, and clinical staff can provide insight drawn from clinical practice, which may not be readily apparent to those further removed from daily hands-on care.

A word of caution is needed: Staff may find it difficult to imagine an orientation different from the one they experienced. A veteran critical care nurse may criticize the orientation as too soft and easy compared to the sink-or-swim method used previously. Others may not believe that learning can occur without lectures. Reluctance to accept change can result in the sabotage of new orientation methods. Only a few critical comments and comparisons to past practices can weaken the faith in CBO of an orientee and even an administrator.

Incumbent staff can help develop the CBO. The staff's areas of strength and weakness should be acknowledged. Critical care nurses are clinical experts, and thus their comments about clinical skills, problem-solving abilities, and patient care situations are invaluable. However, their understanding of educational methodology may be limited. The clinical instructor and nurse manager demonstrate the mutual respect necessary for development of an educationally and clinically sound orientation. Active participation of clinical staff in planning and implementing the successful CBO fosters a sense of staff ownership and responsibility.

Other professional staff may also be helpful. For example, respiratory, occupational, and physical therapists can be asked to collaborate with nursing to formulate and prioritize competencies relevant to their areas of practice. Their input is most useful if it is based on issues arising during the course of clinical interactions. For example, the consultant pulmonologist and chief respiratory therapist may recommend that a higher priority be given to the standard ventilator function competency and alarm troubleshooting than for the ventilator weaning competency, because weaning is not an emergency procedure. Thus, these two competencies are allocated separate time slots on the CBO schedule. Prioritization of competencies allows the nurse to consolidate and practice principles associated with the first competency before progressing to the second.

LEARNING RESOURCE DEVELOPMENT

Once the difficult task of competency identification is accomplished, the next step is to identify the available resources to assist the learner in meeting the competencies. Learning resources come in a variety of formats; some are readily available; others require the investment of time and money to develop.

Written Material

Written learning materials range in format from policy and procedure manuals to journal articles and specially developed learning packages. All may be useful to the orientee, but each is carefully selected and appropriately utilized. For example, it would be unproductive to have an orientee review the critical care policy manual. The quantity of material and the lack of focus would baffle the orientee. A better approach is to match the reading material to a specific competency.

One learning resource for the competency "Able to administer IV-push medication" is the critical care policy on IV-push medications. By reading this policy, the orientee learns that some medications can be administered by IV-push, and others cannot. The acquired knowledge can be validated by a simple posttest. In addition, the orientee now knows that a policy is available for reference in case memory fails.

Journal articles that are used as learning resources must be carefully selected. Only certain sections of an article may be necessary. The nurse manager and instructor can distinguish between the "nice to know" and the "need to know" orientation materials; the orientee independently probably cannot. The orientee's attention can be focused on important sections by underscoring, writing specific directions, highlighting, and developing study questions. Since mastery of the basic material is expected, it is important to limit the quantity of articles to the essentials. Additional articles can be provided for enrichment and clarification of the basic content, but they must be clearly identified as optional reading.

Learning Packages

Learning packages often need to be developed to teach hospital-specific information that is unavailable in any other format. A learning package is a self-instructional program that includes directions, objectives, content, exercises or drills, pretest, and posttest. It may also include equipment and audiovisual resources. Learning packages are designed to guide the learner carefully until the content is mastered. The content is carefully selected to meet the specific objectives of the learning package. Exercises and drills reinforce learning. A final posttest measures the achievement of mastery.

For example, orientees are expected to master documentation skills. A general familiarity with the information will not suffice. This learning package would include samples of all documentation forms, guidelines for using the forms, and practice sessions to complete samples.

A learning package standardizes and guarantees uniformity of the presented content. The amount of time required to develop a learning package is substantial, but if the learning package is used by a large number of orientees, it is worth the investment.

Video Programs

The advent of the affordable and easy-to-operate video camera has allowed educators to create an abundance of video programs. Video programs of complex procedures such as "Nursing actions needed when setting up for a Swan Ganz catheter insertion" are invaluable to an orientee. Since the importance of this competency is recognized, the orientee's eyes are glued to the TV screen. The tape can be replayed until all the steps of the procedure are learned. If the tape is accompanied by a learning package and equipment, the orientee can practice the manual skills.

Although less stimulating than demonstration videos, *talking-head videos* (where a speaker stands and gives a lecture) can deliver content consistently and on demand to any number of learners. The talking head on the video never tires of delivering the same lecture again and again. Although most learners would prefer a live presentation, the video version makes up in availability and consistency what it lacks in spontaneity.

Commercially produced video programs are also useful learning resources for orientees. Careful selection of programs appropriate to the setting is necessary, because they must be consistent with the policies and procedures of the institution. Free programs provided by equipment manufacturers can teach the operation of a specific product, but these programs require screening. On occasion, the equipment manufacturer's video wastes time emphasizing the values of the device. It may be necessary to cut out the commercial and stick to the instructional portions. Other commercially produced programs are generic in nature and excellent for teaching basic principles of practice.

Slide and Filmstrip Programs

Slide and filmstrip programs with audiotapes are cumbersome audiovisual resources. Most learners find it difficult to operate the hardware needed to view the program — it takes longer to learn to operate the projector than it does to learn the content! However, filmstrip and slide programs are somewhat useful. If these programs are the only available resources, use them until they can be replaced by more user-friendly media, such as videocassettes.

Computer-Assisted Instruction

Computer-assisted instruction (CAI) can be excellent for self-instruction because computer programs require a great deal of user interaction. The best CAI programs let the learner progress at their own speed. Poorly designed CAI programs consist of boring text sprinkled with questions and answers in pretense of being interactional.

The cost of CAI can be expensive. Not only are the programs costly, but the computer itself is too. Costs may be prohibitive for small organizations. If an organization already has equipment and educators skilled in this area, cost is less of an issue. However, each CAI takes many man-hours to produce, especially if the educator is learning how to create the product. In these instances, a cost-benefit analysis would be beneficial before moving in the direction of CAI.

Staff Input

The nurse manager and her staff work closely with the nurse educator to select or develop the learning resources for a CBO. Staff confidence in resource quality and appropriateness coincides with satisfaction with CBO. Audiovisual resources cannot be expected to meet all the learning needs of orientees. Time must be provided for questions, concerns, and clarifications of content presented in the prerecorded programs. The instructor and nurse manager are responsible for facilitating the initial acquisition of critical care knowledge, and also for helping the orientee integrate this information into daily practice.

VALIDATING LEARNER COMPETENCY

An important component of a CBO is validation of the orientee's competency. CBO starts with a clear explanation of the required competencies; the learner understands these expectations from the very first day. This eliminates an orientee's commenting, "I didn't know I had to learn that." If appropriate learning resources are provided, the orientee cannot say, "I was never taught that." Instead, CBO fosters a sense of responsibility for learning.

Preassessment Testing

A baseline assessment of critical care knowledge and skill validates whether the orientation program has been successful. Critical care knowledge can be tested with the Basic Knowledge Assessment Tool (BKAT), a statistically reliable and valid test.[12,13] The BKAT has been used in a number of hospitals to standardize cognitive testing of new critical care staff. Ideally, comprehensive, entry-level, minimum-performance competencies will eventually be developed by a recognized professional group such as the American Association of Critical Care Nurses. Until then, the BKAT can be reviewed by the nurse manager and educator to determine its applicability to the individual institution.

In addition to assessing cognitive abilities, a basic skills assessment like the one in the following box is completed by the orientee at the start of orientation. The skills assessment identifies areas of strengths and weaknesses, and helps guide the orientation process. The orientee is recognized as an adult who knows her own personal needs. The skills assessment helps the orientee determine what skills need to be learned to complete orientation.

At the start of orientation, some orientees express a wish to challenge competencies by passing the appropriate test or demonstrating competency to the instructor. The process of challenging competencies is encouraged with guidance from the educator and manager. A study guide developed specifically for selected competencies with a carefully selected reference list to assist in independent study is needed. This gives experienced practitioners a sense of self-direction and personal satisfaction about using the CBO because it helps them decide which competencies to challenge.

Ongoing Assessment Testing

Testing and evaluation are continued throughout the orientation. Each segment of learning is posttested or clinically evaluated. The orientee derives a sense of progress that may relieve anxiety about passing the critical care final exam. Any problems with mastery of specific material can be remediated quickly.

NURSING SKILLS ASSESSMENT

This inventory of required competencies shall be completed by the end of your orientation. Have the clinical instructor or preceptor sign each skill/behavior after you demonstrate competency. Keep this document current and present it for evaluation. After orientation this document will become a part of your record.

1. Read each competency and select a code number that best describes your knowledge and/or experience. Put the number you select in the column labeled Self-assess code no.
2. Each time you demonstrate a skill, have the clinical instructor or preceptor initial a code number that best describes your skill level. You are expected to reach the minimum performance standard at the designated level for most of the competencies by the end of orientation. Of course, there will be some skills that require further work due to a lack of opportunity during orientation.

Performance Code
1. Verbalize limited knowledge or experience
2. Perform with assistance
3. Perform under supervision
4. Perform independently

Competency	Self-assess code no.	Observer initials and date under code no. 1	2	3	4	Minimum performance standard code no.
Apply monitoring leads.						4
Initiate cardiac monitoring on a patient.						4
Print an EKG strip.						4
Interpret a strip of NSR.						4
Document a strip of NSR in the chart.						4
Check blood product per hospital standard.						4
Administer blood product per hospital standard.						4
Document blood product per hospital standard.						4
Monitor patient during blood product administration.						4
Document patient's response to blood product.						4

Posttesting

The BKAT and the skills checklist can also be used to evaluate the orientee at the end of orientation. Standards for acceptable performance levels are set; these standards are reasonable and relevant to the clinical setting. For example, it is unreasonable to expect a new graduate to meet all items on the skills checklist at a level that states: "Perform independently." Some advanced skills, such as cardiac output measurement, may still require supervision. The nurse manager and staff identify the level of skill needed to practice safely in the clinical area. Those skills that cannot be achieved during orientation are targeted for ongoing staff development programs.

Many traditional orientation programs include direct observation of selected procedure performance, either in the clinical area or in the laboratory. Often, the format requires that the orientee perform the procedure in its entirety—in the exact order. This rote performance does not measure the nurse's judgment in skill accuracy and appropriateness. Furthermore, this adherence to each minute detail has a negative effect on orientees experienced in critical care. Relearning mastered procedures in a somewhat altered order wastes time. Competency skills statements highlight only those steps fundamental to the procedure. If correct sequencing of the steps is required, it is so indicated.

For example, if the skill competency being observed is drawing blood from an arterial puncture for arterial blood gases, the nurse checks the patient's ID band, provides patient information, and assembles the necessary equipment. Handwashing and glove-donning proceed skin preparation and the actual arterial site puncture. However, some clinicians palpate the radial and ulnar arteries before donning gloves. As long as the nurse washes her hands before and after the procedure, it does not matter if the arteries are palpated with or without gloves; the gloves are worn for handling blood.

In addition to the nurse's skill in arterial puncture, the nurse's judgment must be evaluated. For example, the nurse recognizes the circumstances in which the determination of blood gases is appropriate, and also understands how to interpret the results. This too is included in the competency.

Although sound judgment and priority-setting abilities are required for competent nursing care in the critical care unit, they are the most difficult ones to assess. del Bueno[4] has designated judgment and priority-setting abilities as *critical thinking dimensions*. Some examples of judgment and priority-setting competencies are managing a patient in shock, responding to a fire in the critical care unit, and dealing with an angry family member.

Critical thinking dimensions are tested by presenting the orientee with simulated situations that require responses at selected points. Simulation may be achieved through use of mannequins, medical equipment, audiovisual media, interactive computer programs, or role-playing. CBO allows more instructor time for these workshop sessions than does the traditional didactic orientation. Since traditional lecture time in CBO is minimal, the instructor is available for these practice and demonstration sessions.

Time Frames

An important component of CBO is the time frame for achievement of competency. Each competency requires a target date for completion. This helps the orientee prioritize the competencies and attain each competency in the correct sequence. For example, a competency in basic cardiac life support is completed before a competency in advanced life support is undertaken. Aiming at a week by which the orientee must achieve a competency gives the orientee a framework for an overall plan. The following box lists competencies to be achieved during the first week.

Returning to the case study, the nurse manager determines that an individualized approach to each orientee's CBO can easily be completed.

The medical-surgical nurse with some experience at a different institution may test out on competencies 2, 10, 11, and 12 listed in the box. These include understanding fire safety; knowing patients rights; knowing that hospitals have policies on patient complaints; and understanding professional misconduct.

The psychiatric nurse may be proficient on items 2, 6, 7, 8, 10, 11 and 12 from the box below. In addition to those identified above for the medical-surgical nurse these include state requirements about reportable incidents; application

---

CRITICAL CARE CBO: WEEK ONE COMPETENCIES

1. Verbalize fire alarm and extinguisher location.
2. Answer questions correctly on actions in fire safety packet.
3. Verbalize actions and the number to call if fire is seen.
4. Complete packet on charting.
5. Chart basic nursing notes per standards.
6. Verbalize that certain incidents are reportable to the state and state where to seek help to verify reportable incidents.
7. Verbalize that restraints require MD order and demonstrate ability to apply restraints per standard.
8. Demonstrate ability to assess wrists when restraints used in the clinical setting.
9. Use siderails at all times except when at bedside and providing care.
10. Verbalize concept of patients rights and where rights are posted on the unit.
11. Verbalize the process used for patient complaints.
12. Verbalize what constitutes professional misconduct and repercussions of professional misconduct.
13. Demonstrate ability to use stethoscope to listen and interpret heart sounds and pulse deficit, verbalize relationship to existing pathology if any, and document findings per standard.
14. Demonstrate ability to apply cardiac monitoring leads and initiate cardiac monitoring on a patient.
15. Print, interpret, and document a strip of normal sinus rhythm on a patient.

of restraints; and the assessment of the patient's wrists when restraints are used.

And finally, the pediatric nurse, an in-house transfer with some special care experience, could potentially test out on competencies 1 through 12, and then focus on adult heart sounds and pathology, cardiac monitoring, and taking an EKG strip. In all three of these examples, prior knowledge is recognized.

An orientee would be on target if all items were completed by the end of the first week, regardless of the completion sequence. However, before proceeding to the second week's competency for dysrhythmia interpretation, all the first week's competencies must be met.

Target dates are initially estimated, then validated by testing them on a group of learners. After adjustments are made, the target dates become fairly reliable predictors of average time for achievement. Variances from these target dates are quickly seen in a CBO. The orientee experiencing problems can be identified as early as the first week. This is a tremendous advantage over a traditional orientation where learner problems may be sensed but not clearly identified early in the orientation.

CONCLUSION

In summary, CBO is an alternative approach to traditional critical care orientation. It must be noted that successful completion of a critical care CBO does not guarantee that the individual will always provide competent care. The same can be said of the traditional program. Human nature, stress, and the environment make critical care practice exciting, but problem prone. CBO's greatest strength is that it provides a flexible, individualized, and appropriate orientation in a timely fashion. Knowledge, skill, and judgment abilities are the areas addressed in a CBO. Most importantly, CBO encourages the orientee to take an active role rather than a passive role in the orientation process.

REFERENCES

1. Alspach J, editor: Education standards for critical care nursing, St Louis, 1986, The CV Mosby Co.
2. del Bueno DJ, Barker F and Christmyer C: Implementing a competency-based orientation program, Nurse Educator, 5(3):16-20, 1980.
3. del Bueno DJ, Barker F, and Christmyer C: Implementing a competency-based orientation program, Journal of Nursing Administration 11(2):24-29, 1981.
4. del Bueno D, Weeks J, and Brown-Stewart P: Clinical assessment centers: a cost-effective alternative for competency development, Nursing Economics 5(1):21-26, 1987.
5. Farmer ML: Competency-based orientation proved effective, Journal of Nursing Staff Development 2(3):126-28, 1986.
6. Flewellyn BJ and Gonell DJ: Comparing two methods of hospital orientation for cost effectiveness, Journal of Nursing Staff Development 3(1):3-8, 1987.

7. Hamilton L and Gregor F: Self-directed learning in a critical care nursing program, Journal of Continuing Education in Nursing 17(3):94-99, 1986.
8. JCAHO Accreditation Manual for Hospitals, Chicago, 1990, The Commission.
9. Kieffer JS: Selecting technical skills to teach for competency, Journal of Nursing Education 23(5):198-203, 1984.
10. Knowles M: Self-directed learning: a guide for learners and teachers. Englewood Cliffs, New Jersey, 1975, Prentice Hall Regents.
11. Smith MF, and Altieri MJ: Competence based assessment in critical care nurses, Focus on Critical Care 16(6):17-22, 1986.
12. Toth JC: Evaluating the use of the basic knowledge assessment tool in critical care nursing with baccalaureate nursing students, Image 16:67, 1984.
13. Toth JC: The Basic Knowledge Assessment Tool (BKAT)—validity and reliability: a national study of critical care nursing knowledge, Western Journal of Nursing Research 8(2):181-96, 1986.

SUGGESTED READINGS

1. Alspach J: The educational process in critical care nursing, St Louis, 1982, The CV Mosby Co.
2. Boss LAS: Teaching for clinical competence, Nurse Educator 10(4):8-12, 1985.
3. Canfield A: Controversy over clinical competencies, Heart and Lung 11, p. 197, 1982.
4. Carr MJ: Legal aspects of standards of practice, Dimensions in Critical Care Nursing 8(2):111-12, 1989.
5. Feeney J, Benson-Landau M: Competency-based evaluation: not just for new nurses, Dimensions in Critical Care Nursing 6(6):368-72, 375, 1987.
6. Hardy GR: Ensuring clinical competence, Nursing Management 19(12):46-47, 1988.
7. Houge MC and Deines ES: Verifying clinical competencies in critical care, Dimensions in Critical Care Nursing 6(2):102-9, 1987.
8. Lassiter CK, Kearnery MR, and Fell R: Competency-based orientation—an idea that works, Journal of Nursing Staff Development 1:69-73, Summer 1985.
9. Primm P: Entry into practice: competency statement for BSNs and ADNs, Nursing Outlook 34(3):135-37, 1986.
10. Scott B: A competency-based learning model for critical care nursing, International Journal of Nursing Studies 21(1):9-17, 1984.

Chapter 12

CAREER LADDERS

Marie Folk-Lighty
Kathleen Klock

Those in management positions have two goals: to improve patient care, and to provide flexibility for upward mobility of the nursing staff. Clinical ladders and career ladders can help reach these goals. This chapter describes clinical and career ladders, explains when they are needed, discusses how to implement them, and examines their rewards and pitfalls. A case study will illustrate key points in the text that can be related directly to implementation strategies.

Case Study: Implementing a Career Ladder Program

You are the nurse manager of a 16-bed intensive care unit. The hospital is interested in implementing a clinical or career ladder program and has asked you to be a member of the committee. In fact, the critical care unit will be a trial unit for implementing the project. What should you do?

First you must develop a conceptual framework for the program. Determine which type of ladder would be best (the clinical ladder or the more involved career ladder) and then determine how to integrate the ladder into the hospital's organizational structure. Once this blueprint is prepared, write entry and promotion criteria. Next, develop job descriptions for each position on the ladder. Before the program is implemented, good planning can often help recognize and avoid potentially serious problems. The box on the next page presents a framework for developing a hospital program. The needs of different hospitals may vary and therefore the specific goals for the ladder program may also vary.

> **FRAMEWORK FOR DEVELOPING A CLINICAL LADDER OR A CAREER LADDER**
>
> A. Conceptual Framework
>   1. Identify the difference between clinical and career ladders
>   2. Choose type of ladder
>   3. Develop blueprint
>   4. Define ladder program within the hospital
>   5. Sell the concept
>   6. Financial analysis (1 and 5 years)
>   7. Feasibility study
>   8. Summarize findings
>   9. Project goals for 1 and 5 years
> B. Evaluation criteria and promotion criteria
>   1. Define requirements for experience, education, etc.
>   2. Establish review process
>   3. Establish time frame for each level
>   4. Develop policies, include progression up and across the ladder
> C. Develop job descriptions
>   1. Determine group to write the job descriptions
>   2. Use of nursing process
>   3. Focus on measurable outcomes
>   4. Use action verbs to describe desired performance
>   5. Clearly differentiate all levels
> D. Recognize the titles
>   1. Assignment planning—job description expectations must be integrated into practice
>   2. Identify the number of positions within each level needed to provide the care required
>   3. Develop preceptor program
>   4. Develop peer support system
>   5. Identify administrative expectations
>   6. Plan vacation and leave coverage for levels
> E. Public relations
>   1. Market the program
>   2. Show how ladder fits into the organization

Clinical Ladder versus Career Ladder

The first step is to decide whether a clinical or a career ladder is the best option. Their differences must be understood. At the same time, the hospital's organizational structure must be considered: Will the program be implemented throughout the hospital? Will requirements be adapted and individualized to each unit? How much freedom will the nurse manager have to set criteria and performance standards?

Early in the process it is important to complete a literature search of clinical ladders and career ladders.[4,7-10,12,13,16] Most of the literature concerns clinical ladders that address professional growth for nurses delivering direct patient care. Career ladders are more comprehensive; they comprise two to three subdivisions, or *tracts*, that allow for movement in the clinical fields, as well as movement in the management and education fields. Alt and Houston[1] described the career ladder program of the University of Texas, M.D. Anderson Hospitals and Tumor Institute at Houston, and included specific job descriptions for all levels in the career ladder. Although they did not detail a step-by-step method of implementation, they do explain how the career ladder was implemented in a variety of nursing units in the same hospital.

Sanford identified the beginnings of the clinical ladder program.[15] The need for a program that addressed the development of professional practice at the bedside was first described by Creighton in 1964, and Zimmer presented the first model for a clinical ladder in 1972.[17] Zimmer's model was developed to provide an environment that would result in professional growth and recognize clinical practice. Throughout the literature a number of clinical ladder program goals are consistently identified: to recognize advancement (monetary and title) of the nurse practicing at the bedside; to allow for growth of, and reward to the RN who remains caring for patients; to foster professional growth; to provide role models for new practitioners; to incorporate peer review to improve the quality of patient care; and to emphasize the RN's growth and promotion in practice settings rather than in education or management settings.

The career ladder provides a much broader scope. Its purpose is to recognize advancement in the areas of clinical practice, education, and management.[6] Many of the clinical ladder components are found in the clinical tract of the career ladder. The career ladder allows the nurse to choose an administrative, clinical, or education tract with clear steps to follow (each tract incorporates the different backgrounds and academic preparations); encourages decentralization of the decision-making process for staff advancement; to encourage independence and career mobility; identifies ways for allow participation and self-direction in management; and encourages nurses to stay in hospital settings.

The focus of the literature has been on the clinical ladder rather than the career ladder. This may be the result of hospital-developed frameworks that already promote advancement in education and management. Advancement of nurses in clinical positions is a more recent concern.

When planning the career ladder, review the current organizational structure to identify the existing levels of education and management, and then determine the number of levels for your ladder. Table 12-1 illustrates a three-tract, five-level career ladder that was developed as the pilot for the case study. The required experience at each level of the education and management tracts must be correlated with that of the clinical tract. The major points to consider when matching experience are found in the following box. The most important of these are years of practice, specialty experience, and education. These should be comparable

> **LEVEL EVALUATION CRITERIA**
>
> - Number of years in nursing
> - Number of years in specialty
> - Number of years at this institution
> - Degree requirements
> - Expectations for practice (clinical performance, committee work, and quality assurance activities)
> - Written contract for accepting level

Table 12-1. THREE-TRACT CAREER LADDER

LEVEL	CLINICAL	EDUCATION	MANAGEMENT
6 months	Probation	Probation	Probation
I (Entry)	Clinical Nurse I	N/A	N/A
II	Clinical Nurse II	N/A	N/A
III	Clinical Nurse III	Unit Educator I, Staff development	Asst. Nurse Manager
IV	Nurse Clinician	Unit Educator II	Nurse Manager
V	Clinical Nurse Specialist		Asst. Director

across all three tracts. In Table 12-1, the clinical and education tracts merge at Level V, culminating in the clinical nurse specialist. Above the assistant director level, management positions are not expected to have analogs on the clinical and education tracts. If the education and management levels of the current organizational structure comprise a flattened system, changes should be made before matching it with the clinical tract.

A well-developed ladder can advance currently employed staff; reward the nurse practicing at the bedside; enable peer review; maintain and improve high standards of clinical practice; increase job satisfaction; and support a decentralized nursing management model.[3]

Potential Problems

The cost of implementing and maintaining the program can be high. Once implemented, however, the program can enable considerable growth over the first two or three years. In addition, if the program decreases turnover, there will be more employees in the higher salary ranges. Access to higher ladder levels can be limited in order to stay within the budget, or the money saved in orientation and recruitment costs can be transferred to pay salaries. If the financial implications are not anticipated, cost-limiting changes can negate the staff's acceptance of the program.

Determine how the effect of the ladder program on the system will be identified. Effects on nursing practice, changes in patient outcomes, and the nature of interactions between nurses and other health professionals require evaluation.

The system must be maintained once it has been implemented. Clear guidelines are needed to ensure that staff meet the standards of the program and continue to grow. If standards are not consistently maintained, staff will readily identify this.

Relating the Ladder to the Hospital's Structure

The clearly stated program objectives are reviewed in the context of the hospital's organizational structure. Consider the type of facility, the amount of freedom each unit has to develop new methods of delivering patient care, whether the staff has been unionized, and the extent of control the union has over practice issues. Consider the effect that seniority and rules for staffing might have on implementation, and whether the expectations for performance and advancement are similar from unit to unit. If there are different expectations, the rationale for differences are clearly identified to the staff. This is incorporated into the model before implementation.

PLANNING A LADDER

The categories of employees that will be included in the ladder program must be decided. Alt and Houston[1] described how a wide range of employees (RNs, students, and others) can be integrated into a career ladder program. This decision should reflect the hospital's philosophy for care within critical care units.

Several questions are considered specifically for the clinical ladder or the clinical tract of the career ladder. How many levels should be incorporated? By what mechanism do nurses transfer from one unit to another? How many positions for each level will be budgeted per unit? Will the limits of participation at each step be based on financial constraints? At this time, identify the numbers of positions at each level that will be required to deliver quality patient care and meet the other objectives of the ladder.

A literature review has shown that the usual number of levels for a clinical ladder and for each tract of a career ladder is four to five.[11] The authors support a ladder with at least five levels. Additional levels might be considered in larger organizations or ones that have joint practice arrangements with colleges or universities. A ladder with less than four levels could constitute a flattened system. Since Level I is usually the entry level, there would only be two levels for advancement. This does not provide for appropriate recognition of advanced clinical practice, such as a master's degree level of a clinical specialty. For a career ladder program, fewer than five levels would not allow for advancement in clinical, management, or education areas. Since the education and experience requirements for education and management positions are usually at the master's degree level with at least five years experience, a limited career ladder would not provide appropriate recognition for experienced practitioners.

Once the number of levels has been selected, determine what effect this number will have on the existing system before expectations and requirements for each level are formalized. For example, how are patient care assignments made? What is the level of experience of current nursing personnel?

Several financial considerations must be addressed: Is there an opportunity for all appropriate individuals to participate in the program? Can the institution support an increase in use of certain benefits? How will their placement on the ladder affect staff use of existing programs, such as tuition reimbursement, conference funds, and hospital educational offerings?

Will the program be voluntary? The literature has so far reported only voluntary programs. If the program is voluntary, the differences between requirements for employment and those for involvement in the ladder program are clearly identified. Staff may request a step downward or a temporary removal from the ladder because of increased involvement in education programs, family commitments, or some other activity. Will options to contract temporarily for a lower position on the ladder be available? The literature has not yet addressed these issues. However, experience with several programs indicates that flexibility enhances the program. The positive aspects of flexibility include increased staff commitment to the concept, increased support of the program even by staff who are not actively involved, and maintenance of quality care.

Developing a ladder program requires considerable time and finances. Before progressing further, consider whether the ladder will truly be useful. Dorothy del Bueno has identified several concerns, in particular, the lack of research to support the effectiveness of clinical ladder programs.[5] Since 1982, the literature evaluating their effectiveness remains sparse.

Professional nursing practice must be recognized and developed in clinical settings, as well as in management and education settings. This can be achieved by using either a clinical ladder, or preferably, the clinical tract of a career ladder. The career ladder is more comprehensive; the entire hospital organization consistently recognizes professional growth in all settings. Regardless of the type of ladder planned, commitment to growth of practice must be clearly identified in the program purpose.

There are institutions that have been able to attract and retain nursing staff. These institutions have designed systems that recognize the importance of the professional nurse and allow the nurse to grow professionally and personally.[14]

When designing the program, it is imperative that the evaluation criteria be developed as the program is being formulated. Objectives for the program can vary from increasing recruitment and retention, to recognizing and developing professional practice. It is important to recognize that although both extremes can be achieved, without careful planning goals can easily become confusing.

Another aspect is the management of ladder entry. What does the system expect of the nurse? Are the nurses expected to demonstrate a higher level of practice when they are in a Level III or IV position? (See Table 12-1 on p. 192 and the box on p. 197.) How is achievement of these higher practice levels evaluated?

The individuals who will constitute the review board are identified. The review board determines whether requirements for the different levels have been met. Membership includes representation from clinical, education, and management positions.

IMPLEMENTATION

Once the program is clearly defined, and the goals, objectives, and evaluation criteria are in place, the concept should be shared with appropriate members of the organization. This process will vary by institution. It will depend on where the ideas for the program originated and who will be making decisions about the ladder. Support for implementing such a program is obtained before initiating any further activities.

Before the ladder is implemented, a budget is projected for one year and for five years. Included in the budget are:

1. The financial resources available.
2. The numbers of nurses projected for each level.
3. The position limitations at any level.
4. The number of positions at each level assigned to a specific unit.
5. The projected growth of the program for at least the first five years.
6. The projected savings (from the anticipated decrease in staff turnover, which decreases recruitment and orientation costs).
7. Salary spread between levels.

By now the feasibility of the proposed program should be apparent. Prior to implementing the ladder program, a written proposal following the outline in Table 12-1 must be completed. This plan includes the persons to be involved, the time frames for developing the evaluation criteria, the requirements for levels, and the projected dates for implementing the project. In addition, the ladder is incorporated into the long-range planning activities of the nursing department and the overall hospital organization for at least five years.

The way the individual enters the ladder must be clearly identified. The requirements that need to be met for an employee to retain position must be addressed. What needs to be done to advance up the ladder must be defined. There can be many requirements. The employee completes an application that will be used to determine which level requirements have been met. In addition, peer evaluations, performance, and other support documents can be additional requirements.

The individuals involved in reviewing the applications were determined during the planning phase. The board reviews all applications to determine if the requirements have been achieved, and forwards its recommendations to a designated administrator, usually the director of nursing services. The outcome of the review will depend on the recommendation of the review board and position availability.

EVALUATION CRITERIA

When the requirements for each ladder level are established, the purpose and goals of the ladder must be kept in mind. The box on p. 197 lists the criteria that must be addressed for each level. Note that experience, education, performance expectations, and a written contract are included. The contract clarifies the expectations of the individuals on the tract in their new positions.

In reviewing Table 12-1 on p. 192, note that there is an opportunity to enter the clinical tract at Levels I and II. Entry for the education and management tracts occur at Level III and above. The specific expectations for the Level III clinical, education, and management tracts are presented in the box on the next page. This is an example of how each criterion can be defined for each tract. It is expected that the specific number of years of experience and educational preparation for each level will vary depending on the institution. The entry criteria for each level must be clearly defined.

The time it takes to achieve each level will vary with the number of levels, and organizational factors such as budget, turnover, level requirements, and position availability on the ladder. The probation period for new employees is usually a maximum of six months. Following probation, the time to enter the ladder program can vary from the end of probation to one year. When considering the progression up the ladder, identify potential restrictions in movement (for example, lack of experience, lack of formal education, budget limitations). The rate at which the staff can progress must be considered, remembering also that there must be continual growth opportunities for all employees. For example, a ladder with five levels would require the registered nurse at Level III to have at least five years experience in nursing, with two to three years in the specialty. To advance to the next level, there would be a minimum of three years' additional experience at that level. Advancement would require formal education and demonstration of desired behaviors of Level IV prior to promotion.

Though it is expected that each institution will develop a ladder that considers its own specific resources, requirements for the middle to higher levels of the clinical, educational, and management tracts should be comparable to the levels of other institutions. When education requirements for each level are determined, the philosophy of the institution, as well as the expectations of the nursing profession, must be considered. Although to progress up the ladder in

LEVEL III CRITERIA

Clinical
1. RN with current licensure
2. Number of years in nursing (5)
3. Amount of time in specialty (2-3 years)
4. Amount of time at institution (6 months)
5. Formal education. Baccalaureate in Nursing preferred. If the employee does not have a baccalaureate degree a statement can be included in the contract so that they will begin work on a degree within 6 months—one year. A tentative completion date will also be agreed on.
6. Expectations for practice including but not limited to:
   A. function as a primary nurse
   B. function as patient/family advocate
   C. collaborate with other health care professionals
   D. serve on a committee, unit or nursing department
   E. demonstrate successful use of nursing process
   F. demonstrate professional accountability
   G. implements findings of nursing quality assurance activities into practice
   H. participates in quality assurance studies

Education
1. RN with current licensure
2. Number of years in nursing (5)
3. Amount of time in specialty (2-3 years)
4. Amount of time at institution (6 months)
5. Formal education baccalaureate in Nursing
6. Expectations for practice meet requirement listed under clinical
7. Demonstrate understanding and ability to assess learning needs of others
8. Demonstrated ability to teach

Management (Assistant Head Nurse)
1. RN with current licensure
2. Number of years in nursing (5)
3. Amount of time in specialty (2-3 years)
4. Amount of time at institution (6 months)
5. Formal education Baccalaureate in Nursing
6. Expectations for practice—meet requirements listed under clinical
7. Demonstrates problem solving skills
8. Demonstrated leadership skills

the clinical area without formal degrees may be acceptable, it is not acceptable for the education or management tracts. In the initial levels, where formal education is preferred but not required, the attainment of certain degrees can be included as a contract item for maintaining and advancing up the ladder. This allows for recognition of individuals who provide excellent patient care while supporting the advancement of the profession of nursing.

For employees placed on the ladder, maintaining a position requires a periodic review that includes a complete application, peer review, and compliance with expectations of the position and contract agreements, (for example, completion of an education program). The time between periodic evaluations varies from one to three years.[1,5] Two year intervals are suggested for a voluntary program. This allows staff an opportunity to meet the additional requirements. After the review, the employees renegotiate a contract to determine their position on the ladder and other specific requirements.

Policy Development

To ensure that the integrity of the program is maintained, policies must be determined and written before implementing any phase of the program. For example, what happens to the employee at one level on a clinical ladder or tract who transfers to another unit? If the ladder program has clearly defined policies, one can easily determine to which level on the ladder the employee will transfer. In addition, the employee will know in advance if there will be a decrease in salary for a period of time until new criteria are achieved. Some institutions allow a grace period during which the employee receives the same salary while meeting the new requirements. If one of the goals of the ladder program is retention of staff, this policy would be appropriate. Policies minimally should include:

1. Philosophy of the nursing department
2. Philosophy of the ladder program
3. Purpose of the ladder program
4. Goals of the ladder program
5. Organizational charts reflecting all positions and relationships of the ladder within the institution
6. Structure and function of the review committee
7. Application process to the ladder program
8. Advancement up, down, and across the ladder (movement from one specialty unit to another; e.g., critical care unit to the post-anesthesia care unit, or medical-surgical unit to a critical care unit)
9. A grace period in which salary remains the same for a nurse transferring from one unit to another, to allow time to achieve new skills and knowledge
10. Job descriptions for each level

JOB DESCRIPTIONS

The job description defines the requirements and provides an overview of the position and the expectations for practice. The job description integrates much of the material previously discussed. The group developing job descriptions includes those functioning in the position, as well as positions above the level. The scope of the ladder and function of each position can thereby be recognized. For clinical Level III, for example, the job description group might include staff nurses with at least five years experience, clinical nurse specialists (CNS), a nurse manager (Level IV management), and possibly an assistant director (Level V management).

When the job description is written, the components of the nursing process provide a guide. One way to define clinical Levels I, II, and III might be to define expectations under the headings of Assessment, Planning, Intervention, and Evaluation. Unfortunately, this format might restrict the job description of a head nurse or clinical specialist. For the role of the CNS, the components recognized by the American Nurses Association and others (clinical expert, consultant, educator, and researcher) are more effective.[2]

Performance expectations identified in the job description are written in measurable terms. Action verbs are used to define the desired performance. Although the job description will define performance expectations in terms of process and outcome, whenever possible, desired patient outcomes should be identified: for example, "The patient demonstrates understanding of the teaching program presented." In the following box, the process expectations for Level III management include, "Coordinates patient care on a daily basis," and "Plans clinical orientation with the unit education nurse." An outcome statement for the same level might be, "Staff are able to successfully meet job description expectations following completion of orientation." A process statement for Level III clinical is, "Evaluates and revises patient education activities." A patient outcome statement for the same level is, "Patient on ventilator demonstrates decreased anxiety and agitation following education related to the need for ventilatory support."

If the ladder program is going to serve as more than an opportunity to provide additional salary, the pivotal factor is integrating the roles and desired performance changes into the job. To enhance self-esteem and recognize ladder position, individuals should be recognized with name pins, personal achievement portfolios, nursing support groups, and committee positions.

To ensure ladder success, support must come from the participants on each level, as well as from the institution. The peer support system should be formalized. This group can provide a mechanism for problem solving. As a nurse progresses up the ladder, the number of nurses in each level decreases. To prevent isolation, a formal program can include nurses from various specialty areas. A mentor program could be developed, in which nurses at a higher level can serve as resources to help nurses identify how they can plan for and achieve the requirements for advancement.

INTEGRATING THE PROGRAM INTO THE ORGANIZATIONAL STRUCTURE

Changing behaviors, expectations, and responsibilities requires that the entire organization understand the program and commit to its objectives. A clear plan is

> **LEVEL III JOB DESCRIPTION EXCERPTS**
>
> **Clinical**
> 1. Identifies patient care concerns to be studied
> 2. Uses quality assurance studies to evaluate patient care concerns
> 3. Provides direct patient care
> 4. Functions as a primary care nurse
> 5. Functions as shift coordinator
> 6. Evaluates and revises patient education activities
> 7. Develops education programs that demonstrate a change in patient compliance with therapy
> 8. Serves as a preceptor for new employees
>
> **Education**
> 1. Provides clinical orientation to organization and unit
> 2. Provides contracted number of hours of direct patient care
> 3. Assesses staff needs for unit education activities
> 4. Collaborates with HN, AHN, and other Level IV and V
> 5. Focuses on unit level activities
>
> **Management**
> 1. Coordinates patient care on a daily basis
> 2. Cares for own patients
> 3. Plans clinical orientation with unit education nurse
> 4. Participates in evaluation of staff
> 5. Represents head nurse in absence
> 6. Evaluates direct practice and performance of employees
> 7. Develops staff in charge position
> 8. Responsible for time schedules for all shifts
> 9. Staff are able to successfully meet job description expectations following completion of orientation

needed to involve all levels of nursing personnel in the acceptance of the job description expectations for each position on the ladder. Within the organization, both formal and informal structures must be revised to incorporate the changes. Once the job descriptions have been formalized, the nursing department's organizational chart and its relationship to hospital organization is reviewed and revised as necessary. This is crucial to the program's success. However, the ease with which it is accomplished will vary considerably from organization to organization.

A test of success in changing attitudes and behaviors is found on the units. How are individual patient care assignments made? The master staffing plan for the unit is developed to ensure that based on patient acuity, adequate numbers of each level are available. Although limiting the number of positions because of financial restraints is not desirable, planning the minimum staffing—specific numbers of each level on the tract to provide a predetermined level of care—can be determined for each unit based on patient population and acuity. This would help ensure that the ladder is an integral part of the organization, and not merely a recruitment and retention tool. If staffing patterns are determined only by available staff, rather than the required levels of nurses, then individual assignments can never be made to ensure that there will always be consistency in care. For example, if there are only a few Level III clinical nurses, are patient assignments based on the complexity of the care required or the personnel available? There must be enough Level III nurses to provide care seven days a week, 24 hours a day. In addition, the program must not fall victim to the cyclical requests for holiday and vacation time. If the purpose of the program is to improve patient outcomes, the institution must demonstrate its commitment by providing enough of each level of staff. The maxim "A nurse is a nurse" is inappropriate. A Level I nurse cannot be expected to provide the scope and type of practice that a Level III nurse can.

Once the program has been established, its perpetuation can only be guaranteed by the quality of the staff who apply for the ladder. A strong commitment to patient care excellence must be woven into the framework of the organization starting from employee orientation. An effective way to integrate new staff is to use Level II and especially Level III nurses as orientation preceptors. A successful program depends on collaboration of the clinical preceptors and the educational and management positions within the organization .

One of the downfalls of ladders is the lack of peer support within each level.[3] Peer support can take a variety of forms; a formal support group led by a CNS is an interesting venture. Monthly meetings are listed on planning calendars and assignments. This group's purpose is to provide support for the ladder program and for each individual's growth. In addition, courses of thirty minutes to an hour could be offered periodically to provide support and growth for staff. Informal networking is as important as formal programs. Programs can be offered outside the institution where small group discussions and networking during meals and free time occur.

MAINTAINING THE PROGRAM

In reviewing the literature, all programs were voluntary, at least to the extent that staff were not required to advance past Level II on the ladder. To ensure that the goals of improved outcomes of care and advancement of nursing practice are achieved, the program must be viewed as desirable by participants and by the organization. A variety of techniques can be used to demonstrate the value of the program. Success depends on the active commitment of the organization, and the value the nurse places on the program goals.

Marketing techniques include those listed below.

1. Publicity about the program in recruitment materials, orientation program, hospital newsletters, and patient orientation materials.

2. Recognition of participation in the program (name pin includes level; level position used when individuals are recognized within the organization).
3. Request participation from various levels of nurses in developing policies and procedures for the nursing department and hospital.
4. Provide opportunities for staff nurses to present their experiences to others within the department and hospital.
5. Foster clinical studies and include Level III and IV clinical nurses.
6. Encourage nurses to describe their practice in nursing and hospital publications.
7. Select department and hospital committee members so that various levels are represented.
8. Provide extra conference and educational benefits for participants on the ladder.
9. Have management formally and informally recognize the contributions of individual participants.
10. Have the organization demonstrate its commitment to the ladder by formally communicating results and evaluation data of the ladder to the medical staff, executive staff, and board of directors.
11. Formalize relationships with schools of nursing and choose liaisons to include representation from Levels III and IV clinical in addition to the CNS, education, and management levels.

CONCLUSION

A clinical ladder or career ladder program presents an opportunity for professional growth of staff and improvement in the quality of patient care. A clinical or career ladder may not meet all of a unit's needs, but it is a viable way to provide job satisfaction for staff. The program provides a way to meet the requirements for care of the critically ill patient. The added benefits for the nurse manager include a way to provide for staff growth while allowing the staff members to continue delivering direct patient care; use of experienced staff for orienting new staff; and the potential for a structured advancement into education and management positions within the critical care unit. To enhance the potential for success of the program, it is necessary to clearly define the goals of the program while the formal evaluation process is developed.

REFERENCES

1. Alt JM and Houston GR: Nursing career ladders, a practical manual, Rockville Md, 1986, Aspen Publishers, Inc.
2. Benner P: From novice to expert, American Journal of Nursing 82(3): 402-407, 1982.
3. Broad J and Derby V: Development of a clinical nursing advancement system, Nursing Administration Quarterly 6(1):33-37, 1981.
4. Collins M and Moyer K: Integrating a critical care internship with a career ladder, Continuing Education in Nursing 18(2):51-53, 1987.

5. del Bueno D: A clinical ladder? maybe! Journal of Nursing Administration 12(9):19-22, 1982.
6. Gassert C, Holt C, and Pope K: Building a ladder, American Journal of Nursing 83(10):1527-1530, 1982.
7. Hartley P: Ladders expand nursing opportunity, American Nurse 20(7):24, 1988.
8. Hartley P and Cunningham D: Staff nurses rate clinical ladder program, American Nurse 20(8):13, 1988.
9. Heatherly S and Sebilia AJ: Recognizing clinical excellence, Journal of Nursing Administration 16(10):34-38, 1986.
10. Hougaard J: Clinical ladder program builds self-esteem, American Nurse 20(8):12, 1988.
11. Huey FL: Looking at ladders, American Journal of Nursing 83(10):1520-1526, 1982.
12. Levine-Ariff J: The clinical ladder: the rungs of implementation, Nurse Management 18(12):63-64, 1987.
13. McKay J: Career ladders in nursing: an overview, Journal of Educational Nursing 25(8):272-278, 1986.
14. Peters JP and Tseng S: Managing strategic change in hospitals, ten success stories, Chicago, 1983, American Hospital Association.
15. Sanford RC: Clinical ladders: do they serve their purpose?, Journal of Nursing Administration 17(5):34-37, 1987.
16. Taylor S, Walts L, Amling G, and Cavouras C: Clinical ladders: rewarding clinical excellence, Anna Journal. 15(6):331-334, 1988.
17. Zimmer JJ: Rationale for a ladder for clinical advancement in nursing practice, Journal of Nursing Administration 2:18-24, 1972.

Chapter 13

NURSE INTERN PROGRAM

Kathleen Daley White

The debate between academia and service over the responsibility of preparing nurses to become practicing competent nurses is one that will continue for years to come.[17,18] One fact that representatives from both sides will agree on is that new graduates are not prepared to practice in a critical care area on graduation unless significant support, training, and resources are available. This chapter will describe a postgraduate program that prepares new graduate nurses to become competent critical care practitioners. In this program, the primary responsibility was assumed by the service area in collaboration with representatives from the school of nursing. This chapter will focus on the establishment, evolution, and development of a critical care intern program over a three year period. Our experience will be shared in a chronological and historical perspective in the hope that it may help others establish similar programs.

BACKGROUND OF AN INTERNSHIP PROGRAM

In February 1987 we were a 543-bed tertiary care facility with 32 beds closed because of the nursing shortage. Most of the closed beds were in the critical care areas. During the seven years the institution had been accepting patients, the nursing department had developed various programs to teach experienced nurses the specialization necessary to work in a tertiary care facility. Until February of 1987, we were able to recruit and train experienced medical-surgical nurses. Suddenly, however, our recruitment pool had diminished sharply, and we had to look toward innovative methods to attract nurses.

The results of the American Hospital Association (AHA)[7] survey reflected our plight. An increase in unfilled nursing positions was reported by 59 percent of the hospitals—at least 14 percent of all nursing positions were unfilled. Particularly disturbing was a reported 30 percent decline in enrollment to schools of nursing and a 50 percent decline in the number of college freshman interested in pursuing nursing as a career.[2] More recently the Secretary's Commission on Nursing[23] published findings that further validate the AHA survey. This data documented that the current nursing shortage is unlike previous cyclical shortages and, as such, would have a tremendous impact for years to come. Facing the possibility of closing more beds, thereby decreasing revenue as well as destroying established referral patterns, we considered the one large applicant pool available: new graduates.

Before 1987, critical care leadership agreed (with rare exceptions) not to hire new graduates to work in intensive care and specialty areas. Our own study in 1986 found that only 48 percent of the 444 nurses who responded to our survey had had student "experience" in critical care nursing, and their reported experience averaged 12 clinical days limited to observation. It was rare that a nurse had had a clinical practicum that included hands-on experience.[15] Hughes[12] said, "Newly graduated nurses who lack clinical experience may find themselves unable to apply knowledge rapidly and appropriately in stressful and critical situations," or in other words, in the daily life of a critical care nurse. Searle[22] as AACN President announced an upcoming study of actual critical care content in BSN programs and cited numerous inconsistencies in present programs. Before our acute need for critical care nurses, we felt strongly that new graduates should begin their careers in an acute care setting to solidify the foundation of clinical practice upon which their specialty of choice could be built. In February 1987, we had come to the crossroads of what was ideal and what was possible. We realized we could no longer limit the selection of critical care and specialty practitioners to experienced nurses only.

Being fully aware of new graduate nurse competency over the past five years, we knew that a support program was necessary for new graduates to safely make the transition from student nurses to practicing nurses. We had three months to plan a program if we were to aim at the next graduating classes of nurses in the spring of 1987. We had a group of interested leaders and staff who really wanted to recruit the best candidates and train them in critical care nursing. This group of nurses formed the internship planning committee, which had the goal of providing an educationally and clinically sound program to support new graduates in the transition from students to critical care nurses. The committee members included the director of critical care services, the assistant directors of nurses, unit educators, instructors, interested staff nurses, representatives from the school of nursing, and the clinical nurse specialist in critical care as chairperson. There were no additional lines or resources to plan and initiate this program, just motivated individuals who put in extra hours accomplishing this goal.

Operationalizing the concept was no easy task; we were under incredible time constraints. The planning committee identified seven areas to be investigated before offering a program:

1. Review of the literature
2. Program content
3. Recruitment and marketing
4. Criteria and selection process
5. Collaboration with the school of nursing
6. Personnel issues and contracts
7. Research and evaluation

In retrospect, these were paramount to our development of a solid program. To keep within the time frame, the main committee met each week, at which time each subcommittee reported the week's accomplishments. By meeting weekly, we kept on schedule to reach our goal of accepting candidates in the program in May 1987.

REVIEW OF THE LITERATURE

The review of the literature was done by a graduate student working with the chair of the main committee. Most of the literature on internship programs was considered old because the last time these programs were needed was in the late 1970s and early 1980s. Nonetheless, the information was extremely valuable, because nursing shortages, regardless of the decade in which they occur, elicit similar issues and concerns. The importance of providing consistent preceptor support was continually addressed, as well as devoting resources towards developing preceptors.[1] The program lengths ranged from six weeks to a year,[20,24] offered annually or semiannually. A few programs[19] recommended a medical-surgical orientation before specializing in critical care, while even more programs[6,20] did not specify internships specific to critical care. Recent literature[12] has indicated that clinical practicums in non-critical-care areas can facilitate the transition to specialty practice and, therefore, should be considered when planning a program. Most of the literature supports that during the independent portion of the internship, the interns should not be included in the staffing pattern.[5,13] Depending upon the length of the program, this nonproductive time burdens administrators' limited budgets. Therefore, we searched for data to justify the expense to administration. Craver[10] reported that interns had fewer absences and less attrition during the first 18 months of employment. She also reported that the initial cost of the program was more, but had a much smaller nurse replacement cost than the general orientation program. Many institutions were able to offer interns salaries less than that of non-intern hires.[20]

Mims[16] reported that before a work commitment from participants was required the retention rate of nurse interns at the completion of the program was 81 percent, and that only 53 percent remained an additional year or longer. Since retention would be a measure of positive outcomes, we considered requiring that intern candidates complete letters of intent or contracts to remain. Rufo[21] reported that most programs did not, because the contracts simply did not hold up in litigation. Tuition fees on the program were another possibility; they would be paid by the nurse's working at the institution for a specific amount of time after the internship. The fee would be prorated for nurses who left earlier, and they would then be obligated to pay the tuition.

During nursing shortages, programs tended to admit graduates of all three basic nursing education programs,[20] because no data has yet demonstrated that critical care experience can be gained by educational preparation.[14] Once a facility establishes an applicant pool, it can optionally institute preferred criteria for nurses with baccalaureate degrees. Overall internship program evaluations were positive,[4,20,21] but Craver[6] reported that reliable evaluation tools were unavailable. Although the literature did not provide ample ammunition to justify a program, it did provide a positive direction for our morally defeated staff who saw no alternative.

PROGRAM CONTENT

What would we be able to offer these candidates, when we had less than three months to develop an internship program? In the interest of time, we looked first at what was available and what credentials were required of nurses entering our adult critical care units. As mentioned before, we were pleased with the results of seven years of didactic and clinical training programs for medical-surgical nurses who were entering critical care, so we used these programs as a foundation on which to build. Specifically, within three months, a nurse entering adult critical care was required to successfully complete the general orientation (JCAHO, DOH mandates), a critical care course (104-hour didactic lecture, including EKG interpretation, critical care courses, and pharmacology course), and the critical care clinical competencies on a specific unit. Nurses with ICU experience were given the option of challenging the course by taking the exams.

Based on the literature and previous experience with senior nursing students and new graduates, we determined that these requirements should be completed within six months and these additional supports would be needed:

- Medical-surgical didactic
- Medical-surgical clinical competencies
- Learning lab (includes simulated clinical case studies and physical assessment review)
- Postconferences
- Guidance by non-line faculty

This guidance consists of rap sessions, which are confidential postconferences held by CNSs for interns to discuss any subject they bring up, including clinical, administrative, educational, and ethical issues; and one-to-one CNS follow-up to ensure completion of credentialing elements and to identify problems and concerns.

Although we required all interns to complete these credentialing elements within their first six months, we also expected them to complete a second six-month period as an independent practicum, thereby officially making the program a one-year internship. This would ensure that they remain at least six more months at the institution, and would provide them with valuable clinical experiences in adult critical care. No certificates of completion would be given to those interns who left the program before they had been in it for one year.

During the first year, we thought it best to offer ICU rotations to all interns after completion of the 6-month credentialing. Each intern had been assigned to a particular ICU for the first six months (they were not counted in the staffing pattern). During the second six months, they rotated through three other ICUs for 6-week periods and returned to their original unit for the last six weeks, thereby completing one year. For example, an intern might be assigned to SICU for the first six months, and then spend six weeks in CCU, in MICU, and in the burn center before returning "home" to SICU for the last six weeks. At that point, the intern would apply for a permanent position in an adult ICU. At the original unit, the preceptors could see the tremendous professional growth of the intern—and they had the last shot at recruiting the intern to their unit.

We expected the interns to have a well-rounded view of critical care nursing from the variety of their experiences. The participating interns gained in terms of adaptability and assertiveness. Unfortunately, they did not learn the nuances of individual specialties as we had hoped they would. In retrospect, it was a rather high expectation to place on new graduates. Through feedback in conferences, in rap sessions, and from staff leaders, we discovered that a high level of anxiety was negatively affecting their ability to function. In addition, different values of some clinical competencies were held by the various units, which was confusing to the interns. These issues were insignificant to patient care delivery, but not to the interns' ability to function and socialize into a particular unit.

Our program has now evolved into a one year program. Each intern is assigned to a medical-surgical area for the first two months, and a critical care unit for the next four months. The 6-month independent practicum is in the same unit, but usually on a different shift. At the end of the year the intern may apply for a permanent position. The independent practicum in the same ICU allows the repetition of clinical experience necessary for the interns to learn the intricacies of ICU specialties as they progress in their careers. This method has proven to be beneficial to interns, patients, and staff.

Myrick[18] stated, "Responsibility for clinical teaching rests squarely on staff nurses." We echo this thought in our belief that the success of the program is totally dependent upon the quality, strength, and availability of the preceptors. These are the clinical teachers of our future nurses and thus the foundation of the program. Nursing leadership recommends nurses as preceptors. It is strictly voluntary. We do not yet have a way to reward these nurses financially for their efforts. These nurses are professionals who view mentoring as a responsibility. Donius[9] believed that the willingness to be a preceptor is evidence of professional commitment, which is ultimately reflected in quality patient care. This is true of our preceptors.

We provide two types of preparational courses for preceptors each spring before the new graduates arrive: one for new preceptors, the other for experienced preceptors. Adult learning theories, role responsibilities, and concrete direction regarding the internship program are covered. Both courses involve the active participation of experienced preceptors and faculty, and adequate time is permitted for discussion, role playing, and guided workshops. These programs have been tremendously successful over the past few years.

We are currently developing a clinical ladder to give these preceptors the recognition they deserve. It will be a voluntary system modeled after the "Professional Recognition System" in place at Children's Hospital of Los Angeles.[8] Many of our preceptors teach in the didactic portions of our critical care and medical surgical courses. Those who teach and have masters degrees are recommended for nonsalaried joint faculty positions in the school of nursing, which is one small way we can recognize them.

The coordination of the program is done by the Critical Care Institute faculty, which currently consists of the director; five clinical nurse specialists, three of whom are on joint faculty with the school of nursing; and one secretary. The number of faculty positions should not increase greatly as the program expands. The object of the program is to utilize bedside nurses as teachers and mentors of future nurses; the Critical Care Institute faculty supports and helps them develop on the path towards excellence in practice. Myrick[18] recommends guiding preceptor education and selection. Additional duties of the faculty are in administration and coordination of programs, weekly follow-up of interns, pointing out difficulties that may be encountered, and working with staff leaders to resolve problems. As a result, we are constantly revising the program based on need and feedback.

Many smaller institutions with limited resources are unable to provide training for new graduates or for those new to critical care. Small institutions could ask nearby institutions or schools of nursing if they can provide critical care classes and experiences for a fee. Many of these institutions and schools are considering consortiums in which resources are pooled to train critical care nurses.

Various programs throughout the country reward their preceptor staff in different ways. One institution offers preceptors one day off for every six weeks they are preceptors. This day can be used freely, it does not have to be used for educational or professional purposes. If the nurse manager is unable to grant the day off within six months, the nurse receives time-and-a-half for this rewarded 8-hour day. Another institution sponsors its preceptors' annual AACN membership dues. Our institution's reward was a 3-credit course at the school of nursing for interns and preceptors who participated in the program's first year. Many institutions lack the financial resources necessary to provide adequate recognition and reward.

RECRUITMENT AND MARKETING

Once we knew we were planning a solid program, we investigated ways to market our program in recruitment. Members of the marketing subcommittee met with the hospital's nurse recruiter and the school's assistant dean of student affairs. Both were extremely knowledgeable and able to guide us in our investigation. First we identified our target groups as nursing schools from which we have recruited many nurses historically. For example, we found out that our Long Island institution attracted local graduates, as well as graduates from northern New York. We did not attract New York City graduates as we had thought we would. Once our target groups were identified, we concentrated on those areas. We participated actively in target job fairs. We found that new graduates wanted to talk with "real nurses," not nurse recruiters or nurse managers. When establishing our first program, we sent critical care nurses to these job fairs. Now we send interns and former interns as our representatives, and this method is highly received. Our interns are our best marketing tools, which speaks highly of the program. It is advisable to match interns to their alma mater when assigning job fair assignments. Once again, participation is strictly voluntary and the individuals are paid for that day as a regular working day.

We wanted a brochure and learned the key to developing a brochure is to keep the language as nonspecific as possible. The philosophy of the program, the minimum selection criteria, the areas of experience covered, and the application information should be included. We avoided details of program content and time frames to increase the longevity of the brochure and to allow for flexibility in the program.

We then mailed these brochures to the target students. We now have the addresses of students' "favorite instructors," or instructors who give our brochures directly to the students. (I had written letters directly to them, identified the nurse who referred them to me, and requested that the enclosed brochures be distributed.)

Finally, we advertised locally. The first year, one ad in the local paper drew 50 new graduates who applied for 20 positions. Well-organized efforts in 1988 yielded almost 200 applicants for 40 positions. In 1989, minimal advertising due to a hiring freeze drew about 540 inquiries. This incredible response allowed us to hand-select our candidates. In addition, there were many candidates that were hired for other units of the hospital. In 1988, when we had close to 200 applicants for 40 positions, we hired a total of 99 new graduates. The large applicant pool generated by the internship program marketing enabled us to select a quality group of new graduates.

CRITERIA AND SELECTION

In the planning stage of our program, we had to determine candidate selection criteria and to organize and coordinate the interviewing process efficiently. We expected large numbers of candidates who would need to be interviewed in a relatively short period of time, probably within four to six weeks.

In the midst of the worst nursing shortage we had ever experienced, we did not envision large numbers of candidates vying for these positions; therefore, we initially made the qualifications minimal: successful completion of an accredited nursing school program and two references from clinical instructors or preceptors. Our preferred criteria were a BSN, GPA of 3.2 or higher, and, most significantly, clinical experience in direct patient care.

In our three years of experience, we have identified key elements that are somewhat prognostic for the candidate's success in the program. Most significant is the amount of clinical experience prior to graduation. Additionally, BSN candidates were more successful. These candidates progressed through the program within the expected time and without supplemental supports and resources. They were able to digest and integrate quickly and thoroughly the large amounts of information necessary for them to care for critically ill patients. Upon further investigation, most of our BSN graduate interns have had a clinical practicum as part of the educational requirement of their senior year—a block of time dedicated to independent practice. The associate degree programs in our area lack this. Our experience with diploma graduates is almost nonexistent as there are very few diploma schools left in our target areas.

In addition to these two qualities, we place heavy weight on the candidate's interview. We look for enthusiasm, ability to adapt, and overall eagerness. Since the program is clinically based, changes occur frequently and rigidity and inflexibility in a candidate do not bode well.

In our first year, we accepted candidates from all three programs, all with varying clinical experience. We now emphasize the clinical experience as a strongly preferred criteria, and refer associate degree and diploma candidates without clinical experience to a medical-surgical unit. If they express a very great interest in critical care, we encourage them to apply for a transfer after they spend a minimum of six months in the medical-surgical units, and preferably, after one year.

The interviewing process is coordinated in the nurse recruiter's office. The specific selection process is coordinated by the Critical Care Institute director. All leadership staff participates in interviewing the candidates. The Critical Care Institute distributes a fact sheet with specific information about the program so that all candidates receive the same information from the interviewers. The interviewers must fill out a preprinted interview sheet which has the same questions for each candidate. Thus when the selection process begins, we have a collection of the same information on each candidate. We ask each interviewer to rate the candidate on a scale of 0 to 5, with 5 as the highest rating to show how interviewers rate the applicant compared with others.

After all candidates have been interviewed, interested leadership personnel, the nurse recruiter, the Critical Care Institute faculty and the director sit together and select the candidates, based on the criteria. The interview sheets, the transcripts, and the clinical references are reviewed; the pros and cons discussed. The interviewer is contacted directly if more information is needed, or a second interview is arranged, this time by the director. Three years of candidate selection has proven this method successful.

COLLABORATION WITH THE SCHOOL OF NURSING

As it is part of the State University of New York, University Hospital is physically connected to a sister nursing school. Initially we contacted the dean, explained our plan for the internship program, and asked if the school would like to participate. She was eager to take part in it for two reasons: The faculty could help us develop a quality program, and the dean could draw candidates for baccalaureate and graduate programs from the resulting large applicant pool. Furthermore, the dean suggested that we work toward developing a program that could offer academic credits. This would help marketing and recruitment at both the hospital and the school.

Today, we have two courses approved for 6 elective graduate credits in the school of nursing: Critical Care Concepts, and Parent-Child Critical Care Concepts. The interns must complete one full year of the program, and meet the requirements with a passing grade of 75 percent or higher before they are eligible to petition the school for these credits. Most interns do register for these credits, and the offering of academic credits has proved an effective recruitment tool as well.

Since we began our program we learned that Creighton University in Omaha, Nebraska, offers academic credit for its internship program, a 10-week course that offers 9 graduate credits for $2,000 tuition. Nurses are often sponsored by a hospital that requires 12 to 18 months of employment.[24]

The deputy director of nursing and the dean supported the establishment of joint faculty positions in the Critical Care Institute. It was agreed that two clinical nurse specialists would divide their workload: from September to June, they would work part-time for the hospital and the school; and July and August they would work full-time at the hospital. This worked out well because support for the internship program was most needed during the summer. The role of the faculty has been primarily one of intern support.

The collaborative effort has been invaluable because of its impact on education and clinical practice. Suddenly, we had faculty who were preparing and receiving new graduates, and who as a result were able to identify the interns' strengths and weaknesses and relate them to their education. Curriculum issues have been addressed, based on the evaluations and feedback from the internship programs. Additionally, joint faculty can identify program candidates at an early stage. We are confident that we are making a difference where it counts: in the educational preparation of nurses.

PERSONNEL ISSUES AND CONTRACTS

The possibility of letters of intent or contracts to remain working at the facility upon program completion was researched. Because a tremendous amount of money and resources is consumed training these persons, and because an incredibly marketable commodity is produced, the hospital wanted a return on its investment. The possibility of lower intern salaries their first six months was also researched. Both possibilities were denied by the state and the union. A few institutions can offer tuition waivers for nurses participating in training programs.

We were able to insert an important sentence in the letter of employment: "Hours and units will be subject to change based upon your learning needs." This sentence proved invaluable as the year progressed, as it enabled the Critical Care Institute to control intern schedules. Once hired, it took the interns very little time to negotiate with the system for time off, shift requests, and unit assignments. Since patient populations and preceptors are constantly in flux, program planning is difficult. We wanted the authority to change intern assignments so that learning needs would best be addressed. To be sure that each intern met the criteria, we needed control without seniority demands of outside (state and union) forces. We work hand-in-hand with our human resources department in development and implementation of our internship programs, and because our rules are consistent and our assignments fair, we have had no problems. The interns have the option of applying for a position outside of the internship program at any time if they are unable to meet our requirements.

RESEARCH

The literature search had demonstrated the lack of reliable evaluation tools in past internship programs. One of the nurses on the committee was in graduate school looking for a master's thesis project.[10] She measured the intern's knowledge and competency during the first year of the program using the national critical care test to measure knowledge, and the Dyer Tool[11] to measure competency.

The critical care knowledge gained by these nurses from the program was easily measured. All failed the test upon date of hire, and all passed the test within three months. The test results at three months, six months and one year were similar to the national results.

Measuring competency proved to be as difficult as we thought it would be. The Dyer Tool is filled out by the preceptors, who rated their intern's level of competency. All interns were competent within six months of hire, 80 percent were competent between 20 and 26 weeks. However it took the preceptor an hour to complete the tool, and in spite of all our efforts (including offers of breakfasts and luncheons), preceptors could not fill out these forms in the allotted time. After a year of this, we stopped using the tool. All interns in the program are expected to be competent in their area within six months of their hire date. After three years, this is a reasonable expectation.

RETENTION

Hospital administration and the finance department constantly want to know about our retention rates. In the first year we hired 24 nurses. One year later we had an 83 percent retention, two years, 71 percent. Our nonintern turnover rate in these years was 26 percent.

In 1988, we hired 38 nurses and offered both adult critical care and parent-child critical care programs. At the end of one year, our retention was 86 percent (turnover of 14 percent). At this point, our nonintern turnover rate has dropped to 23 percent, so we are doing well.

At about the two-year mark, interns sometimes seek experiences at other institutions, because they have never worked anywhere else. Fortunately, after they transfer to other hospitals, we have an increase in rehires about 6 to 13 weeks later. We hope that over a period of five to ten years, our overall retention rate remains high.

Other hospitals have discovered our highly trained pool and are actively recruiting our interns who complete the program. Since one of our goals as a tertiary care facility is to give nurses a high level of critical care proficiency, we should be honored and pleased that our high calibre nurses are so desired by these community hospitals. After all, these nurses should improve patient care, encourage referral patterns, and even help our institution's recruitment simply by role modeling. For the sake of the morale in our own institution, however, we would prefer that they stay with us longer.

In 1989, we were under a state-imposed hiring freeze in the heavy recruitment month of April. Even without recruitment efforts, we had over 500 inquiries about the internship programs. In May, we were given permission to hire 34 new graduates into the program. Because of the limited number permitted, we assessed the institution's needs and identified the areas most in need of new graduate hires. We hired 13 into adult critical care, 15 into medical-surgical critical care, 4 to acute pediatric critical care, and 2 into gynecological surgery. We merged resources so that all 34 interns went through the same first eight weeks of the program, which we called "Acute Care Foundations." If the candidates successfully completed this portion of the program, they were permitted to continue with their specialty. Our goal is to continue this for all new graduates and to enlarge the pool of nurses in our acute care areas so that we will always have a group of experienced non-critical-care nurses from which to draw.

COSTS

Most of the opposition to internship programs is related to costs. To counter this opposition, three factors must be considered: First it is difficult to recruit any nurses except new graduates; next, with decreasing staff, the possibility of closing beds increases, which decreases revenue; and finally, the hospital's average replacement cost of one nurse is very high. It has been reported that it costs a minimum of $20,000 to replace one nurse,[7] which is a low estimate that does not include costs of decreasing services and closed beds.

At our institution, it costs approximately $8,842 to orient an *experienced* nurse into her area of specialty. At least three or four months of orientation passes before the nurse is considered "productive" by her peers. The "warm body" method of staffing, in which the nurse's ability is not considered, is not practiced in this hospital. One reason our program is so successful is that administration supports the program and allows interns the time necessary to complete the credentialing requirements. If you accept that it takes four months to orient and train an experienced nurse in a new specialty of critical care, the cost of training is already $14,083.

Our data show that it takes four to six months for a new graduate to reach competency in critical care. Therefore, the cost per intern is $14,083 to $19,824. Out of context, this may sound prohibitively expensive, but an institution would invest in this program only if all other recruitment alternatives were exhausted.

Although we are still unable to justify the program statistically, the intangibles of the program have done much to improve morale. In addition, even during the nonproductive phase of their training, the interns could help with patient care by assisting on road trips to diagnostic labs, or by bathing patients. This was helpful to staff and provided learning opportunities for interns.

We have been able to demonstrate that intern sick-time use is far less than that of noninterns up to 24 months post-hire date. At four months, the intern calls in an average of 0.4 days, the nonintern, 4 days. At six months, the intern uses 1.5 days; and the nonintern, 6 days. In time intern sick time use begins to increase, but at two years it is still 3 days less than that of nurses who were noninterns.

We believe that the decreased abuse of sick time is the result of attention to the needs of a specific group of individuals. High expectations are defined in advance and are placed on these individuals; and with support they effectively meet the challenge.

Overall, the program has been a success. When the program was implemented staff morale was at an all-time low. The interns brought an enthusiasm to the units that had been lacking. In the midst of a national nursing shortage, our nurses had a program they could be proud of—a program that was making a difference. In addition, the interns keep the staff on their toes. The healthy competitiveness was due to the interns' insatiable appetites for more information. Senior nurses were opening books, reading current journals, and looking for more information on all topics to "keep ahead of the intern." This enthusiasm had a positive effect on the quality of care given to the patients.

The program had tremendous support from all members of the interdisciplinary team. A positive socialization occurred that first year. Attending physicians, medical residents and interns, clergy, and allied health professionals understood what it meant to be teaching someone at the bedside.

The limitations of the program involved the use or misuse of the intern. Interns cannot be relied upon as the core of any staff. Interns can give care to critically ill patients, but do not have the credentials needed to provide total care for patients requiring intraaortic balloon pumping or other extreme measures, unless they have additional training. The nurse with ten or fifteen years of experience cannot expect interns to be as proficient as she is without all those years of experience. An understanding of nurses progressing from novice to expert,[3] especially by unit staff leaders must exist. The ability to continue learning and developing in a chosen career must be emphasized, and this goal should be supported.

CONCLUSION

We are currently expanding our program's critical care focus. Critically ill patients are in all areas of the hospital, and in the home as well; they are no longer restricted to the ICU. Each hospital area has its own specialty, and as a result, we must address this need. Our goal is to have a variety of internship programs for all new graduates coordinated by the Critical Care Institute and using the proficient and expert bedside nurses as the clinical teachers and faculty. In this way, we are building a secure foundation for all new graduates. The clinical staff will have the same expectations of all new graduates at the end of a designated time frame. In addition, these programs will enable us to utilize our limited resources in the best way possible.

Finally, we want to spring forth from the internship program into all areas of post-graduate clinical education for nurses. We know from the surveys done across the nation that recognition, respect, and salary[7] are the three most important values. It was our goal in establishing a Critical Care Institute to provide a clinically based learning center for nurses at all levels of practice from novice to expert.[3] These offerings will be planned and implemented in collaboration with the school of nursing, so that many of them will offer academic credits. We hope that in providing these educational and professional opportunities, we will be better able to recruit and retain quality clinical practitioners.

Florence Nightingale described nursing as "an unending series of learning experiences."[2] We embrace this philosophy and support our nurses. Our goal is acceptable to both academia and practice: to develop clinical nursing as the practice profession it should be, and to continue postgraduate development through our service-supported programs. In this way, nurses actually will move through the unending series of learning experiences; and with each experience, they will complete a part of their quest for clinical excellence. In supporting this philosophy, we also support the model of the professional nurse who gives the ultimate in patient care.

REFERENCES

1. Alspach JG et al: From staff nurse to preceptor: a preceptor training manual, Secaucus, NJ, 1988, Hospital Publications Inc.
2. Astin A et al: The American freshman: twenty year trends, 1966-85, Los Angeles, 1987, University of California, The Higher Education Research Institute, Graduate School of Education.
3. Benner P: From novice to expert: excellence and power in clinical nursing practice, Menlo Park, Calif, 1984, Addison-Wesley Publishing Co.
4. Bullas J and Anderson P: Establlishing a critical care unit orientation program. Critical Care Nurse 2(4):72-76, 1982.
5. Clough J: Developing and implementing orientation to a critical care unit, Focus on Critical Care 9(5):224-29, 1982.
6. Craver M: Investigation of an internship program, Journal of Continuing Education in Nursing 16(4):114-18, 1985.
7. Curran C: Hospital research and education trust of AHA Commission in Chicago, Illinois, March 7, 1988.
8. Davis S: A professional recognition system using peer review, Journal of Nursing Administration 17(11):34-38, 1987.
9. Donius MA: The Columbia preceptoring program: building a bridge with clinical faculty, Journal of Professional Nursing 4(1):17-22, 1988.
10. Duffy MC: Evaluating knowledge and performance of critical care interns, Unpublished Mater's Thesis, State University of New York at Stony Brook, School of Nursing, 1989.
11. Dyer ED: Descriptive scales for nursing performance, Form 2, 1967, Salt Lake City.
12. Hughes L: Employment of new graduates: implications for critical care nursing practice, Focus on Critical Care, 14(4):9-15, 1987.
13. Jiricka MJ et al: Critical care orientation: a guide to the process, Newport Beach, Calif, 1987, American Association of Critical Care Nurses.
14. Landmark study confirms nursing shortage problem, American Association of Critical Care Nurses Newsletter 14:1988.
15. Manchester, P: A study of professional developmental needs in critical care nursing, Stony Brook, NY, 1987, Division of Nursing.
16. Mims B: A critical care internship program, Dimensions in Critical Care Nursing, 3(1):53-59, 1984.
17. Mundinger MO: Three dimensional nursing: new partnerships between service and education, Journal of Professional Nursing 4(1):10-16, 1988.
18. Myrick F: Preceptorship: is it the answer to the problems in clinical teaching? Journal of Nursing Education, 27(3):136-38, 1988.
19. Penny M: Recruitment and retention of nurses in critical care, Nurse Management 19(2):72, 1988,.
20. Rosell S: Nurse-intern programs: how they're working, Nurse Educator 6: 29-31, 1981.
21. Rufo K: Termination of successful internship program, Journal of Nursing Administration 14(6):33-37, 1984.
22. Searle L: President's message: preparing critical care nurses: an essential need, Focus on Critical Care 16(2):157-58, 1989.
23. Secretary's commission on nursing final report, Vol. I and II, Washington, DC, 1988, U.S. Department of Health and Human Services.

24. Thielen J: Internship course helps prepare new graduates for practice, American Association of Critical Care Nurses Newsletter 14:1988.
25. Toth J and Ritchey K: The basic knowledge assessment tool for critical care nursing, Heart and Lung 13(3):272, 1984.

SUGGESTED READINGS

1. Aggleton P et al: Models of nursing, nursing practice and nursing education, Journal of Advanced Nursing 12(5):573-81, 1987.
2. Aiken L: Special report: the nursing shortage, myth or reality, New England Journal of Medicine 317(10):645-51, 1987.
3. Alspach JG et al: Education standards for crticial care nursing, St. Louis, 1986, The CV Mosby Co.
4. Beaulieu LP: Preceptorship and mentorship: bridging the gap between nursing education and nursing practice, Imprint 35(2):111-15, 1988.
5. Bolton J: Educating professional nurses for clinical practice, Nurse Health Care 5(7):384-389, 1984.
6. Cary AH: Preparation for professional practice: what do we need? Nursing Clinics of North America 23(2):341-51, 1988.
7. Dear M: Nursing internship: asking the right questions, Imprint 30(4):12-17, 1983.
8. Farrell J: The changing pool of candidates for nursing, Journal of Professional Nursing 4(3):145, 230, 1988.
9. Friesen L and Conahan B: A clinical preceptor program: strategy for new graduate orientation, Journal of Nursing Administration 10(4):18-23, 1980.
10. Hamilton JM: So you're graduating...now what, Imprint 34(6):89-90, 1987.
11. Harvey E: Nursing shortage remedies, Current Concepts in Nursing 2(5):10-16, 1988.
12. Huey F and Hartley: What keeps nurses in nursing? American Journal of Nursing 88(2):181-88, 1988.
13. Lachance-Everhart R: Transfer orientation: developing a retraining program, Journal of Continuing Education in Nursing 17(4):122-24, 1986.
14. Marchette L and Merker A; The effect of a nurse internship program on novice nurses' self-evaluation of clinical performance, Journal of Nursing Administration 15(5):6-7, 1985.
15. Meissnir JE: Nurses: are we eating our young? Nursing 16(3):51-53, 1986.
16. Metzger N: Revisiting the preceptor concept: crosstraining nurse staff, Journal of Nursing Staff Development 2(2):70-76, 1986.
17. Neathawk RD et al: Nurses' evaluation of recruitment and retention, Nursing Management 19(12):38-45, 1988.
18. Piemme J et al: Developing the nurse preceptor, The Journal of Continuing Nursing Education 17(6):186-89, 1986.
19. Prescott P: Shortages of professional nursing practice, a reframing of the shortage problem, Heart and Lung 18(5):436-443, 1989.
20. Ramprogus VK: Learning how to learn nursing, Nurse Educator Today 8(2):59-67, 1988.
21. Samuelson L: Retention in critical care nursing, Heart and Lung, 17(1):107-8, 1988.
22. Shamian J and Inhaber R: Concepts and practice of preceptorship in contemporary nursing: a review of pertinent literature, International Journal of Nursing Studies 22(2):79-88, 1985.

23. Shamian J and Lemiceux B: An evaluation of the preceptor model versus the formal teaching model, Journal of Continuing Education in Nursing 15(3):86-89, 1984.
24. Smith MF and Altieri MJ: Competence-based assessment of critical care nurses, Focus on Critical Care 15(16):17-22, 1988.
25. Tuggle D: Metamorphosis of a critical care nurse: the first year, Critical Care Nurse 8(2):14-15, 1987.
26. Turkett SM: New graduate nurses: the answer is yes, Imprint 35(2):91-94, 1988.
27. Weissmian JK et al: The impact of the nursing shortage on clinical practice: challenges and opportunities, Imprint 34(4):36-37, 1987.
28. Wood V: Nursing instructor and clinical teaching, International Nursing Review 34(5):120-5, 1987.

Chapter 14

ROLE OF THE CLINICAL NURSE SPECIALIST

Barbara Leeper

Specialization in nursing has been occurring since Florence Nightingale helped nurses develop special skills to care for the wounded in the Crimean War. The role of the critical care clinical nurse specialist (CNS) has evolved with the need for applied knowledge, teaching, clinical expertise, and research in critical care practice.[3] The American Association of Critical Care Nurses (AACN)[1] defined the role of the CNS in critical care in 1987, and this is used as a frame of reference for delineating the CNS role. This chapter analyzes how the CNS facilitates advanced practice, knowledge, and research in the unit. Various dimensions of the CNS role are discussed, including the place of the CNS in the organizational framework and strategies for measuring the effectiveness of the CNS. A case study demonstrates how the role of the CNS can be incorporated in the critical care unit.

The working relationship between the nurse manager and CNS is the key to the success of delineating this role within a unit. A nurse manager who seeks out and uses the CNS facilitates quality care. Recognition of the expertise and the contributions of the CNS augments professional practice within the unit.

DEFINITION OF THE CNS ROLE

The title of CNS is earned by the individual when a master's level of study that focuses on a specific patient population has been completed.[8] There are various graduate level nursing programs that are designed to prepare a CNS for critical care specialization.[3] These programs offer a masters of art (MA), master of nursing (MN) or a master of science (MS) degree. The focus can be age-specific, such as adult or pediatric critical care; disease-specific, such as cardiovascular critical care; or generic to a wide range of critical care practice settings. However, each program provides an opportunity for the experienced critical care practitioner to learn advanced practice concepts in a university setting. Thus, the CNS gains advanced knowledge and can provide scientifically based nursing care with a high level of competence.[24]

The American Nurses Association[2] stated that the CNS must have a client-based practice. Beecroft and Papenhausen[4] reported that the CNS's practice is focused on the patient and family in the clinical setting. Hamric[13] added that the CNS's practice is directed toward improving patient care and nursing practice. Despite all of the literature defining it, the role of the CNS is still often misunderstood, and causes confusion for nursing administrators and staff. This confusion results when the responsibilities of the CNS are poorly defined.

Each CNS interprets and develops her own role. The personality of the CNS directs her interactions with people. Specialized skills provide the CNS with career direction and security; they include the ability to be a clinical expert, an educator, a consultant, a researcher, and an executive.

The Clinical Expert

The clinical expert role is seen when the CNS is involved in several activities that are beneficial for the unit. "The CNS uses high-level assessment and problem-solving skills to plan patient care."[22] The CNS assists with nursing interventions to facilitate individualized care. Use of problem-solving and decision-making skills and theory-based expert practice are all part of the CNS's functions in the critical care unit.[22]

In direct patient care, the CNS uses advanced skills that the general nursing staff have not developed.[10] Through this direct care, the CNS experiences the obstacles met by staff nurses daily, and can develop realistic methods to deal with these patient care problems. Direct care enhances the visibility and the accessibility of the CNS, who can then serve as a role model for the staff by demonstrating independent judgment skills. The CNS helps staff define nursing care by formulating appropriate nursing diagnoses. Through direct patient care, the CNS establishes and maintains credibility with the nursing staff.

Metcalf and colleagues[20] suggested that the CNS who works with staff to provide care can be more effective. Most nursing administrators and CNSs view direct patient care as part of the CNS role, but acknowledge that it limits CNS accessibility to the staff nurses.[20,27] The heavier demands placed upon the CNS providing patient care may ultimately affect quality care. And, finally the risk that the CNS role be viewed as the same as the staff role raises questions about efficient resource use. A master's prepared CNS should offer more than direct patient care to the unit.

Noble[22] suggested that the CNS is a role model for modifying staff communications. The CNS teaches the principles of therapeutic communication by demonstrating to staff that talking away from the bedside is appropriate behavior and that communication with patients is improved by offering reassurance and explanations.

The CNS interacts with patients and families, offering support, answering questions, and providing counseling. The CNS spends time with families, clarifies information they have received from physicians, and answers questions about this information. The CNS's availability provides an avenue for the family to express their frustration and grief. In addition, the CNS communicates family desires and needs to physicians and staff.[22] The CNS takes the time needed to communicate effectively and has the expertise to be a patient advocate.

When problems occur with a specific patient because the CNS is removed from the situation, she can more easily identify probable causes, communicate these to the staff, enlist staff involvement in solving the problem, and help resolve the issue. The CNS often responds innovatively to patient care problems by introducing other methods or equipment that would simplify a particular procedure, provide more information, or improve patient outcomes.[14]

The Educator

Buchanon and Glanville[6] describe the CNS in the role of the staff educator as facilitator, coach, and promoter of educational development and professional growth. Working with the unit instructor, the CNS provides a wide range of topics that spans introductory classes to continuing education. The CNS coordinates critical care internship programs, including preceptor and intern follow-up. Orientation for experienced critical care staff is also developed and coordinated by the unit instructor and the CNS. Many facilities rely upon preceptors for the actual clinical orientation; however, it is within the role of the CNS to oversee the program.

In the staff educator role, the CNS has both supportive and creative endeavors. Supportive endeavors include participating in patient care conferences, teaching and coordinating review courses for critical care certification, helping with classes for advanced cardiac life support certification, and facilitating the programs that are mandated by the individual institution. Creative endeavors include applying research outcomes to the practice setting, conducting nursing grand rounds, promoting the development of a nursing journal club, and identifying state-of-the-art practice changes for the unit.

The CNS is encouraged to have a joint appointment with an affiliated academic institution in the undergraduate and graduate nursing programs. Many

CNSs assist with teaching critical care to undergraduate nursing students and serve as preceptors for graduate students. Other health professionals also benefit from the expertise of the CNS when they attend programs taught by the CNS.

The Consultant

The CNS serves as a consultant to many individuals. Staff nurses seek out the CNS to assist with solving patient problems that require expert assistance. For example, the CNS works with the staff nurse who is unsure of her interpretations of EKG changes on a patient experiencing chest pain, interprets the EKG, and helps her decide whether to administer medications. The CNS supports her (appropriate) decision to notify the physician, and stays with her to reinforce this new learning. Beyerman[5] found that the clinical specialist provided information to other people (staff and patients) almost twice as often as any other activity. Menard[19] stated that a major role of the CNS consultant is to help develop and refine problem-solving skills of those requesting assistance.

Nursing staff outside the critical care unit use the CNS to help solve technical patient problems. In this era of rising acuity, activities such as setting up chest tube drainage systems and managing mechanically ventilated patients out on medical-surgical floors are becoming routine. The CNS easily demonstrates, teaches, and assists; and assures that these activities are well done. In addition, the CNS provides emotional support to the medical-surgical staff by assisting them with problem-solving as they learn these new skills.

The CNS works very closely with nursing and ancillary staff to facilitate critical care unit patients' recovery in the unit and discharge from the hospital. For example, the CNS may collaborate with social service to develop discharge planning protocols that are implemented on the patient's admission to the critical care unit. The CNS works closely with the respiratory therapy department to identify and select appropriate methods for arterial blood gas sampling, suctioning, and managing mechanical ventilation.

The Research Role

A major component of the CNS role is focused on research. The CNS may communicate research outcomes published in the literature to all personnel. Working with the nurse manager and the instructor, the CNS may suggest modifications to nursing practice based on these research findings. For example, research demonstrating the necessity of hyperventilation and hyperoxygenation when suctioning patients led to the addition of a policy and procedure requiring both of these activities for suctioning. The CNS might also identify problems that could be researched. Unit-based research directed by the CNS may involve quality assurance or may validate nursing practice within the unit.

The Executive Role

The executive role of the CNS is seen in involvement with various committees that oversee interdisciplinary critical care, cardiac arrest code team review, nursing care standards, peer review, and other activities. Regarding peer review, the CNS uses clinical expertise to determine outcome standards for the institution. The CNS facilitates change by defining and communicating the practice of nursing to other members of these committees. Other aspects of the executive role include reading and preparing reports, corresponding with other departments and agencies, and participating in decisions to purchase new equipment.

The various components of the CNS role are all related to the educational process. Beyerman[5] summarized the role, and said that the CNS "provides information to the staff, recommends interventions, motivates the nurse to think by asking questions, and stimulates thinking by data collection."

ORGANIZATIONAL DEVELOPMENT

The critical care CNS is qualified to provide support for the organizational development of the unit. The CNS, in collaboration with the nurse manager, defines nursing's role to the staff, physicians, administrators, and other health care workers. McDougall[17] stated that it is important for the CNS to articulate the role of nursing to the nursing staff, in addition to other health care providers, particularly where professional boundaries may become blurred, as in the critical care setting. For example, a staff nurse may notify a physician about a patient's pulmonary artery catheter that has migrated back into the right ventricle. The physician, who is busy elsewhere, tells the nurse to pull back and readvance the catheter. The staff nurse consults with the CNS for assistance with this procedure. The CNS comes to the unit, explains to the staff nurse that this task is not within the practice of nursing in this setting, instructs the nurse to notify the physician and remains with the staff nurse until the problem is resolved.

Together, the nurse manager and CNS create a positive working environment, identify problems and appropriate problem-solving methods, and evaluate the results. The nurse manager and the CNS consult separately and together with other health professionals—such as physicians, respiratory therapists, pharmacists, social workers, laboratory technicians, and quality assurance coordinators—to define and improve the standard of care in the critical care unit. Both consult with administrative representatives to inform them of unit needs and appropriate standards of practice.

The nurse manager and the CNS collaborate to make decisions about policies and procedures that affect patient care. The CNS who identifies an infection control problem in the unit works with the nurse manager to select the best way to minimize the related nosocomial infections. In addition, the CNS collaborates with the nursing staff to make decisions about clinical practice. For example, the

CNS consults with the staff to determine the best method to care for a patient with complex problems.

McDougall[17] said that the CNS demonstrates leadership qualities by role-modeling her problem-solving and conflict-resolving expertise. This has an effect on staff behavior in the unit. In addition, the CNS is active in nursing organizations and hospitalwide committees, which encourages the staff to participate and promotes a professional climate within the unit.

Communication skills are very important. McDougall[17] stated the CNS's power is based on the ability to influence the behavior of others through excellent interpersonal communication. The CNS who communicates effectively with all individuals entering the critical care unit thus has power to influence others.

PLACE IN THE ORGANIZATIONAL FRAMEWORK: DEFINING AUTHORITY

Within the hospital organization there are two types of authority: administrative and professional. Administrative authority is associated with a line position that gives an individual the power to hire and fire staff beneath them in the line. The power inherent in a line position is granted by the structure of the organization regardless of the individual filling the position. Note that Figure 14-1 is a repre-

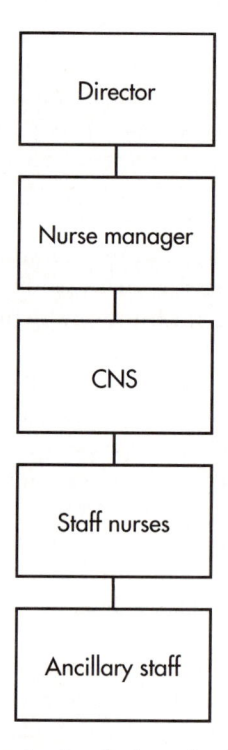

FIGURE 14-1. Organizational chart depicting line authority.

sentative organizational chart in which the CNS has line authority and responsibility over staff. On this chart, the CNS answers to the nurse manager.

Professional authority is that authority granted to the CNS who is in a staff position. In nursing management the term *staff position* is used to describe those upper-management-level jobs that have a set function but do not carry line authority. Professional authority is earned by the CNS because staff and others recognize the CNS's expertise and leadership abilities. Figure 14-2 depicts the CNS in this type of staff position. On this organizational chart the CNS answers directly to the director and has a broken line to the nurse manager, which represents indirect authority at the level of the line. This means that the CNS is on the same level as the nurse manager.

Placement of the CNS within an organization varies greatly. The trend is moving toward pulling them out of education departments and placing them in administrative line positions.[29] There is debate over line versus staff authority of the CNS's position in the organization.[17] Wallace and Corey suggested placing the CNS in a middle management position, particularly if budgetary cuts are an issue.

The CNS in a line position is accountable for a limited number of patients within a given specialty. The management component of this line position includes responsibility for other employees and using management skills to achieve administrative responsibilities.[17,26] For example, the CNS may be responsible for hiring and evaluating staff, budgets and capital equipment expenditures, and unit representation at the administrative level. The CNS in a staff position works with line managers to achieve unit goals. The CNS is responsible for a specific caseload, acts as a consultant, provides needed education, and serves as a role model.

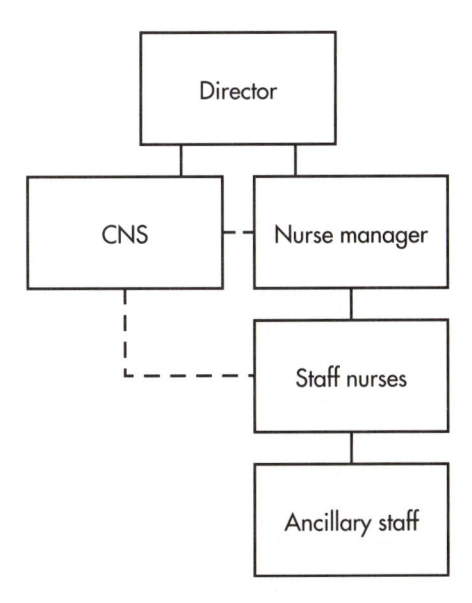

FIGURE 14-2. Organizational chart depicting professional authority.

A CNS with professional authority exerts influence through strong interpersonal skills that are used to promote a positive working environment and collegial relationships in the unit. These skills affect decision making.[17] Regardless of the position, the CNS utilizes formal and informal power to influence others.

Centralized versus Decentralized Location

A CNS is held accountable for a predetermined set of functions as determined by the institution. For reporting mechanisms and for evaluation, the CNS is held accountable for achievements in one of three ways. The first occurs when the CNS reports directly to the chief nurse executive with no other person in direct line between them as in Figure 14-3. The second occurs when the CNS reports to the director of nursing for critical care (see Figure 14-2). This is called a *decentralized system* because the CNS in each nursing department develops independent functions. The third occurs when all of the CNSs in the organization answer to one person, such as the director of education. Figure 14-4 shows this *centralized approach* in which all of the CNSs and their functions are centralized within one department. There are advantages to all three of the approaches.

When the CNS reports directly to the chief nurse executive, one advantage is the close working relationship that enables critical care unit goals to be easily shared and identified. Solutions can be discussed and approval to move ahead with projects is readily given. This is more advantageous for the CNS if the nurse manager and CNS do not have similar philosophies or if the nurse manager does not understand the role of the CNS. A disadvantage is that the nurse manager may perceive that the CNS has more power, which may promote a negative climate between the two individuals.

In centralized facilities where all of the CNSs report to the director of education, advantages include the existence of a support group for each other. This is important, especially for the recently hired CNS. This support group consists of others who are well acquainted with the problems inherent in role transition. This system promotes the sharing of ideas, facilitates problem solving, and encourages sharing educational offerings throughout the facility. Lastly, there is more effective communication from one unit to another regarding educational

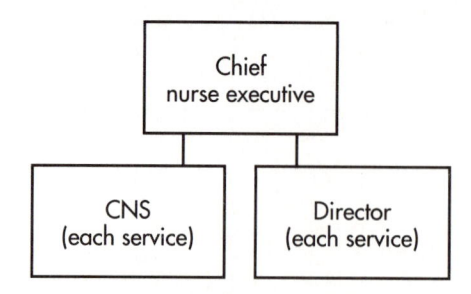

FIGURE 14-3. Organizational chart depicting CNS answering to chief executive.

offerings, projects, research, and day-to-day business. A major disadvantage to the centralized approach is that the CNS may be perceived as having only an educational role, which could result in less visibility and participation in the clinical setting. The CNS may spend too much time organizing and teaching the nurse internship classes, advanced cardiac life support courses, and other inservices. In the centralized system, the CNS is often asked to participate in other general programs targeted for the entire facility. All of these responsibilities require time and limit the availability and visibility of the CNS in the critical care unit.

A decentralized system is advantageous because both the nurse manager and the CNS answer to the same director of critical care, are on an equal level within the organizational structure, and are perceived as having an equal power base. The disadvantages to this system are related to the director's understanding of the CNS role. The director may attempt to use the CNS as an assistant to help solve problems, complete projects, or fill staffing vacancies. All of these will dilute the CNS's ability to accomplish goals within the unit. Similar problems may exist when the CNS reports to the head nurse of the unit.

Problems associated with having more than one director occur when the CNS is shared by more than one unit (see Figure 14-5). Most of these problems arise from differing opinions of the line managers about the role of the CNS and the way the CNS is expected to spend her time. This can be overcome by an experienced CNS, but for a new CNS struggling with role identity, it is a major hurdle.

Orientation: The Unit Preceptor or the CNS

Many CNSs in critical care are responsible for organizing and conducting new staff orientation. Once the didactic component of orientation is completed, the new hires are assigned a preceptor with excellent clinical and communication skills. The preceptor facilitates the clinical component of the orientation process. The CNS communicates with the preceptor and new staff member at frequent intervals to provide direction and determine progress.

In some settings, a critical care educator conducts the classroom portion of the orientation and critical care course. The CNS assumes the preceptor's responsibilities for the new staff member during the clinical experience. This approach is advantageous because the CNS is the clinical expert and serves as an excellent

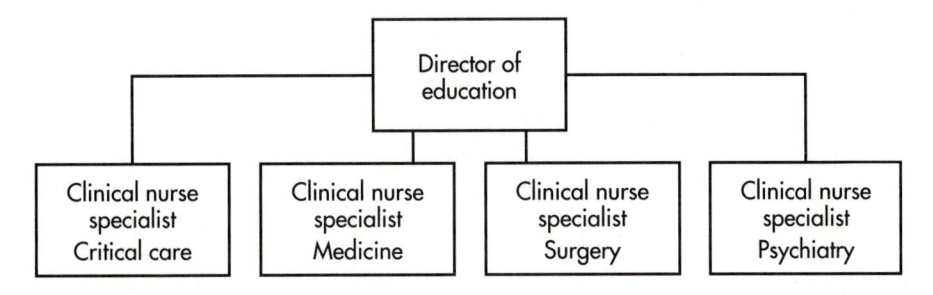

FIGURE 14-4. Organizational chart depicting CNS answering to director of education.

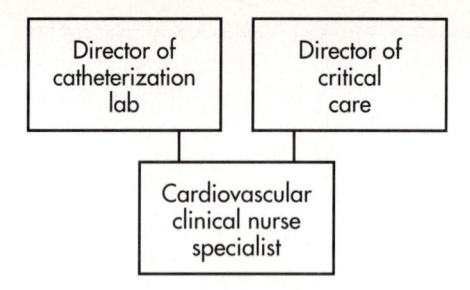

FIGURE 14-5. Organizational chart depicting CNS answering to several directors.

role model. All new staff then receive the same information about institutional protocols and procedures. Scheduling problems arise when the CNS is active in other projects and has to be absent from the unit.

Assessing Staff Needs

High visibility on the unit is important. Gleason and Flynn[12] reported that the staff consult more often with the CNS when immediately available and visible rather than when accessible by beeper. As the CNS works with the staff, strengths and weaknesses of individuals are identified. After discussing the findings with the nurse manager, a plan is formulated to assist the individual in attaining a particular goal or change in practice.

Trusting Relationship

The nurse manager and the CNS must have a sense of mutual trust for this system to work well. Both must collaborate to attain and maintain optimum levels of patient care. The nurse manager focuses on managing the unit and the CNS focuses on enhancing clinical practice.[12] Together, they facilitate and ensure quality care.

Complementary Leadership Styles

Through mutual trust and respect, understanding, and support, the CNS and nurse manager complement each other's role in the unit. Both positions are associated with a certain degree of autonomy, respect, and professional expertise. If they are comfortable and open with each other, a true sense of collegiality will be present; one is able to support and fill in for the other during an absence from the unit. Conversely, the nurse manager and the CNS can sabotage each other's success. If one chooses to be antagonistic and verbally expresses dissatisfaction and hostility towards the other, there will be disharmony within the unit. The staff note this disharmony and choose sides, and often the quality of patient care declines. These undesirable outcomes are avoided through scheduled weekly work meetings, and open and honest communication.

MEASURING OUTCOME

Robichaud and Hamric[25] suggested using a framework to evalute the CNS's activities, which is based on structure, process, and outcome. *Structural* criteria specific to the individual institution are evaluated by listing those administrative activities expected of the CNS. *Process* criteria examine the CNS's role of facilitating and coordinating patient care activities. *Outcome* criteria are based on the effects of nursing interventions on patient care.

Hotter[16] presented the list of strategies in Table 14-1 to measure CNS effectiveness in the critical care unit. These strategies were developed by the CNS Special Interest Group of the American Association of Critical Care Nurses. Note that these strategies focus on the clinical component of the CNS role. Additional strategies regarding other aspects of the CNS role within the critical care unit can be obtained from that publication.

Goals and objectives set for the CNS, and appropriate time frames for reaching them, need to be realistic. The time spent in practice is not as important as the outcome of patient care. This author finds that time commitments to the various components of the role vary according to patient census, and acuity, educational needs of the staff, administrative requests, and consultation activities. The ultimate goal of all activities is high quality patient care.

Many CNSs play a very active role in the quality assurance program in the critical care unit. The impact of the critical care unit on patient outcomes is determined by both clinical and administrative management of resources. Clark[8] suggested that the CNS does not need to do actual audits for quality assurance, but instead should focus on actual delivered care. Specific outcomes to be evaluated might be length of stay, reduced expenditures, and nurse retention.

Short and Long-Range Planning

The CNS works very closely with the nurse manager to establish the short- and long-range goals of the unit. Generally, the CNS focuses on goals related to clinical practice while the nurse manager concentrates on administrative goals. The CNS incorporates current trends in practice, education, and research to meet these goals.

Nursing Research

Hodgmen[15] stated that specific goals for conducting and promoting nursing research frequently receive a low priority because the CNS becomes so involved in the other roles. Several reported studies identified situations that block

Table 14-1. STRATEGIES FOR MEASURING CLINICAL EFFECTIVENESS

CLINICAL PRACTICE	OUTCOME	SUGGESTIONS FOR MEASUREMENT
Conduct routine patient care rounds to assess patient progress and appropriateness of therapy, as well as demonstrate advanced clinical decision-making skills.	Decreased length of stay Decrease or no increase in iatrogenic complications Improved level of critical thinking of staff	Anecdotal records on individual patients Complication rates Monitor length of stay
Identify/implement cost-saving methods of care delivery, e.g., change in equipment for cardiac output measurement, IV tubing changes.	More efficient use of equipment without increase in complications Decreased equipment expenditure	Consult purchasing for actual cost of supplies Calculate cost of nursing time spent/saved on procedure Add care and supply costs, multiply by number of patients per year
Identify/implement practices and procedures that decrease risk of liability, e.g., falls, self-extubation, infection.	Decreased incident rate Decreased complication rate Decreased length of stay Decrease in threatened or actual lawsuits	Consult with facility's risk manager, QA coordinator, or legal counsel to determine frequency, pattern
Develop, revise, and implement documentation standards to maximize reimbursement.	Increased revenue retrieval Compliance with accreditation standards for documentation	Consult with facility's prospective payment department to identify documentation deficiencies and impact on reimbursement
Coordinate/facilitate support groups, e.g., patient, family, and staff.	Improved patient compliance and satisfaction Decreased RN turnover	Calculate compliance and patient satisfaction with reliable and valid research tools Calculate nursing turnover and retention

From Hotter AN: New strategies to measure CNS effectiveness, *AACN News*, March 8, 1989. Reprinted with permission of the American Association of Critical Care Nurses.

nursing research. These blockers include lack of time and knowledge about the research process, lack of administrative support, and difficulty disseminating information.[7,9,11,23] Wabschall[28] suggested that the CNS is the logical person to incorporate clinical aspects of research to define the practice of nursing. Douglas, Hill, and Cameron[9] agreed, suggesting that a collaborative approach be used with nursing administration and doctoral nursing fellows.

The CNS may conduct original clinical research or may promote the spirit of inquiry among the staff. It is important that the staff nurses be involved with the research process from beginning to end to achieve this goal. For example, Medoff-Cooper and Lamb[18] used a clinical specialist–staff nurse research team to study infants with bronchopulmonary dysplasia. The CNS assumed the responsibility for developing the initial proposal. The staff nurse developed a small pilot project that represented a segment of the larger study. The staff nurse, using the CNS as a mentor, collected the data and wrote the draft of the report. This model represents one approach the CNS can use to facilitate the involvement of the staff nurse in research.

Education

The CNS creates the climate for the educational process within the unit. As the health care system continues to change rapidly, educational goals need to be flexible and attainable. Educational goals address patient and family education, staff education, advanced practice issues, and managerial overlap.

Patient and family education may begin with the CNS initiating the education and counseling, and continue with the staff nurses reinforcing the information. Meyer[21] suggested that the CNS initially assume all responsibility for patient education. Serving as a role model, the CNS demonstrates how, what, and when to teach. The CNS is responsible for developing teaching outlines, providing audiovisual aids, and writing patient information materials. A long-range goal is for the staff's active initiation and participation in patient and family education using the CNS as a role model and consultant. Meyer[21] cautioned that if the CNS always assumes responsibility for all education, the staff nurses will have little opportunity to assume any responsibility for teaching.

The nurse manager, the unit instructor, and the CNS collaborate on staff education. The nurse manager is responsible for cost issues related to program implementation; the instructor and the CNS determine the content for formal courses. Inservices are shared and assigned based on expertise and need.

An important aspect of the CNS's role is to develop the staff's potential to teach. Meyer[21] stated that not all staff nurses have the desire and confidence to formally teach. However, interested staff should have the opportunity and the assistance to do so. Many staff begin by teaching CPR and advanced cardiac life support and progress to giving lectures about critical care in formal courses. The CNS and instructor continue to act as role models and remain accountable for the teaching, but the staff have the opportunity to develop new skills and experience professional growth.

Standards of Practice

Goals for advanced practice include the establishment of standards of nursing practice, consultation within nursing or other disciplines, and role-modeling. The CNS is often asked to write formal nursing care plans that define nursing practice. The institution often approves these as standard care plans, especially if they address a high-volume type of patient. The CNS then teaches staff how to implement and use the care plan. Staff are often doubtful about the need for care plans. The CNS encourages staff to work together to incorporate care plans into daily nursing practice. This practice helps set high standards, complies with regulatory requirements, and establishes the CNS as an expert.

Obviously there is some managerial overlap between the nurse manager and the CNS. Together, they are responsible for solving problems, improving patient outcomes, promoting professionalism within the unit, and refining nursing practice. Specific goals for each of these can be defined with one assuming more responsibility than the other for a specific project. The focus is always improved quality patient care, higher staff satisfaction and retention, and demonstrated professional growth of all individuals.

Case Study: Orientation Planning for the CNS

You are the nurse manager for an 8-bed critical care unit. The hospital has hired a master's prepared CNS to work with patients before cardiac catheterization and to be the educator for the inpatient cardiac rehabilitation program. You have been asked to help orient the CNS. You recognize that you can develop a unique relationship for future mutual endeavors. What plan would you try and why?

The orientation of a CNS is organized jointly by all first-line managers who will interface daily with the CNS and who have line authority for staff who will work under the CNS. These efforts are coordinated by the unit instructor and approved by the director of critical care.

As the unit's nurse manager, you suggest the following plan: meet with the CNS to define her role together; schedule direct patient care time for the CNS, initially with a senior preceptor, and then independently; schedule time for the CNS to meet cardiologists and selected surgeons; arrange for the CNS to observe procedures in the cardiac catheterization laboratory, and include and introduce the CNS at the CCU staff and department meetings. The orientation phase lasts about six weeks, but the role transition takes minimally six months.

Thus, you, as the nurse manager, ask the CNS to evaluate current practice standards gradually, and are open to new ideas that may be applicable to that setting. As the CNS role evolves in that institution, the nurse manager and CNS continue open communication to identify problems, discuss proposed changes and evaluate patient outcomes.

The CNS is expected to develop patient education materials for cardiac catheterization and other high-volume procedures. Once the CNS is familiar with the procedures at that facility, the CNS develops care plans for the cardiac catheterization patient, which are then implemented in the CCU and on the appropriate medical units. The CNS then works on developing discharge planning tools such as drug information sheets. The CNS teaches staff what, when, and how families and patients are given information. This includes questions to anticipate and discharge information for patients with and without medically treated disease. After a period of time, the CNS and nurse manager choose a research project to measure the effectiveness of the patient/family education program.

CONCLUSION

The CNS plays a vital role within the critical care unit and the institution. Professional staff development becomes apparent as the CNS develops each component of the CNS role (clinical practice, educator, researcher, consultant, and executive). As the nurse manager and CNS work together to promote mutual goals, the atmosphere within the unit becomes collegial. The outcome of this is a working environment where competent practitioners provide quality care to patients and family.

REFERENCES

1. American Association of Critical Care Nurses: the critical care clinical nurse specialists: role definition, Newport Beach, Calif, 1987, The Association.
2. American Nurses' Association: Council of clinical nurse specialists: the role of the clinical nurse specialist, Kansas City, Mo, 1986, The Association.
3. Amos-Taylor RP and Elberson KL: Quality care: the emerging role of the CNS, Critical Care Nurse 9:28-37, 1988.
4. Beecroft PC and Papenhausen JL: Who is a clinical nurse specialist? Clinical Nurse Specialist 3(3):103-4, 1989.
5. Beyerman KL: Consultation roles of the clinical nurse specialist: a case study, Clinical Nurse Specialist 2:91-95, 1988.
6. Buchanon BF and Glanville CI: The clinical nurse specialist as educator: process and method, Clinical Nurse Specialist 2:82-89, 1988.
7. Cason CL and Beck CM: Clinical nurse specialist role development, Nursing and Health Care 3:20-25, 1982.
8. Clark S: The clinical nurse specialist in critical care, Critical Care Quarterly 5(1):51-89, 1982.
9. Douglas S, Hill MN, and Cameron EM: Clinical nurse specialist: a facilitator for clinical research, Clinical Nurse Specialist 3:12-15, 1989.
10. Felder LA: Direct patient care and independent practice. In Hamric AB and Spross J, editors: The clinical nurse specialist in theory and practice, New York, 1988, Grune & Stratton, pp. 58-71.
11. Girouard S: Implenting the research role. In Hamric AB and Spross J, editors: The clinical nurse specialist in theory and practice, New York, 1988, Grune & Stratton, pp. 33-39.
12. Gleason JM and Flynn KT: The surgical clinical nurse specialist as consultant in a tertiary care setting, Clinical Nurse Specialist 1:129-132, 1987.

13. Hamric AB: History and overview of the CNS role. In Hamric AB and Spross JA, editors: The clinical nurse specialist in theory and practice, New York, 1988, Grune & Stratton.
14. Harrell JS and McCullough SD: The role of the clinical nurse specialist: problems and solutions. Journal of Nursing Administration 16:44-48, 1986.
15. Hodgman EC: The CNS as researcher. In Hamric AB and Spross J, editors: The clinical nurse specialist in theory and practice, New York, 1988, Grune & Stratton, pp. 78-82.
16. Hotter AN: New strategies to measure CNS effectiveness, American Association of Critical Care Nurses Newsletter 15:March, 1989.
17. McDougall GJ: The role of the clinical nurse specialist consultant in organizational development, Clinical Nurse Specialist 1:133-39, 1987.
18. Medoff-Cooper B and Lamb AH: The clinical specialist–staff nurse research team: A model for clinical research, Clinical Nurse Specialist 3:16-19, 1989.
19. Menard SW: The CNS as a consultant. In Menard SW, editor: The CNS—perspectives on practice, New York, 1987, John Wiley & Sons.
20. Metcalf J, Werner M, and Richmond TS: The clinical nurse specialist in a clinical career ladder, Nursing Administration Quarterly 9:9-19, 1984.
21. Meyer JS: The CNS as a teacher. In Menard SW, editor: The CNS—perspectives on practice, New York, 1987, John Wiley & Sons, pp. 101-26.
22. Noble MA: The critical care clinical nurse specialist: need for hospital and community, Clinical Nurse Specialist 2:30-33, 1988.
23. Oberst MT: Integrating research and clinical practice roles, Topics in Clinical Nursing 7:45-53, 1985.
24. O'Rourke MW: Generic professional behaviors: implementation for the clinical nurse specialist role, Clinical Nurse Specialist 3(3):128-32, 1989.
25. Robichaud AM and Hamric AB: Time documentation of clinical specialist activities, Journal of Nursing Administration 16:31-36, 1986.
26. Stevens BJ: Accountability of the clinical specialist: the administrator's viewpoint, Journal of Nursing Administration 6(2): 30-32, 1976.
27. Tarsitano BJ, Brophy EB, and Snyder DJ: A demystification of the clinical nurse specialist role: perceptions of clinical specialists and nurse administrators, Journal of Nursing Education 25:4-9, 1985.
28. Wabschall JM: The CNS as researcher. In Menard SW, editor: The CNS—perspectives on practice, New York, 1987, John Wiley & Sons.
29. Werner JS, Bumann RM, and O'Brian JA: Clinical nurse specialization: an annotated bibliography, Clinical Nurse Specialist 2:14-15, 1988.

Unit III

Developing Administrative Skills

Chapter 15

BENEFITS OF EVOLVING TECHNOLOGY

Mary-Michael Brown

Picture yourself as the nurse manager of an active 10-bed critical care unit. As you walk onto your unit, you see that the patient receiving extracorporeal membrane oxygenation (ECMO) following coronary artery bypass surgery remains stable. You observe the CNS and the cardiac perfusionist explaining the ECMO circuit to several nurses and physicians. You move to the patient's bedside computer and retrieve the latest data about hemodynamic parameters, medications, and laboratory studies, which have been entered automatically during the night. As you visit the next patient, you listen to nurses and intensivists discussing the merits of administering estrogen conjugates (Premarin) to control postoperative bleeding; and you hear one nurse's intention to consult with the pharmacist about this use of this drug.

You return to your office, sort your mail, and see that an article written by two of your staff members has been published in the current issue of a nursing journal. You take a telephone call from the nurse recruiter who wants to arrange yet another interview for a staff nurse position (that makes three interviews this week alone). At the end of the day, you attend the monthly educational meeting of your local chapter of the American Association of Critical Care Nurses, where you are greeted by two colleagues from another hospital. They tell you that nurses and physicians from their hospital have been commenting favorably about your unit and that they would like to meet with you to discuss the operation of your unit in more detail.

Too unrealistic? Perhaps not. This scenario represents some of the benefits derived from rapidly changing technology and the dramatic applications of new drugs and recent research. This scenario also reflects the work of an astute critical care nurse manager who has made these benefits work effectively.

The first part of this chapter will describe the benefits of evolving technology and knowledge, as well as some of the problems associated with this rapid technologic evolution, and will consider some ways to maximize benefits and minimize problems. The last part of the chapter explores the contribution of a patient data management system in critical care.

BENEFITS OF TECHNOLOGY AND KNOWLEDGE

Today's critical care unit is rapidly changing, and is complex and dynamic, which reflects spectacular advancements in technology.[8,12,18,20,29] Closed-loop administration of vasoactive medications, computer-driven ST-segment monitors, oximetric pulmonary artery catheters, and in-line capnography are only a few of the additions changing the critical care landscape. Even the patient's bed has not escaped modification. Now, electric beds may also include hydraulically powered controls for bed position changes during patient transport as well as roentgen film holders and in-bed scales to minimize repositioning unstable patients.

The influence of this rapidly changing critical care environment can clearly be seen by the topics of continuing education courses. Today these include advances in intra-aortic balloon counterpulsation, automatic internal cardioverter defibrillators, dual-chamber temporary pacing, autotransfusion, ventricular assist devices, the total artificial heart, coronary sinus retroperfusion, cyberphysiology, intraosseous infusions, extracorporeal membrane oxygenation with carbon dioxide removal, high frequency jet ventilation, and invasive and noninvasive monitoring of the mechanically ventilated patient.[2]

A review of recent nursing and research literature reveals that remarkable progress has been made in twentieth century critical care, that a cornucopia of new technology exists, and that a new technologic age is here.[13,16,20] In the evolution of critical care, the benefits of technology are striking and exciting. These benefits fall into at least four major categories: patient care, morale and teamwork, recruitment and retention of nurses, and public image of the institution. The box on the next page contrasts the benefits of evolving technology and knowledge with some potential problems that will be discussed in this chapter.

Patient Care

Improved patient care is one important benefit of new technology and knowledge. New technology allows nurses and physicians to monitor patients more accurately with a clearer and more timely picture of the patient.[24] Nurses collect

> **POTENTIAL EFFECTS OF TECHNOLOGY AND KNOWLEDGE**
>
> **Benefits**
> Improves patient care.
> Encourages morale and teamwork.
> Enhances nurse recruitment and retention.
> Improves institution's public image.
>
> **Problems**
> Contributes to iatrogenic patient injury.
> Favors nurse overdependence on technology.
> Increases nurse's liability.
> Imposes stress.
> Depersonalizes patient care.

more data, detect more subtle changes and trends in the patient, intervene more rapidly, and thus prevent complications—and promote and restore life.[20,24]

The findings of current medical and nursing research have also enhanced patient care. Drug research has given patients more choices and opportunities for pharmacologic interventions and control of illness. For instance, the introduction of calcium channel antagonists, tissue plasminogen activators, and cyclosporine have revolutionized the care of patients with coronary heart disease and organ transplants.[23]

Nursing research projects study the effects of new technology in a variety of settings. Nurse researchers look at the benefits and problems inherent in adding devices to facilitate patient care. Nursing research illustrates nursing's attempt to adapt technology and new knowledge to derive maximum patient benefit.

Morale and Teamwork

New and sophisticated equipment can improve survival rate; however, it can also complicate patient care. Nurses and physicians must master this new, sophisticated equipment while simultaneously caring for the patient. More than ever, a team effort has become necessary.

Nurses, physicians, respiratory therapists, and other health professionals recognize the necessity of teamwork to obtain the best possible outcome for the patient.[30] A smoothly run resuscitation effort, in which everyone knows her own job but anticipates others' needs, will maximize patient survival, recharge the group, and help team members appreciate each other's individual contributions. For example, consider what can occur when a postoperative cardiac patient arrests: The bedside nurse alerts a charge nurse, who summons help. The respiratory therapist ambues the patient. The bedside nurse relinquishes chest compressions to another nurse or physician. While anticipating intravenous access ports, she prepares the defibrillator. The charge nurse obtains the open chest tray and prepares medications requested by the intensivist. The perfusionist manages the intra-aortic balloon pump and assists with obtaining blood samples. This type of teamwork now is necessary to manage critically ill patients, and it can positively influence staff morale while it improves patient outcomes.[3]

Recruitment and Retention

A recent study describing the nursing shortage indicated that 40 percent of hospital-employed nurses work in critical care.[21] Patients supported by the technologic advances in today's critical care units require more intensive nursing attention and a higher nurse-to-patient ratio than in times past.

Despite their inherent stressors, critical care units and their ever-changing environments can also be attractive to nurses.[12] Critical care nurses work on the cutting edge of technology, thrive on fast-paced activity, and are satisfied by using their intellectual skills constantly in this dynamic setting.[18] The intensity of the work experience in this environment and the opportunity to affect people emotionally is profoundly satisfying to many critical care nurses.[18]

The critical care units with state-of-the-art equipment, dynamic, challenging environments, and evident teamwork philosophies can be used as recruitment tools. Additionally, a progressive and innovative unit can help retain nurses by accepting nurses who transfer from other units, rather than letting them seek employment at a different institution.

Public Relations

In this era of prospective reimbursement and cost containment, consumers and insurers seek acute care facilities that offer the most services for their dollars. Favorable patient outcomes, low surgical mortality rates, up-to-date equipment, and physician recommendations are all reasons that patients choose one hospital over another.

A critical care unit that can treat specialty patients with advanced technology, coordinated teamwork, high staff morale, and nursing staff interest in working there has a good effect on patient outcomes and promotes confidence in the community. Referring physicians are convinced that their patients are receiving the best possible medical and nursing care. Patients and their families are reassured that the most current treatments and compassionate attention will be received. Patients, families, and physicians discuss their experiences with a critical care unit with neighbors, friends, and colleagues, thus enhancing the hospital's public image and increasing the number of patients seeking its services.

Improving patient care, enhancing teamwork and staff morale, recruiting and retaining nurses despite the nurse shortage, and increasing patient referrals by a positive public image are benefits of evolving technology and knowledge. Unfortunately, these benefits can also give rise to problems.

POTENTIAL PROBLEMS OF TECHNOLOGY AND KNOWLEDGE

Potential problems that accompany the tremendous growth in technology and knowledge can be considered grouped in five areas: iatrogenic injury, overdependence on technology, increased liability, stress, and depersonalized patient care.[24] Tomasik[29] estimates that more than 15,000 medical devices marketed under about 50,000 different brand names are available for use—nurses are introduced to a new piece of equipment almost every week. In addition, the number of individual pieces of equipment that accompany each patient may be staggering: On a single patient, some nurses care for up to fifteen infusion devices, each delivering a different medication.[29] Given the diversity, complexity, and the sheer volume of equipment, patient injury and mechanical errors related to improper operation of equipment may occur.[24,29]

Iatrogenic Injury

Approximately 35 percent of all iatrogenic injuries are related to invasive devices; these injuries occur often in critical care units. Equipment malfunctions cause 36 percent of these iatrogenic injuries.[16,24] Heightened injury and risk are often due to inexperienced personnel, constant influx of new equipment, and the invasiveness and complexity of the equipment or therapeutic procedure.[24]

Overdependence on Technology

Nurses in critical care units simultaneously manage the life-sustaining machinery and the biopsychosocial needs of the patient. The nurse runs the risk of becoming overdependent on technology when interruptions occur. Nurses may also ignore their clinical assessments when their findings are incongruent with the machine's results. Nurses who sense that something is seriously amiss with their patient may question their own judgment in the face of "perfect" laboratory studies and "textbook" hemodynamic parameters.

Increased Liability

Because advances in technology enable swift delivery of more precise data, trends in the patient's progress are detected more rapidly. Quick response to data and trends has become paramount. Nurses, physicians, and other health care professionals must assume responsibility, take action, and make decisions as rapidly as the data is produced. Hesitating to collect more data instead of acting on existing findings could result in patient injury. The collector and analyzer of the data is accountable, responsible, and hence liable for negative patient outcomes. Additionally, nurses who fail to assess equipment accuracy are liable for errors resulting from the improperly used equipment.[24]

Stress

Sinclair[24] reports that the demands of proper equipment use, the overdependence on technology, and the threat of liability all increase the stress of the critical care nurse. Additional stress may be experienced when advances in technology impose ethical and philosophical dilemmas upon the clinician. Nurses may perceive themselves as caretakers of irreversibly ill patients whose lives are painfully and unmercifully prolonged by technology and equipment. Critical care units are infamous for their inherent stress; and advances in technology and pursuant changes in nursing clinical practice may compound this condition.

Depersonalized Care

Depersonalized patient care may result from increased technology. Additional tubes, wires, and pumps may limit contact with the patient. Sinclair[24] noted that to reduce technology-related stress, critical care nurses may choose to care primarily for the equipment rather than the patient. The resultant imbalance of "high tech" with "low touch" can result in depersonalized patient care practices.

Despite the potential problems of technologic advances, the nurse manager can utilize three major strategies to maximize the benefits and minimize the problems: emphasize the benefits, consider feedback carefully, and utilize hospital resources.

STRATEGIES TO MAXIMIZE THE BENEFITS
Emphasizing the Benefits

Introduction of new equipment or technology may be planned or spontaneous. Regardless of the situation, before formally introducing new equipment, procedures, or research, the nurse manager determines the effects of this technology—how the technology will affect patients, how it will influence teamwork and morale, how it will maximize nurse recruitment and retention, and how it will be reflected in the hospital's public image.

The nurse manager also estimates the probability of patient injury; the likelihood of the nurses' overreliance on the equipment; and the possibility of increased liability, stress, and depersonalization of patient care. The nurse manager can plan inservices to prevent problems and fears of problems at staff conferences.

The nurse manager compares the benefits of new technology with the potential limitations and risks. Careful consideration helps the nurse manager decide if the benefits outweigh the risks. If they do, the nurse manager is enthusiastic about the introduction of technology into the critical care unit. When the risk-benefit ratio is equivocal, the nurse manager emphasizes the benefits and develops safeguards against the risks. This process is dynamic and also includes careful consideration of staff feedback.

Feedback

Soliciting the staff's response to new technology is essential. However, the experienced critical care nurse manager rarely accepts their comments at face value, but asks more questions, acquires more details, and separates fact from emotion to clarify the issues. For example, the staff's report of their first impression of a new, portable transport monitor may be, "We do not like it." Further questioning may reveal that only one nurse does not like it—and she dislikes it because she did not attend the inservice and has not mastered its use.

Informing staff of your analysis of the new technology prepares them for their own careful analysis. Asking staff for their opinion directly on the merits of a new procedure or technology usually reveals plentiful data. The box below shows an example of a form that obtains staff feedback about a product. It is also important to obtain information about the staff's stress, morale, and ability to view the patient as a person, despite the presence of technology. When staff are aware of the benefits rather than just the potential problems, their anxiety is minimized and their openness to the advantages of technology is maximized.

To acquire the necessary information when considering a new technology, the nurse manager utilizes valuable internal hospital resources. With the direction of her supervisor, the nurse manager consults with hospital committees to successfully lay the groundwork to introduce new technology.

SAMPLE PRODUCT EVALUATION TOOL

Arterial Blood Gas Kit Evaluation

Instructions: Circle the appropriate response for each item. Write comments as appropriate.

1. Does this kit contain all the supplies you need to do the procedure?   Yes   No
   If not, what was missing?
2. Does this kit contain supplies you did not use?   Yes   No
   If yes, which supplies?
3. Does the syringe fill easily?   Yes   No
4. Please rate this product:
   Excellent   Good   Average   Fair   Poor

Used with permission from Dickerson M: Product evaluation: a key to controlling costs, Nurs Econ 50(2):60, March-April 1987.

Hospital Resources

PRODUCTS COMMITTEE

A hospital products committee coordinates most aspects of product evaluation. This includes responding to requests for new products and equipment and for replacement of old equipment, as well as determining which products best meet clinical needs while being most cost-efficient.[10]

While members of the products committee may vary from institution to institution, it should have members that represent major users and involved departments. Typically, the group includes representatives from the departments of nursing, medicine, purchasing, materials management, clinical engineering, and hospital administration.[6,11,19] The products committee generally meets monthly, but frequency may vary depending on the institution's needs.

The objectives of the products committee are numerous, but may be categorized into four main areas: (1) to provide quality supplies, (2) to standardize equipment, (3) to control costs, and (4) to develop procedures for product evaluation.[6,10,19]

The products committee determines criteria for quality. Quality products are those that perform the intended function reliably and accurately, that are user-friendly, and that incorporate patient safety features.

Although it is not always possible to standardize equipment and supplies throughout a hospital, it is usually desirable. Per diem nurses, float nurses, agency nurses, and transferring nurses work in different areas of the hospital and may experience anxiety when faced with unfamiliar equipment and supplies.[6] Standardizing equipment eliminates the need for the biomedical engineering department to learn another manual, reduces the need for the education department to prepare another class, and prevents materials management from micro-dividing their shelves.[7]

A major objective of the products committee is to control costs. The products committee may engineer at least four different types of purchases: *Direct purchases* are items obtained directly from the manufacturer. *Special orders* are custom-designed by the manufacturer for the buyer. Direct purchases and special orders are more costly than other types of purchases because they often involve a small number of items, and the relatively fixed additional charges for shipping.[6]

Routine *distributor purchases* are based on wholesale prices, requisite profit margins, and discounts or promotionals.[6] *Negotiated prices,* another form of volume buying, result when an institution commonly places large orders with a specific manufacturer.[6] This usually is covered by a contractual agreement that has been negotiated to prevent automatic shipments and oversupply of items.[6]

Purchaser consortiums are groups of institutions that negotiate with manufacturers to reduce costs through volume buying.[6] The larger consortiums comprising institutions with similar equipment and supply needs command the best buy for their money.

The process of introducing a new product may be initiated several ways. Nurses may learn about a product at a critical care conference or through informal networks among institutions, and may envision the product's merits in their critical care unit. Nurses and physicians may be awarded research grants that contain provisions for new products. Creative staff members may develop ideas for saving time or money that include new products. An institution's expansion project, such as renovating or developing a new critical care unit, may include plans to purchase or upgrade equipment. Regardless of the way the product is discovered, a member of the products committee is consulted.

Typically, the requested item goes on the agenda of the next scheduled meeting, and the products committee reviews its advantages and disadvantages. Clearly, adequate representation by the nursing department is essential. It is often possible to attend a meeting of the products committee to observe the process of product evaluation or to explain particularly complex products used in critical care units.

When a new product is being considered, several things occur. First of all, a list of needs showing the product's essential features is developed by the products committee with input from high-frequency users. Examples of essential features may be ease of use, patient comfort and safety, product reliability and accuracy, ability to interface with existing equipment, service warranty, and cost.[6] The next box shows an example checklist of essential features that could be used by nurses evaluating several cardiac monitors. When using this tool, the nurse manager or committee representative collects the completed forms, totals the responses, and presents a cohesive report to the products committee.

Product cost, cost savings, and conversion costs are considered. Cost savings represent the actual dollars saved by introducing new equipment or replacing old equipment. Conversion includes the cost of inservicing the new product and the cost of reduced productivity while the staff master the use of the item. The costs of other supplies may increase if the old product was supplied by a vendor who also supplies other products to the institution. Finally, the potential for reimbursement by insurers for the product's cost is considered.[6]

The products committee then determines which companies sell the product and reviews their prices, rental agreements, and evaluation cost policies. A comparison of the products of two to four companies is planned. Sometimes a company representative will give an initial demonstration of the product, which allows early determination of the advantages and disadvantages of each product.[10]

The products committee then develops an evaluation tool to compare the items and their characteristics. This evaluation tool needs to be clear, concise, and easy to complete; and it must reflect the original reasons a new item was considered. The tool also includes closed- and open-ended questions, as well as rating scales. Optimally, the wording of questions is positive and easy to understand.[6] Figure 15-1 is an example of an evaluation tool.

The products committee then plans the product trial. The products committee and the manufacturer negotiate the number of items to be used in the trial,

EVALUATION CHECKLIST

Essential Features of a Cardiac Monitor

	Company X	Company Y	Company Z

1. Visability (screen size, clarity of alphanumerics)
2. Alarms
    a. Audio
    b. Levels
3. User-friendliness
4. Arrhythmia function
    a. Detection
    b. Recall
    c. Levels
    d. ST-segment monitoring
    e. Audio
5. Cartridge for transport
6. Overview function from bedside to bedside
7. Overview function from operating room
8. Educational commitment
9. Service and warranty
10. Captnometer
    a. Separate
    b. In-line
11. Oximeter
    a. Separate
    b. In-line
    c. Skin
    d. Finger
    e. Ear
12. Respiratory rate function
13. Cardiac output
    a. Separate
    b. In-line
14. Telemetry
    a. Two-lead
    b. Three-lead
    c. Five-lead
15. Noninvasive monitor for blood pressure, pulse, temperature
16. Remote housing
17. Cost
18. Ability to interface with patient data management system

Part I. To be completed by evaluation coordinators.
Product being evaluated: _____
Evaluation coordinators: _____
Dates of evaluation: _____ Number of products to be evaluated: _____
Reason for evaluation (check all that apply):
☐ New product ☐ Problems with present product ☐ Improvement over present product
☐ RN request ☐ Less expensive than present product
☐ MD request ☐ Other _____

Areas participating in trial: _____
Approved by: _____ Date: _____

Part II: To be completed by trial participant.
Questionnaire return deadline:
We have conducted a clinical trial of the above product. Please rank the existing product (if applicable) and the new product on a 1–5 scale based on the following criteria:
1 is the lowest (least satisfactory): 5 is the best (most satisfactory).

Criteria	Old Product	Office Use	New Product	Office Use
1.	1 2 3 4 5		1 2 3 4 5	
2.	1 2 3 4 5		1 2 3 4 5	
3.	1 2 3 4 5		1 2 3 4 5	
4.	1 2 3 4 5		1 2 3 4 5	
5.	1 2 3 4 5		1 2 3 4 5	
6.	1 2 3 4 5		1 2 3 4 5	
7.	1 2 3 4 5		1 2 3 4 5	
8.	1 2 3 4 5		1 2 3 4 5	

Check one:
1. Would you recommend changing from the present product to the new product based on product features ☐ Yes ☐ No ☐ Doesn't make any difference
2. Would you recommend changing from the present product to the new product if it would represent an estimated $_____ increse/decrease in cost/year?
3.

4.

Comments:

FIGURE 15-1. Sample product evaluation form. *(Used with permission from Price MS and Wujcik D: Product evaluation in critical care, Crit Care Nursing 8(2):8, March-April 1988.)*

which is the manufacturer's expense. The evaluation coordinator arranges inservices taught by company representatives, nurse educators, and nurse managers.

During the clinical trial, the evaluation coordinator visits the participating areas to answer questions, handle problems, and ensure that enough supplies are available.[6] Staff complete the evaluation tools, and the trial is completed.

The evaluation tools are reviewed and analyzed, and the evaluation coordinator and the products committee prepare a report. The products committee makes recommendations, and hospital administration chooses the company. Introduction of the new equipment is then planned.

This evaluation process may vary depending on the institution and the product complexity. The role of the nurse manager is to facilitate the clinical trials. It is important that the nurse manager support the introduction of the equipment into the critical care unit.

BIOMEDICAL ENGINEER

Equipment in the critical care unit is very complex. The biomedical engineer can give insight into the safety, durability, accuracy, and reliability of equipment. Nurses normally are not educated as engineers, and thus most do not fully understand this technology and equipment. Although some nursing leaders[29] have discussed adding this kind of curriculum to basic nursing education, until things change, nurse managers today consult the biomedical engineer to bridge this gap.

Biomedical engineers are involved in the evaluation of new equipment and know what equipment is already used in the institution.[5] Biomedical engineers help the nurse manager prevent equipment problems by developing preventative maintenance procedures and monitoring repairs and down time.[5] Often, the nurse manager merely describes the equipment problems, and the biomedical engineer (with the help of departmental records) can resolve the problems.

PHARMACY AND THERAPEUTICS COMMITTEE

The pharmacy and therapeutics committee is a hospital advisory group mandated by the Joint Commission on Accreditation of Hospitals.[1] Usually it comprises representatives from pharmacy, medicine, nursing, and hospital administration, but this is variable, depending on the institution or the agenda. For instance, if the committee plans to consider an intravenous admixture program for the hospital, a member of the products committee may be invited to consider appropriate intravenous tubing and materials.

The pharmacy and therapeutics committee is charged with advising hospital staff on the evaluation, selection, therapeutic uses, and costs of drugs; recommending and formulating hospital policies and procedures pertinent to drug use; participating in quality assurance activities that concern drug use, such as monitoring acute drug reactions; planning educational programs to communicate the introduction of new drugs or new uses of drugs; and responding to requests from the hospital's institutional review board and others to introduce experimental drugs or other drugs available commercially.[1]

During the course of daily practice, the nurse manager seeks information and guidance from the pharmacist and from the pharmacy and therapeutics committee on drug actions, doses, compatibilities, and delivery methods. Although pharmacology references are available for routine consultation, the nurse manager encourages staff to utilize the advanced educational preparation and experiences of the pharmacist. Frequently, the hospital pharmacist can answer questions not in the references. Sometimes in emergency situations, drugs are used for unconventional applications. For example, prostaglandin E is used for neonates, but when it is used for adults to control pulmonary hypertension, the pharmacist can outline usual doses, suggest methods of delivery, review potential problems, and encourage the critical care nurses to communicate with the neonatal critical care nurses for practical experiences.

HOSPITAL INFORMATION SYSTEMS SPECIALIST

No discussion about technology and knowledge in critical care is complete without mentioning computers. Computer technology in critical care has been described as ubiquitous and irresistible.[4,14] Understanding the benefits, problems, and selection criteria of computerized patient data management is necessary.

Computers have been almost universally accepted in non–health care industries. Airlines, hotels, insurance companies, and banks routinely use computers; hospitals, on the other hand, have lagged behind in computerizing their departments. In fact, many hospitals continue to record and distribute clinical and clerical data manually.[4]

The complex, labor-intensive work in intensive care units involves collecting voluminous amounts of data.[4] Computerizing patient data can relieve cost pressures, documentation time, and problems of managing enormous amounts of information.[4]

A patient data management system (PDMS) is a computerized system designed to collect, capture, store, retrieve, examine, and analyze data.[4,11,17] A PDMS organizes and manipulates critical care data, presenting it logically and easily for continuous clinical use.[17] Many hospitals use different computer systems in different departments. A PDMS organizes all these systems and functionally replaces the patient's chart.

In many critical care units, the technology automatically captures and documents the patient's vital signs, ventilator settings, and laboratory values.[4,11,14,22,28] Calculation of cardiorespiratory parameters, analysis of waveforms, and detection of arrhythmia are automated.[4,11,15] Microprocessors and software algorithms contained in some bedside computers, intravenous infusion devices, and ventilators can communicate with a PDMS, and data can then be displayed to highlight trends in the patient's condition. Figure 15-2 is a sample flowsheet report generated by a bedside PDMS. Figure 15-3 is an example of a PDMS graphic display of trends.

Nursing assessments, documentation of nursing care, nursing care plans, nursing patient care standards, shift reports, nurse schedules, patient assignments, and quality assurance reports can all be organized by a PDMS. The nurse

Cardiovascular Surgical Unit Record

Patient Name: SMITH, JOHN A **Pt. ID:** 111111

Parameters										
Date:	08-16-89	08-16-89	08-16-89	08-16-89	08-16-89	08-16-89	08-16-89	08-16-89	08-16-89	08-16-89
Time:	07:04:25	07:28:24	07:45:54	08:03:18	08:17:25	08:20:00	09:17:14	09:31:20	09:44:35	10:00:59
Ht	185. cm	185. cm	185. cm	185. cm	185. cm	185. cm	185. cm	185. cm	185. cm	185. cm
Wt-preop	95. kg	95. kg	95. kg	95. kg	95. kg	95. kg	95. kg	95. kg	95. kg	95. kg
Wt-daily	kg	kg	kg	kg	kg	kg	kg	kg	kg	kg
BSA	2.20 m^2	2.20 m^2	2.20 m^2	2.20 m^2	2.20 m^2	2.20 m^2	2.20 m^2	2.20 m^2	2.20 m^2	2.20 m^2
Oral Temp	C	C	C	C	C	C	C	C	C	C
Rectal Temp	C	C	C	C	C	C	C	C	C	C
Core Temp	36.2 C	36.2 C	36.3 C	36.3 C	36.3 C	36.6 C	36.8 C	C	C	36.8 C
Toe Temp	C	C	C	C	C	C	C	C	C	C
Respirations	14	14	14	14	14	14	14	14	14	14
Heart Rate	101 BPM	101 BPM	101 BPM	98 BPM	102 BPM	102 BPM	102 BPM	102 BPM	102 BPM	98 BPM
Rhythm	A PACED	A PACED	A PACED	A PACED	A PACED	A PACED	A PACED	A PACED	A PACED	A PACED
Paced Rate	100	100	100	100	100	100	100	100	100	100
MA	.1	.1	.1	.1	.1	.1	.1	.1	.1	.1
Mode	ASYNC	ASYNC	ASYNC	ASYNC	ASYNC	ASYNC	ASYNC	ASYNC	ASYNC	ASYNC
Threshold										
A1/A2/A3	/ /	/ /	/ /	/ /	/ /	/ /	/ /	/ /	/ /	/ /
V1/V2/V3	/ /	/ /	/ /	/ /	/ /	/ /	/ /	/ /	/ /	/ /
Aline mmHg	104 53	104 53 70.	110 66 80.	110 57 75.	116 62 80.	116 62 80.	126 74 91.	112 66 81.	118 66 83.	118 64 82.
Cuff mmHg	102 102 55			112 112 56			122 122 69			107 107 62
PAP mmHg		32 22 25.	30 18 22.	28 18 21.	24 18 20.	24 18 20.	25 19 21.	27 17 20.	30 18 22.	28 17 21.
RA/CVP mmhg	/	/ 12	/ 8	/ 9	/ 9	/ 12	/ 12	/ 9	/ 10	/ 10
LAP/PCWPmmHg	/	8 /	4 /	5 /	5 /	5 /	7 /	6 /	6 /	6 /
SVO2 (%)	%	66 %	60 %	58 %	58 %	58 %	56 %	62 %	62 %	62 %
CO / CI	71. / 4.8	/ 4.5	/	75. / 4.8	/	/	87. / 4.9	/	/	77. / 5.0
SVR / PVR	/	/ 302	/	/ 266	/	/	/ 228	/	/	/ 240
IV Drugs:										
Amicar	g/hr	g/hr	g/hr	g/hr	g/hr	g/hr	g/hr	g/hr	g/hr	g/hr
Aminophyllin	mg/hr	mg/hr	mg/hr	mg/hr	mg/hr	mg/hr	mg/hr	mg/hr	mg/hr	mg/hr
Amiodarone	u/kg/m	u/kg/m	u/kg/m	u/kg/m	u/kg/m	u/kg/m	u/kg/m	u/kg/m	u/kg/m	u/kg/m
DRUG A	mg/m	mg/m	mg/m	mg/m	mg/m	mg/m	mg/m	mg/m	mg/m	mg/m
DRUG B	mg/m	mg/m	mg/m	mg/m	mg/m	mg/m	mg/m	mg/m	mg/m	mg/m
DRUG C	u/kg/m	u/kg/m	u/kg/m	u/kg/m	u/kg/m	u/kg/m	u/kg/m	u/kg/m	u/kg/m	u/kg/m
DRUG D	u/m	u/m	u/m	u/m	u/m	u/m	u/m	u/m	u/m	u/m

FIGURE 15-2. Sample flowsheet report on a patient data management system. *(Used with permission from Georgetown University Hospital, Washington, DC, 1990.)*

manager explores the benefits and problems associated with a PDMS before promoting it in the critical care unit.

Patient care can improve through timely data acquisition, analysis, and trending. With a PDMS, the nurse spends less time retreiving reports, ordering tests and equipment, and clarifying orders. Her time is for patient care.

The quality of documentation may improve with a PDMS's menu-driven nurse's or physician's patient progress notes. This may be helpful to

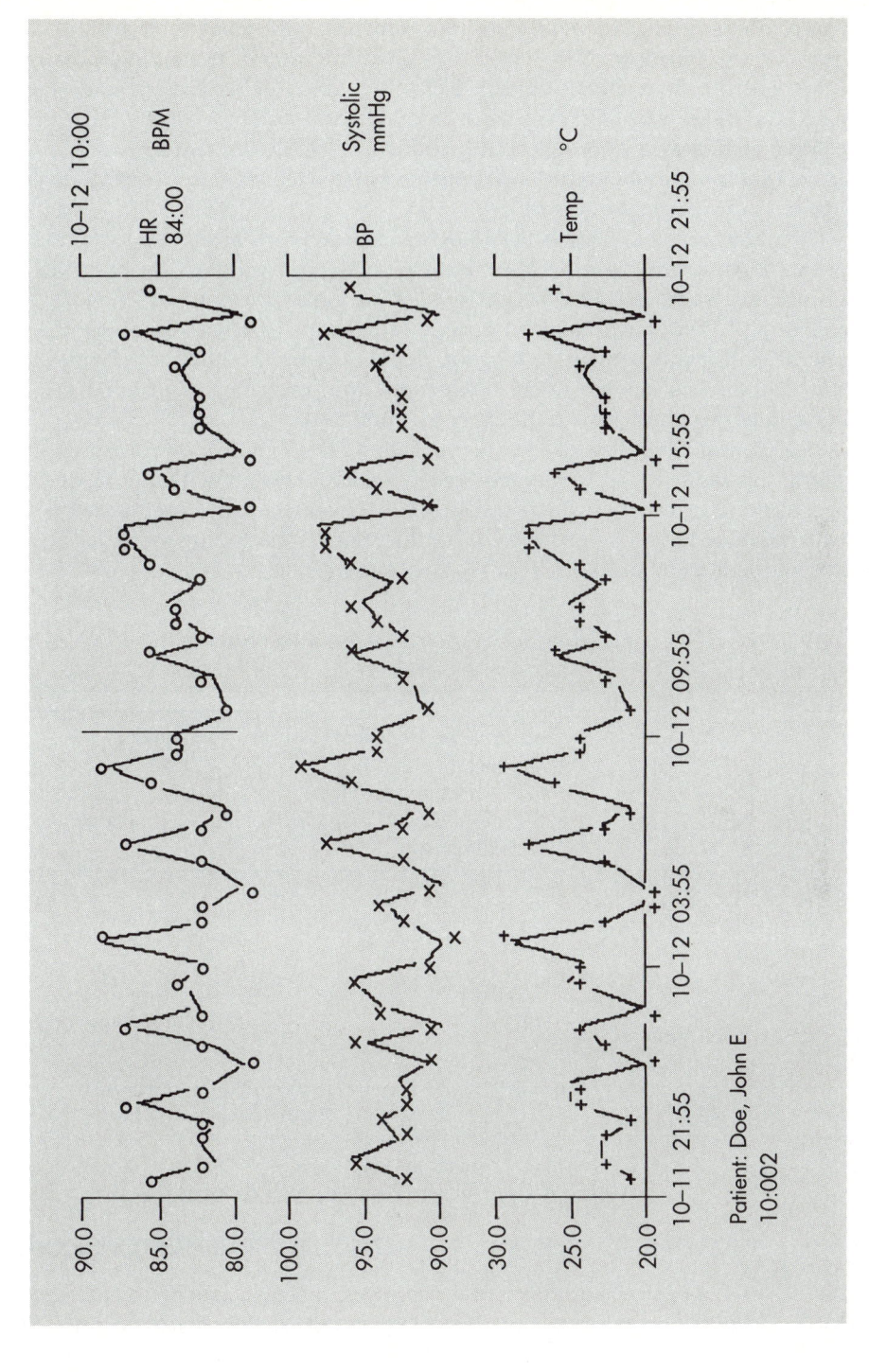

FIGURE 15-3. Sample of a graphic display generated from a patient data management system. *(Used with permission from Trinity Computing Systems, Houston, Texas, 1990.)*

less-experienced practitioners who have difficulty describing their patient's condition clearly. Further, this makes the medical record (including physicians' orders and the flow sheet) more legible,[25,26] which helps reduce transcription errors and time wasted trying to decipher handwriting. A PDMS can increase personal productivity and organization efficiency, while improving patient care.[22] Figure 15-4 is a sample menu from which a nurse may select appropriate descriptions to document patient care.

On a less favorable note, a PDMS demands attention. Automated data that are entered must be validated by the bedside nurse, and routines for entering data that are not captured automatically (such as pulse assessment) can be time-consuming.[15] The time it takes to generate hard copy (such as a printout of a flow sheet or progress note) can be lengthy, depending on the number of pages to be printed. It also takes a long time to view the flow sheet before printing, because only a small part of it fits on the screen at one time.[15]

The potential benefits and problems with a PDMS will vary depending on the system. It is unlikely that any commercially available PDMS will meet all desirable specifications of every hospital department. Hospitals can either develop their own system or they may purchase a commercial PDMS. In any case, the hospital information system specialist (HIS) is consulted.

```
10-31-1991           Intensive Care Support System/Nurses Notes           22:55:56
User: SU                          Nurses Notes
```

			_ Incisional wound without signs of drainage or	—
			_ infection.	
			_ WBC within normal limits:	—
10-31-91	22:55	SU	SYSTEMS ASSESSMENT: ADMISSION NOTE: Patient admitted from:	—

A. OR
B. ER
C. Catch Lab
D. Home
E. Clinic
F. Transportation Mode

```
Patient: DOE, JOHN E          Bed: 1    Ward: CCU    Last Save: 15:28:22
                                                                      =CAP=
                              admfrom. icu
          Select an Option or use Function, Punctuation, or Numeric Keys

      F2FREFMT        F5SAVE        F7EDIT    F8RESUSCF9OPTIONF0DONE
```

FIGURE 15-4. Sample menu from a patient progress note in a patient data management system. *(Used with permission from Trinity Computing Systems, Houston, Texas, 1990.)*

The HIS specialist is the expert on the institution's current computer systems who can advise the nurse manager considering a commercially available PDMS. The HIS specialist translates the nurse manager's questions or requests about a PDMS and explains how data is presented.

The HIS specialist also helps the nurse manager determine requirements, attributes, and characteristics desired in a PDMS. The HIS specialist can assist the nurse manager in reviewing commercially available systems. The HIS specialist and the nurse manager estimate the number of full-time equivalents required for staff training, system installation, maintenance, and upgrades of software and hardware. The box below represents important criteria to consider when purchasing a PDMS. The nurse manager is then better prepared to consult with others before recommending a PDMS.

STAFF EDUCATION

To keep pace with technology in the critical care unit, nurses continuously acquire new knowledge and new skills. In-services and staff development programs can help critical care nurses gain this information.

Inservice classes are instructions given to nurses to acquire and improve skills or to correct practice deficiencies.[9] Inservice classes may be conducted by nursing personnel, but are frequently arranged by a member of the staff education department in collaboration with the nurse manager.

An inservice for a new product is usually a factory representative's or salesperson's review of the product. The representative demonstrates the way the product is used, and answers the nursing staff's questions. These inservices are often limited. Malila[16] noted that representatives often emphasize the virtues of the product and diminish the flaws. The nurse manager asks that the clinical nurse educator and CNS supplement these inservices with staff development programs.

SELECTION CRITERIA FOR A PATIENT DMS

Ability to communicate with other hospital computer systems (laboratory, pharmacy, materials management, dietary)
Ability to be customized to patient population, critical care unit, user
Ability to calculate cardiopulmonary parameters, fluid intake and output totals, and cumulative totals
Clarity of graphic and printed displays
Ease of data acquisition
Location of data entry and acquisition (bedside or central station)
Ability for one-time autotranscription
Ability to capture, store, and retrieve data reliably
Cost of system, of full-time equivalents needed for programming and training, and for hardware and software upgrades
Service and warranty

Staff education programs improve the understanding of technology, including the new product's purpose, design, function, and limitations.[16] Staff education programs involve a staged process of planning, implementation, and evaluation of the nurse's learning. The program objectives are that the nurse understands and uses the new product safely.

The most successful staff education programs include clear and concise statements that help nurses demonstrate competent applications of new knowledge and skills.[16,27] The box below contains a sample statement of a competency-based orientation tool for an intra-aortic balloon pump. The nurse manager works closely with the nurse educator or clinical specialist to delineate competencies, to schedule educational programs, and to facilitate the nurse's patient assignment to accommodate skill acquisition and mastery.

Other options available to the nurse manager to support continuing education growth in the critical care unit are to establish a unit-based clinical practice committee and data resource group. A unit-based clinical practice committee is composed of the nurse manager, nurse educator or clinical specialist, and interested staff with all levels of experience. Its purpose is to review current practices, and to recommend and outline nursing care procedures as new equipment and technology are introduced.

A data resource group is a group of staff who are acquiring advanced PDMS skills to function as resources for other nurses. This group makes recommendations to the nurse manager and HIS specialist during the evaluation and installation of a PDMS.

These are only a few ways to involve staff in implementing new technology and knowledge in the critical care unit. The nurse manager who carefully considers the benefits and risks of new technology, and who consistently communicates with staff and others, maximizes the great contributions of the evolving technology and knowledge to critical care.

SAMPLE STATEMENTS
A COMPETENCY-BASED ORIENTATION TOOL
INTRA-AORTIC BALLOON PUMP

Competency: To safely care for the patient with an intra-aortic balloon pump.

Assesses cannulated extremity for color, temperature, motion, sensation, pulses, and capillary refill.
Demonstrates proper timing of balloon inflation and deflation.
Identifies dangers associated with early or late timing of inflation or deflation.
Identifies possible complications of intra-aortic balloon counterpulsation.

Developed by Kristine J. Peterson RN MSN CCRN.
Used with permission from Georgetown University Hospital, Washington, DC, 1990.

CONCLUSION

This chapter describes the effects of today's technological evolution in critical care. The nurse manager's role is to organize the safe introduction of new technology into the critical care unit. The critical care nurse manager looks forward to using new knowledge to improve patient care, increase staff morale, encourage nurse recruitment and retention, and effect a favorable public image of the institution.

Potential problems associated with new technology are critically analyzed. These include iatrogenic patient injury, nurse overdependence, increased liability, stress, and depersonalized patient care. The nurse manager emphasizes the benefits of technology and knowledge, safeguards against problems, seeks feedback from staff, and diligently pursues resources available in the hospital. With these strategies, the nurse manager creates an environment to assist staff in their mission to promote patient comfort, safety, and recovery from critical illness.

REFERENCES

1. ASHP Council on Clinical Affairs: ASHP statement on the pharmacy and therapeutics committee, American Journal of Hospital Pharmacy 43(11):2841, 1986.
2. Boller J, editor: 1989 proceedings: making the critical difference, Newport Beach, Calif, 1989, American Association of Critical Care Nurses.
3. Bream T and Schapiro A: Nurse-physician networks: a focus for retention, Nursing Management 20(5):74, 1989.
4. Brimm JE: Computers in critical care, Critical Care Nursing Quarterly 9(4):53, 1987.
5. Clochesy JM: Introducing new technology: biomedical engineers and staff nurse involvement, Critical Care Nursing Quarterly 9(4):64, 1987.
6. Dickerson M: Product evaluation: a key to controlling costs, Nursing Economics 5(2):60, 1987.
7. Duff I: Street smarts in hospital purchasing, Journal of Cardiovascular Nursing 2(2):4, 1989.
8. Dunbar SB: Perspectives on critical care nursing: the international arena, Heart and Lung 16(1):18A, 1987.
9. Edwards TJ and Gurley LT: Pro and con: staff development vs in-service training: Applied Radiology 16(8):24, 1987.
10. Enger EL, Mason J, and Holm K: The product evaluation process: making objective decisions, Dimensions of Critical Care Nursing 6(6):351, 1987.
11. Groom D: Automation of the medical chart: Computers in Healthcare 8(14):22, 1987.
12. Hartshorn JC: Reality and vision, Heart and Lung 17(3):29A, 1988.
13. Hicks L, Bopp K, and Speck R: Forecasting demand for hospital services in an unstable environment, Nursing Economics 5(6):304, 1987.
14. Lagler R: Computer technology in the ICU: part 1: the possibilities, Indiana Medicine 79(8):676, 1986.
15. Lagler R: Computer technology in the ICU: part 2: the limitations and precautions, Indiana Medicine 79(9):756, 1986.
16. Malila FM: Caring in a technologic age: education for adaptation, Focus on Critical Care 14(3):21, 1987.

17. Milholland K: Patient data management systems (PDMS): computer technology for critical care nurses, Computers in Nursing 6(6):237, 1988.
18. Pfettsher-Hopper S: Dimensions in critical care. In Holloway NM, editor: Nursing the critically ill adult, ed 3, New York, 1988, Addison-Wesley Publishing Co.
19. Price MS and Wujcik D: Product evaluation in critical care, Critical Care Nursing 8(2):8, 1988.
20. Quaal SJ: Foreward, Critical Care Nursing Quarterly 9(4):7, 1987.
21. Roberts M, Minnick A, Ginzberg E, and Curran C: The commonwealth fund report on the nursing shortage, New York, 1989, The Commonwealth Fund.
22. Schank MJ and Doney LD: General purpose microcomputer software: new tools for nursing professionals, Nursing Management 18(7):26, 1987.
23. Searle L: Milestones, Heart and Lung 18(3):23A, 1989.
24. Sinclair V: High technology in critical care: implications for nursing's role and practice, Focus on Critical Care 15(4):36, 1988.
25. Staggers N: Using computers in nursing, Computers in Nursing 6(4):164, 1988.
26. Stefanchik MF: Point-of-care information systems: prioritizing bedside applications, Computers in Healthcare 8(4):42, 1987.
27. Stewart SL and Vitello-Cicciu JM: Designing a competency-based orientation program for the care of cardiac surgical patients, Journal of Cardiovascular Nursing 3(3):34, 1989.
28. Taylor PL, editor: How computers are improving patient care, Health Technology 2(6):224, 1988.
29. Tomasik K: QA update: nursing and technology, Quarterly Review Bulletin 14(8):254, 1988.
30. Whitney L and Holm K: Nursing care delivery: into the 1990s, Dimensions of Critical Care Nursing 6(5):259, 1987.

Chapter 16

STRATEGIC PLANNING

Nancy J. Gantz

Airline pilots have a strategic goal with a well thought-out plan before they even move the plane. Whether a plane is flown one hundred miles or one thousand miles, the pilot is held accountable for following a charted course. Like the pilot, the critical care nurse manager needs a plan to chart unit direction successfully. Both pilot and nurse manager engage in strategic planning to achieve goals. This chapter describes the process of strategic planning and how a unidirectional focus helps the nurse manager achieve short- and long-term unit goals. Through strategic planning, nurse managers help staff define standards of care, quality outcomes, and parameters that address professional accountability. A case study demonstrates the implementation of strategic planning at the unit level.

AN OVERVIEW OF STRATEGIC PLANNING

Strategic planning is a means by which the nurse manager directs and evaluates the work of the unit. Steps used in the process facilitate participative management, management by objectives, fiscal accountability, and positive patient outcomes. The process helps the nurse manager think through and create a vision of the future with staff input. Strategic planning provides a mechanism by which each unit has a master plan that directs future action. Events of the hospital, the community, and the nation, and changes in the medical and nursing professions—and health care in general—may change and redirect the unit strategic plan.

Strategic planning involves initiative, innovation, and risk-taking. It is consumer driven and encompasses long-term goals directed at providing a service. Christopher[1] defined strategic planning and stated: "It determines how the game will be played or the campaign fought. It's intellectual and imperial, theoretical, and practical. It motivates commitment and common action." Because strategy can win wars, elections, and ball games, nurse managers need to understand how to devise strategies.

Marketing plays a critical part in the success of developing and implementing the strategic plan. Convincing staff of the importance of planning becomes the manager's first task. The nurse manager identifies who the unit "consumers" are, and what they want. Physicians, patients, and families are consumers of critical care nursing service, and they collectively want quality patient care. Marketing a strategic plan directed at this goal is clearly beneficial to all. Strategic planning prepares for the unexpected, encourages staff to be systematic thinkers, and facilitates cooperation between all health care providers. Strategic planning plays a vital part in forecasting, making projections, and creating future vision for the critical care unit.

One of the pitfalls encountered by the nurse manager in this era of cutbacks and short staffing is spending excessive time resolving daily crises and conflicts that occur in the day-to-day unit operations. This expenditure of time and energy can overwhelm a manager, who then is always reacting to external stimuli instead of planning and achieving goals. The risk here is that both manager and staff will loose sight of the unit's focus—providing quality critical care to patients and their families.

Successful strategic planning requires a forum for group discussion. The nurse manager is responsible for assuring that the goals developed and written by the group remain congruous with those of the department and the institution. The nurse manager facilitates group interaction and encourages all staff to participate. If everyone involved in patient care delivery is involved in goal setting, commitment results. These individuals are then called *stakeholders* because they have a vested interest in the process and outcome of the overall plan. Commitment from staff and support from management is necessary to insure plan success. Using strategic planning is a *result-oriented* approach to achieving outcomes.

Within the strategic planning process, goals and objectives are separated so staff see the steps that need to be followed to reach the outcomes. Stakeholders use the mission to identify the goals; these become the unit specific outcomes. Objectives are used as steps to reach this. The strategic plan then becomes the global picture on which the staff focus to insure future progress. Strategic planning is not a *react-and-adapt* approach, if it is well thought-out and documented, and it produces workable goals.

Mason[4] developed a strategic planning process to demonstrate how the nurse manager actually applies theory to practice. This particular process was originally tested in a nonprofit community hospital and found to be highly effective. Figure 16-1 schematically depicts the planning process.

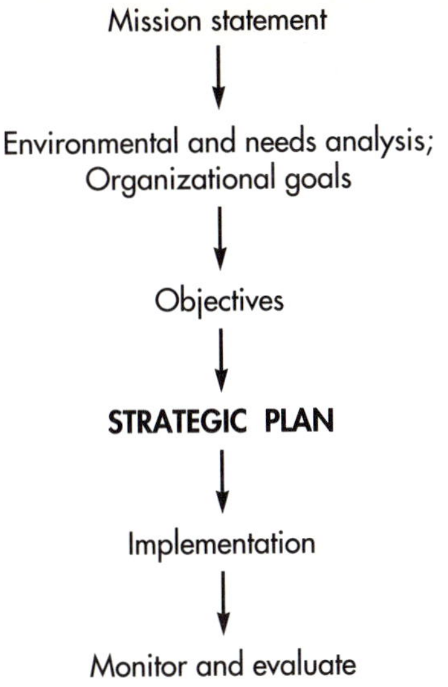

```
        Mission statement
               │
               ▼
Environmental and needs analysis;
      Organizational goals
               │
               ▼
          Objectives
               │
               ▼
        STRATEGIC PLAN
               │
               ▼
        Implementation
               │
               ▼
      Monitor and evaluate
```

FIGURE 16-1. The planning process.

Webber and Peters[6] wrote that an unstated strategy cannot be tested or contested and is likely, therefore, to be weak. This means that the nurse manager is responsible for insuring that this plan is operationalized, well structured, and focused on outcomes.

UNIT CULTURE

The purpose of an organization is to provide a common ground upon which employees can work together toward shared objectives. All organizations are structured in a way that facilitates this process. Part of this structure evolves from the product or services delivered to consumers. Each organization has a culture that influences its employees. The culture also affects the way the organization operates and plans. For example, an individual can learn much about a critical care unit by simply looking at the patient type, the number of patient days, and the staffing plan.

Thomas and colleagues[5] said, "Climate is a measure of individual perceptions or feelings about an organization. Culture is a measure of common thoughts, behaviors, and beliefs." Each critical care unit has a distinct climate and culture. This results from the mingling of these elements in the institution over time. The astute nurse manager recognizes this and uses the staff's shared values, habits, and attitudes when considering the strategic plan. The culture and climate in the unit that provides quality patient care is often noticeable and is identified as a positive, desirable trait. In units without a positive and colleagial climate and culture, quality patient care is not at the forefront of staff efforts. The nurse manager who is new to a unit with a less-than-positive culture recognizes that encouraging staff involvement in the strategic planning process can help reverse this. Staff input at all levels helps effect this change. Staff can do this by working on the mission statement or making suggestions about changing policies and procedures that no longer reflect practice. Although the personality makeup of the staff contribute to the culture and climate, a manager focuses energy on facts and not emotional responses to identified issues when planning for change.

The nurse manager recognizes who the formal and informal leaders are in the unit and uses the assessment of power bases to understand both the unit climate and culture. Power is having the information, support, and resources needed to get others to do what you want them to do. Physicians exert a tremendous amount of power and influence in hospitals. The nurse manager recognizes this and uses all of the power available to her to achieve goals.

The nurse manager gathers data that provide information, which results in power. A nurse manager who wants to exert influence for future change understands power bases, considers the personalities in the unit, and assesses the collective skills of staff. Sometimes, an experienced nurse manager new to a unit can read the existing policies and procedures and gain an understanding of staff strengths and weaknesses. These are related to the focus and wording of these documents. A mature staff requires a less stringent or specific policy. A staff that is not cohesive requires rigid and precise policy to insure adherence. Thomas and colleagues[5] stated,

> The concept of culture is an important tool for understanding and changing the behavior of individuals in organizations.... To relate the two concepts [of culture and climate], when an employee's personal beliefs and values are consistent with the prevailing culture, he tends to perceive the climate as "good." However, a perception of a "poor" climate results when the beliefs and values are in conflict.

Through the use of strategic planning, the nurse manager fosters an environment where a good climate goes hand in hand with a good culture.

THE CHANGING SCENE

In the late 1960s hospitals were like "cottage industries"—each hospital was self-sufficient and each provided multiple services. However, this is no longer true. Health care changes have been rapid and ongoing since the national implementation of diagnosis related groups (DRGs). Hospitals have closed, census figures fluctuate greatly, complexity and acuity of patient mix continue to rise, organizations have changed their modes of operation, mergers and acquisitions are common, rationing of critical care services is openly discussed, who gets the critical care bed is debated, and ethical issues abound. Macrodynamic trends caused great changes. To cut costs and improve efficiency, hospital specialization is increasing.

All of this change necessitated the need to look at more cost-effective ways to operate. In this environment, programs that cost money will receive great scrutiny, and will more than likely be denied. The thrust continues—to do more with less. Statistics that affect strategic planning include the fact that the population 75 years of age or over is projected to increase four times as fast as the average annual rate of increase for persons under 65 years of age.[2] These individuals will more than likely require critical care services in their lifetimes. Despite the difficulties associated with these issues, the nurse manager is challenged to incorporate these constraints into the strategic plan.

Although the public is demanding maximum critical care services with minimal risk and suffering for the critically ill, a balance with reality will emerge; that is valuing saving lives must be balanced with appropriate decisions about quality-of-life issues. Ethical decision-making will need reinforcement at all levels. Staff need to see the broader social issues that demand that sufficient resources be available to provide quality care to patients who will survive. Strategic planning helps the nurse manager deal with the changes and challenges presented by new reimbursement methods, increasing competition for health care dollars, advancing technology, and expanding roles of health care facilities.

INTERPRETING CHANGE TO STAFF

Change is a given in this current era of cost containment. Policies and practices are frequently rewritten in an attempt to provide cost-effective, efficient care. The nurse manager interprets this process of ongoing change to staff in a positive light and accepts change as an opportunity for growth. When change is anticipated, the nurse manager informs staff of the facts as soon as the information is available, to give them time to consider the change. Concern for the staff's response to ongoing change builds their confidence in the nurse manager. This confidence is important to effective strategic planning.

Both the manager and staff need coping strategies to work in an environment of ongoing change. The manager must be available to listen and intervene when necessary, and to make sure there is support for staff problems. The nurse manager becomes a facilitator who interprets staff behavior and determines when staff are having difficulty coping. The manager then ensures that staff are getting appropriate rest breaks, creates new opportunities for rewards, and most importantly, keeps communication networks intact. During this phase of rapid transition, the nurse manager uses strategic planning as a mechanism for directing efforts in a positive manner, focusing on goals, strengths, and values of critical care practice.

MISSION STATEMENT

The mission statement of the unit is centered on patient care. It incorporates the hospital's mission and philosophy with those of the nursing department, and is specific to unit service. This mission statement is developed by staff and communicated to all. The mission statement identifies a purpose that builds institutional strength and supports the specific unit objectives. The mission statement reflects the positive, progressive, innovative, and caring environment of the critical care unit. It expresses what makes the unit unique and valuable to the hospital and to the health care system. The statement reflects sound business practices, recognizes the community it serves, focuses on excellence and service in patient care, and identifies key concepts that foster a positive working environment, including mutual respect, trust, thoughtfulness, accountability, compassion, and ethical standards.

An overly broad mission statement makes planning difficult, while a narrow statement overlooks important needs and opportunities in the unit. A mission statement distinguishes one institution from another through the provisions and services outlined in the statement. For example a statement can read: "The mission of this critical care unit is to meet the needs of the sick or injured and their families in a quality-driven, cost-effective, and outcome-centered environment that recognizes the values, dignity, and needs of employees." The focus of this statement is twofold: patients and staff are given equal consideration. Thus, this type of mission statement indicates the interrelationship of the two parties—care receiver and care giver. This statement can be expanded to include more information on health care outcomes, quality of care, and unit financial solvency, if desired.

The nurse manager realizes it takes time to develop a mission statement that incorporates all desired elements. This statement is not the idea of the nurse manager, it comes from the staff. Group work is needed. The nurse manager assures that a representative cross section of the unit participates in a steering committee. Personnel of every level become stakeholders in this process, which insures the output will adequately reflect the purpose of the entire unit. The nurse manager can suggest that the mission statement focus briefly on a specialized type of care and service provided for the community, if appropriate.

This steering committee needs some structure and guidelines for success. An assessment of the current position of the unit leads to analyzing the position desired in the future. In other words, the gap between actual and desired is assessed and used to develop the plan. This is not easy. Staff need encouragement and examples to help them identify where they personally and professionally want to be in five years. Similarly, vision about the unit takes the same type of effort. Meetings are held regularly, and the minutes of all meetings posted for staff review. Any drafts of statements, goals, or objectives require staff input, feedback, and discussion. The committee makes no unilateral decisions. Once a draft is accepted by the staff, the committee moves to implementing it by moving to the next step. The mission statement needs to be reevaluated yearly and rewritten if the focus or philosophy changes. The quality of a mission statement is the hallmark of good management. The mission statement is completed before strategic planning is begun, because the mission statement provides a focus for the overall plan.

IDENTIFYING GOALS

The mission statement and the goals of the organization and department should be given to the staff, with instructions to incorporate them into the unit plan. Next comes the planning phase, in which institutional strengths, weaknesses, opportunities, and threats are identified. These are unique to the institution and unrelated to external factors. An example would be the mission of an institution that services the inner city poor: to provide care, and to reach out and address community needs. This type of institution provides nondiscriminatory service (strength), usually has a limited budget (weakness), welcomes innovative ideas that provide community health care (opportunity), and tends to be subjected to media criticism (threat). A critical care nurse manager in this type of institution analyzes and considers these factors when developing the unit strategic plan.

Input from other managers, patients, families, physicians, and staff nurses is needed. The nurse manager also seeks out and communicates with ancillary departments that provide services to the unit, and with other units directly affected by the critical care unit. For example, if the unit receives patients from the post-anesthesia care unit and transfers patients to surgical units, both of these areas are sought out. As the manager of a critical care unit, this process insures a greater understanding of the way care is provided and perceived, and could be called "having a finger on the pulse of the unit." The information gathered is sorted and stored to provide direction for areas needing change. The nurse manager now asks the immediate supervisor to provide hospital and nursing department goals for the future. Before the unit can develop specific goals, the broader goals defined by upper management must be incorporated into the unit-specific plan. These upper-level goals are posted and openly discussed with staff, so staff also know the direction the institution and department are heading. During the planning process, the manager considers the various roles assumed by staff and other personnel who provide care in the unit.

The next step is to develop unit-specific goals and objectives. A goal is a generalized statement of what the unit would like to obtain within a specific time frame. These are both short- and long-range. Immediate goals are those obtainable within the year. Short-range goals are achieved during a one-to-three-year time frame; long-range goals can take six years to come to fruition. When goals are written, each is placed in its respective category of immediate, short- or long-range. The nurse manager introduces the concept of playing out scenarios to make sure each goal is placed in a time frame where it is likely to be achieved. Goals on a time line, when identified with objectives, make it possible to assess progress. The different levels of goals provide realistic stepping stones for staff. Each health care team member plays a contributing role in the strategic planning process. Goals take on a different direction when assigned to various individuals. Staff grow with responsibility and need encouragement to work on a plan when they have had limited previous experience. The nurse manager constantly assesses the planning process and identifies when staff are floundering. The manager then acts as a coach, offering support so the staff can move ahead.

OBJECTIVES AND STRATEGIES

Objectives used to meet goals must be clear, specific, measurable, realistic, and obtainable. As each objective is written, the nurse manager looks critically at the feasibility and makes suggestions for needed modifications. Only achievable goals relevant to the overall plan are used. This step is achieved by starting with a small group of key staff. This group of stakeholders develops a preliminary draft. Then strategies are developed that put guidelines and policy into place. Before deciding on the actual goals, all alternatives are discussed, and the path that leads to the most desired outcomes is used. A draft of this is presented to the staff collectively at a staff meeting, suggestions are made, and the group meets again later to finalize the draft.

Pretesting the alternatives comes next. The developed objectives are pretested to validate their effectiveness. The operational plan needs appropriate support systems in the form of budget justification. And finally, the entire strategic planning process is reviewed and evaluated. Once the plan is written, the goals are reevaluated quarterly and posted in the unit for all staff to review. The nurse manager considers the value of discussing specific aspects of the plan at staff meetings and insures that all physicians and other health care providers know what the goals are. As each objective is enacted, the goal is reached, and understanding of the purpose of strategic planning is enhanced. This provides greater credibility for the nurse manager and expands her power base. The group presents this revised strategic plan at a subsequent staff meeting for staff approval. The nurse manager ensures sufficient communication about the plan. A copy is posted and returning staff who were absent are asked by the nurse manager to read the plan. A copy of this plan is shared with the immediate nursing supervisor, physicians, other appropriate administrative staff, and ancillary departments impacted by the strategic plan.

The outcome of the strategic plan depends on the values and beliefs within the culture. The manager who focuses on providing a caring environment and emphasizes the unit mission, goals, and objectives contributes to the long-term survival of the unit and ultimately the organization. Once a plan is written, the nurse manager assesses patient care outcomes, and when problems are identified with individual staff practice, the manager rapidly moves in, provides guidance or education so goals are met. This intervention is needed to keep the direction focused and aimed at outcomes. Nurse managers do need a flight plan just as a pilot does in order to direct the unit. Strategic planning provides a mechanism for developing this plan.

PRODUCTIVITY AND THE FUTURE

Donovan and Lewis[3] stated: "It is said that nurses are clearly more productive and cost effective than is generally acknowledged." Productivity means getting away from the short-term, quick-fix methods used in the past, and focusing on the long-term effects of change. In progressive organizations, nursing productivity is viewed as a challenge and an opportunity, with all staff working smarter, not harder. High productivity is associated with high staff morale. A nurse manager who understands the concept, "feeding opportunity and starving problems," can achieve all of these goals with effective strategic planning.

Critical care managers use strategic planning to increase the effective use of resources that facilitate patient care outcomes. Managers need to have astute business skills to survive in the current environment, since no one is exempt from external pressures to cut costs. A focus on research to keep up with trends in high technology helps the manager and staff adapt to change. Reimbursement, available resources, reorganization, the state and federal governments, and society will play a part in reshaping critical care units. A savvy manager is aware of these changes and faces the future knowing the unit can adapt and grow with the times because of the influence and experience all staff have with strategic planning.

Case Study: Moving the Unit Forward

You are the nurse manager of a 12-bed mixed medical and coronary care unit. Because the unit is in a small community hospital that transfers difficult patients, most patients do not require high technology invasive therapy. However, the hospital wants to expand and specialize in cardiac care. The revised mission statement includes this information, and a cardiovascular surgeon specializing in laser angioplasties has just been recruited and has joined the staff. You think services in the unit may need to be expanded to include the use of intra-aortic balloon pumping. You have discussed this with the medical director and the nursing director, both of whom are supportive.

You, as the nurse manager, initially start the strategic planning process by sharing the revised hospital mission statement with staff. Feedback and input about the potential impact of this change is solicited. The concept of balloon pumping is introduced. A task force is formed of the medical director, the nurse manager, the instructor, and five interested staff nurses. This task force revises the unit mission statement to be congruous with the hospital statement. This committee starts meeting weekly to discuss planning and identifies that balloon pumping is very likely to be instituted. The logistics are discussed: how this will be done and who will be responsible for pump-setting changes, since there are no house staff. This discussion is taken to staff for their input. The staff determines that use of the intra-aortic balloon pump will facilitate effective cardiac care. The staff become excited about the challenge.

Before going ahead with any further action, the task force evaluates the current practice in the unit. To generate discussion, the nurse manager presents a scenario: "In 12 months, a patient is admitted for routine angioplasty. During the procedure, major vessel occlusion occurs. What happens to this patient?"

Without ballooning it is surmised that the patient will not survive long enough to be transferred for coronary bypass surgery. The staff believe that with ballooning and helicopter transport services, this patient would have a chance of surviving. They conclude that the ability to provide ballooning decidedly makes a difference. Specific plans are needed to enable this staff to implement intra-aortic balloon pumping.

The task force reviews unit protocols, policies and procedures. Several would need revision, and specific standing orders and a pump protocol would need to be written. The task force feel additional dialog is needed with the cardiovascular surgeon, the laser angioplasty nurse, bioclinical engineering, and central stores — departments identified in a brainstorming session in which the group recognized that they would be directly involved in providing care for this type of patient.

After discussion with these ancillary services, the task force brings additional information to the staff. If the program moves ahead, the items identified in the box on the next page will be addressed.

After staff review the objectives, many questions about the feasibility of all staff attending the proposed all-day workshop on balloon pumping arise. Alternatives are quickly discarded, given the intensive nature of this invasive technique. Therefore the staff requests that monetary compensation be included in the plan, to ensure that all staff attend. The nurse manager was initially reluctant to do this because staff were already overworked. However, since it had been openly discussed at staff meetings, the manager agrees that if the plan is implemented, all staff will be assigned a workshop day and paid for that day.

The nurse manager brings this information to the attention of the chief nurse executive. Support for implementing the plan is obtained. An operational plan and a budget is now needed. Two staff members of the task force, the instructor, and the nurse manager work together to determine the monies needed for balloons, two pumps, and an all-day workshop for all staff. This subgroup scrutinizes the plan to insure that it is complete and feasible as written. The group develops a flyer that outlines the proposed new service. This is inserted in the hospital newsletter and sent to all physicians on staff.

The expected outcome of this type of strategic planning includes the fact that all staff would have the necessary knowledge to care for patients on intra-aortic pumps. Additional factors that are identified include writing quality assurance monitors and providing follow-up discussion after the first patient was cared for by the staff.

CONCLUSION

Strategic planning is critical to the success of any unit in the hospital system. Strategic planning involves initiative and risk-taking. It is proactive and directed. Strategic planning includes identifying, formalizing, implementing, and evaluating unit plans on an ongoing basis. These plans demonstrate specific areas of unit growth. The process provides a potential far beyond what could have been imagined ten years ago. Nurse managers committed to strategic planning expend energy communicating, creating, encouraging, and reevaluating performance so that goals are met by target dates. Strategic planning is a statement about the output efforts of the individual unit. Future planning challenges all critical care

OBJECTIVES AND TIME FRAME

Objectives	Time frame
A literature review on pumping	One month
Cost-benefit analysis of two pump brands	Two months
Staff inservice	Nine months
Protocol and standing orders with medical board approval	Six months
Written policy and procedure	Eight months
Revision of flow sheet	Twelve months
Standard care plan	Five months
Family information sheet	Seven months

managers, and using the strategic planning process puts the manager in a position of power and control: Real, measurable accomplishments are identified. Maraldo[3a] said, "The time is now for nursing to assume responsibility . . . to exert badly needed leadership for shaping a bold new vision for healthcare." Strategic planning is the process used to achieve goals.

REFERENCES

1. Christopher NF: Management of the 1980s, Englewood Cliffs, NJ, 1980, Prentice Hall, Inc.
2. Coile R and Grossman R: Tomorrow's macrotrends, Healthcare Forum Journal, (6):51, 1988.
3. Donovan M and Lewis G: Increasing productivity and decreasing costs: the value of RNs, Journal of Nursing Administration. 17(9), 1987.
3a. "Executive Director Wire." Winter 1989. NLN, NY. Pg. 2.
4. Mason SA: The multiple hospital development process and strategic planning, Hospital & Health Services Administration 26(6):60, 1981.
5. Thomas C et al: Measuring and interpreting organizational culture, Journal of Nursing Administration 20(6):17, 1990.
6. Webber JB and Peters JP: Strategic thinking—new frontier for hospital management, Chicago: American Hospital Association, 1983.

SUGGESTED READINGS:

1. Bice M: Employee orientations should stress core values, Hospitals, (3):72, 1990.

Chapter 17

BUDGETING CONCEPTS

Carole Birdsall

Nursing budgets account for 25 to 50 percent of the hospital's total budget. Since the enactment of federal legislation in the early 1980s to curtail expenditures for health care, hospitals have moved to reduce spending and control costs. Nurse managers are responsible for monitoring the way dollars are spent and for creating cost-effective strategies. Thus, there is pressure from all sources to find ways to increase both the efficiency and effectiveness of the way money is spent and budgets are kept.

Budgets are used to plan and control resource utilization. These resources include manpower, major equipment, and disposable items used in everyday bedside practice. The nurse manager understands how supplies and equipment are used by practitioners, and provides vital input into the budget process. The nurse manager is crucial to the effective utilization of funds.[2] The budget is a plan of the resources (personnel and supplies) needed to accomplish unit goals. The nurse manager can best articulate the plan for these needed resources; when numbers are attached to the plan, this plan becomes the budget. The reason nurse managers are involved in budgeting and fiscal planning is their expertise in planning for patient care.

Most hospitals have sophisticated departments that deal exclusively with set monetary functions. For example, the accounting department usually collects and pays bills, keeps its own records and provides analyses about the financial state of the institution. The finance department provides long-term projections, obtains funds needed to operate, develops specific rules and regulations for various departments, deals with reimbursement issues, and decides the in-house policy on departmental expenditures.

Historically, there was little interaction between nursing and other financial departments. Times are changing, however. Nursing departments and nurse managers are becoming increasingly sophisticated; they provide invaluable insight for finance departments. Thus, the need for understanding budgets now rests at the unit level. This chapter will provide a basic introduction to budget concepts and practices. A nurse manager with limited budget experience or a practitioner who wants to understand the budget process will gain broad knowledge about budget preparation. A case study will be used to help explain specific aspects of each type of budget.

TYPES OF BUDGETS

Budgeting is a skill acquired by spending time doing it and by understanding the basic concepts. Much like using sophisticated technology in bedside practice, budgeting for the nurse manager requires attention to detail and the acquisition of new terms. Hospitals divide the budget into two distinct entities: the capital budget and the operating budget. The *capital budget* is concerned with the acquisition of major equipment; the *operating budget* is directed at the day-to-day costs of running the unit. The operating budget is further broken down into two subbudgets: the personnel budget and the nonpersonnel operating budget. The personnel budget is that portion of the budget spent for salary. The nonpersonnel operating budget refers to the money used for all the other operating costs except major equipment and labor costs. Both the capital and operating budgets are planned and executed in different ways. Thus, discussion for each will be separate.

Capital Budget

The capital budget is the easier budget to understand. Costs due to acquisition of new equipment or services, real property, and architectural renovations are considered capital expenditures. New equipment is defined by most institutions as major purchases that cost more than a preestablished amount (usually $200 to $500) and that have a life expectancy of more than one year. (The amount varies from state to state and from institution to institution.) *Equipment* includes major moveable items, such as cardiac monitors and intra-aortic balloon pumps, and discrete items, such as new magnetic resonance scanners that are installed and considered fixed capital items.

Real property includes land, buildings, and other discrete real estate owned outright by the institution. Buses, vans, trucks, schools, affiliated health maintenance organizations (HMOs), sister institutions, apartment buildings, and other major properties are considered real property in the capital budget.

Architectural renovations of existing space, modifications to the current space, and additions to owned property also fall under capital budgeting. The term *plant* is often used to refer specifically to the physical building. Thus, a renovation to the plant means a renovation to some part of the hospital building.

CAPITAL APPROVAL PROCESS

Some states legislate the approval process that a hospital must use before spending capital money for major renovations or for adding new services. The cost of renovation must exceed a certain amount (usually $25,000 to $100,000) before this system is used. (This figure also varies from state to state, but in regulated states, any renovation exceeding the limit must wait for approval.) For example, a renovation of the critical care nurse manager's office costing $9000 would not require state approval. However, a renovation of the critical care treatment room that involved the installation of an operating room table complete with lights, a gas scavenge system, an x-ray tray and a C-arm for radiology procedures, costing $230,000, would require state approval. This approval is needed even if the money for the renovation is donated by a rich patron.

The following box provides a schematic outline of the capital approval process for renovations. Note that a time line indicating months depicts an approximate 12-month time period from initial in-house budget approval to the beginning of renovation. This reflects the minimum amount of time that any renovation would take in states where capital expenditures are regulated.

The state approval may include an appeal process, a community hearing, and a variance passed by a special board functioning in this capacity. For example, some community boards decide if and when an institution can purchase a new computerized tomography (CT) scanner or add a helicopter transport service in a particular geographical area. Any new major projects, such as the addition of a

---

CAPITAL APPROVAL PROCESS FOR RENOVATIONS

		Months
Cost < $9,999	**Cost > $10,000**	3
↓	↓	
In House List	State approval	6
	↓	
	Community Board or Health Department	9
	↓	
	Justification warranted	
	↓	
	Approval	12
	↓	
	Renovation would begin	12

cardiac rehabilitation program, are considered capital investments. This is related to a change in existing services and the long-term benefit the institution will derive from the addition. All major service changes, especially in highly regulated states, must go through a capital purchase approval process.

Capital budgets give rise to long-lived assets whose benefits accrue over a long period of time. In other words, capital purchases are future-oriented. Think of this as you would your own home. Each time you fix, improve, and renovate some aspect of your home, you increase the real property value. This is the same for capital budgets in the hospital. The capital budget is used to plan the institution's future investments in plant and equipment.

THE CAPITAL PLANNING PROCESS

The process for planning and buying capital items is also different. Most institutions have a one-, a three-, and a five-year plan. As each year passes, an additional year is added to the end of the capital budget. One major problem associated with capital budgets is predicting what new equipment is coming on the market and how vital it will be for the unit to own this equipment. Each service usually resolves this by using tradeoffs from other existing items in the capital budget. However, this system of tradeoffs is limited to items on the existing capital budget and has nothing to do with the operating budget.

Capital purchases often require written justification. It is in this realm that an astute critical care nurse manager is a definite asset to long-range planning. The nurse manager who attends major critical care conventions, sees new equipment, and reads about new items in research journals remains current in her field; this manager knows about equipment before it really is needed. As soon as the nurse manager envisions how the new technology will be used in the unit, that item is then costed out and a written justification of the item's necessity is prepared. When capital budget planning comes around, this new technology item is then added to the existing capital cue list, even though true unit application may not be necessary for two or more years.

Capital budget planning involves exploring and defining the benefits of the new equipment, including improved patient care, enhanced patient safety, lower operating costs, and reduced lengths of stay. Any item that can be justified by one of these benefits is usually purchased. However, Stevens[3] advised that stating how many man-hours will be saved with the equipment be avoided because the wage budget could be cut according to the savings predicted.

When planning equipment or projects, the cost of outright purchase, delivery fees, installation, maintenance contracts, added personnel, training, and other hidden items are identified. These hidden costs include potential expenses to other departments that interface with nursing. For example, when the nursing department buys a new type of hypo/hyperthermia machine that requires new probes, the central stores department responsible for buying, sterilizing, and storing the probes is consulted. If more money or personnel is needed, it is added to the capital budget. Each of these costs must be justified. The justification for new items often requires the cost of repair for existing equipment, the necessity for the service to be provided, how and when the equipment is used, and who will use the equipment.[4]

For projects, capital costs are only incurred at the inception of the program. For example, if the unit expanded services for temporary pacemaker insertions to the entire hospital, the cost of the radiology C-arm for the treatment room and any other added equipment would be part of the original capital purchase. Any additional equipment for this project would not be a part of capital planning for at least three years. Thus if a computer was needed next year for billing, its cost would be approved in this year's budget for next year. If the manager forgot to put the computer in the budget, the unit would have to do without it and wait three years.

Consideration is given to item impact on the personnel and nonpersonnel operating budget. For example, if the nurse manager requests new cardiac monitors that require a special type of ECG paper or electrodes, the cost of these new items is determined and included in the supply budget.[2] Whenever additional personnel are needed to operate new equipment, this also is identified. The project costs for inservicing the new item, including the costs of inservicing the bioclinical engineering staff who will maintain the equipment, is built into the budget.

Capital equipment is requested on special forms reserved specifically for this purpose. These equipment forms require a description and estimated cost of each item; a proposed vendor; the use of the item; the nature of the capital item such as replacement, renovation or addition; the year needed; the justification; and often a priority ranking (See Table 17-1, p. 283). Since all capital purchases are considered together, the nursing department is usually all part of one budget. The astute critical care nurse manager is aware that the competition for capital monies is fierce; thus she uses clear, concise, clinically-based, easily understood language in preparing the budget. Administrators understand state-of-the-art high-technology equipment when they know how it will be used. Thus, the manager prepares the justification with these laypersons in mind.

The nurse manager involved with capital planning also recognizes the need to keep a chronological list of all equipment purchased. The date of purchase is extremely useful in planning replacement as equipment wears out. Generally speaking, each institution is guided by in-house rules usually determined by the purchasing department about planning replacement equipment. A good rule of thumb is to break equipment replacement down into five, seven, and ten year cycles. A five-year cycle is for mechanical devices that get heavy wear and tear, such as wheelchairs and bed scales. Seven-year cycles are used for intravenous pumps and other type of high-volume, high-use electrical equipment. The ten-year cycle is reserved for expensive equipment that is carefully maintained, such as cardiac monitors.

DEPRECIATION

As stated earlier, capital costs benefit the institution in the future. This is because capital items can be depreciated over time. *Depreciation* is an on-paper reduction in value of fixed assets. For example, as a building gets older, the building is worth less money even if the real estate is worth more money. Whenever a capital asset loses usefulness or gets older, the value decreases. Depreciation is the way the institution's records demonstrate that equipment and buildings wear out. The amount of depreciation is based on the item's lifespan, its salvage value, and its age when no longer useful. Depreciation is kept on a balance sheet. This process has strategic value to the institution, and thus a clear distinction is made between capital costs and operating costs.[1]

Through depreciation, capital costs can be converted to operating expenses. For example, if the unit purchases an intravenous pump that is used 300 days a year for five years, the $2000 purchase price is depreciated over the five years based on the amount of use and salvage value, if any, of the pump at the end of this time. This is not necessary at the unit level unless a cost per use is calculated into the patient charge. Furthermore, the institution, not the unit, derives the benefit, so from the manager's perspective, depreciation is nice to know about, but really irrelevant to budget planning.

Thus, the nurse manager plans capital equipment as new innovations and technology emerge. Justification is written and stored until the capital budget annual update. Unit goals, changes in services, and state-of-the-art practices influence planning. An inventory of equipment is kept and used to update and plan future purchases.

Operating Budgets

All operating budgets function in one-year cycles corresponding to the hospital's fiscal year, which may or may not be a calendar year. Each year is divided into four quarters of three months each. Unlike capital costs and budgets, operating costs and budgets are ongoing, with expenses spread out over the length of the budget period. Thus the operating budget is related to the current period of time and, therefore, is focused on current costs. Institutions usually plan the budget six or more months in advance of the fiscal year. Some institutions use ongoing budgets, in which this month's budget is dropped off as they move into next month, always keeping a balance associated with twelve months of the year. Although this type of continuous budgeting is sometimes useful, it is not normally used for routine budget planning.

The budget process in hospitals includes budget planning, preparation, review, and final approval. Both budget monitoring and control become a part of the budget once it is activated. Therefore the entire process is put on a timetable so that all departments and managers know in advance what pieces of the process are due on what dates.

The operating budget tells the organization how much money it costs to maintain operations for the planned year. As mentioned earlier, this budget is divided into personnel costs and nonpersonnel operating costs. However, the nurse manager responsible for a budget associates both personnel and nonpersonnel operating budgets with individual unit costs.

The cost to operate the unit is usually expressed as the expenses of a cost center. Levine-Ariff and colleagues[2] defined *cost center* as the smallest functional unit that generates costs within an institution. For example, in some hospitals the psychiatric unit is a cost center, the obstetrical service is a combined cost center, the critical care unit is a separate cost center, and the two medical units under the direction of the same nurse manager is a single cost center. Therefore, some nursing units are not complete cost centers, because their budgets are combined with those of other similar units. For clarity, we will define the critical care nursing unit as a separate cost center.

Both expense budgets and revenue budgets are part of the budget process. Expense budgets include the personnel and nonpersonnel operating budgets. Revenue budgets will be briefly discussed at the end of this material.

THE PERSONNEL BUDGET

The personnel budget is the largest part of the operating budget and includes the salary and fringe benefit package for all employees working within the cost center. The benefit package is 23 to 30 percent of the budgeted salary and includes money for orientation, continuing education; vacation, sick and holiday pay; overtime, shift differential, experience differential; and other salary programs.

The goals associated with the personnel budget include keeping the salary scales equitable and competitive within the organization and the geographical area; attracting and retaining staff for the unit; planning for salary increases; directing and controlling utilization of the benefit package; and foreseeing and planning for staffing changes as needed.

To appreciate the complexity of planning personnel budgets, the nurse manager thinks in terms of staffing the unit. Staffing includes regular staffing, replacement staffing, emergency situations, and incremental increases. Regular staffing is based on the daily table of organization needed to provide 24-hour coverage. Replacement staffing is systematically planned for vacation, holiday, and sick call coverage. Emergency situations include contingency plans for personal emergencies or unit crises. Money must be built into the budget to pay for supplemental staff when these emergencies arise. In addition, each personnel budget projects incremental increases associated with the experience differential that may be needed before the year is over.

Table of Organization. To begin building the unit budget, the nurse manager starts with the *table of organization,* or the number of approved positions that compose the core of the regular staff. Most institutions control the table of organization. A process of position control is used by the department of human resources to prevent each cost center from hiring more than the approved number of positions for each category of staff.

The table of organization is expressed in the number of full-time equivalents (FTEs). An FTE is a hypothetical full-time position equivalent to 40 hours of work per week, or 80 hours per pay period. In institutions where nurses work 12-hour shifts, 72 hours per pay period may constitute 1 FTE. Paid hours include productive time, or hours actually worked. However, because of fringe benefits, each employee receives pay for hours not actually worked. This is called *nonproductive time* and includes vacation, sick, and holiday time. The amount of nonproductive time actually built into each budgeted FTE position varies with each institution. For budgeting purposes, the nonproductive time is an expense that must be covered by additional paid productive hours either through agency, overtime, or additional staff.

Of the FTEs on staff, there are two types of staffing positions: variable and fixed. Variable staffing positions are the bedside care givers. The number of staff needed to provide care is variable, depending on patient acuity and census. Fixed staffing positions are those personnel needed to operate a unit independent of patient census. For example, the unit clerk, the instructor, and the nurse manager all have fixed staffing positions. Fixed positions are added into the budget over position control. Since fixed positions are not usually replaced when the employee is off duty, each position is simply budgeted as 1 FTE.

A unit is considered to have a stable occupancy rate if on average the beds are occupied at least 90 percent of the time. When occupancy is considered stable, staffing and budgeting are more consistent and easier. Flexibility in staffing can be achieved by planning monies for all budgeted positions whether they are vacant or not. Another helpful strategy is to calculate the turnover rate, subtract the orientation phase from productive hours, and budget replacement staff for the projected number of vacancies and the orientation time for new hires.

For each level or category of personnel (management, staff, or ancillary) employed by the cost center, a different calculation is used to determine the fringe benefit package and wages. For example, the nurse manager with LPNs (vocational nurses) in the critical care unit prorates the shift differential for these personnel when it is different from the differential paid RNs. In fact, different categories of personnel have different salary and benefit packages.

Nonpersonnel Operating Budget

The nonpersonnel operating budget, also called the supply and expense budget, is used to plan, direct, assess, and control all expenditures for supplies and noncapital equipment needed by the unit. This is an expense budget that includes all of those items purchased by the unit from inside and outside the organization, including ancillary departments, general stores, and central service. Monies needed to pay for specific unit services are calculated as part of this budget. For example, the cost of journal subscriptions (an outside purchase) for the nursing lounge is budgeted here.

Budgets are based on incremental increases from last year's expenses (budgeting-by-exception approach, see also Chapter 18) or as a zero-based system. Zero-based budgeting requires the nurse manager to justify every expense on the budget regardless of what was on last year's budget. Zero-based budgeting is not commonly used for the nonpersonnel operating budget.

All budgets are calculated based on units of service. The unit of service in nursing is based on the number of patient days for which service is provided for each cost center. The census, patient acuity, and hours of care per patient are significant in critical care. Therefore, all of these are considered in budgeting.

Most institutions base the nonpersonnel operating budget on the previous year's use of supplies and adjust for inflation. The nurse manager obtains the annual inflationary factor from the finance or purchasing department. This factor varies item to item, but generally ranges from 4 to 7 percent. Monthly expense reports may be used to make projections of annual expenditures.

Budgets that are reported monthly or quarterly have year-to-date (YTD) expenses. Often these YTD figures are annualized and used by the institution to project expenses. Annualized budgets are those that are calculated based on the spending trend. The actual year-to-date costs are multiplied by the spending factor, which is the number of months remaining in the year divided by the number of months that have already passed, plus 1.0. For example if the actual YTD costs covered 7 months,

$$\text{Spending factor} = (5 \text{ [months remaining]} \div 7 \text{ [months passed]}) + 1.0$$
$$= 1.7.$$

If the YTD costs covered 9 months,

$$\text{Spending factor} = (3 \text{ [months remaining]} \div 9 \text{ [months passed]}) + 1.0$$
$$= 1.33.$$

TYPES OF COSTS

For the remainder of this section terms generally used in budget preparation will be defined. *Direct costs* are those directly connected to the delivery of patient care. Salaries for variable staff and the cost of medical-surgical supplies are direct costs. *Indirect costs* are necessary, but they are not directly related to patient care. For example, the medical records department is an integral part of the hospital, but the costs incurred by this department cannot be charged to patients directly, thus they are indirect. These indirect costs may be called standard costs if they are part of the fixed overhead of the institution, prorated (based on budget size), and passed along to each cost center.

Transfer prices are used for transactions within an organization when service to one department is provided by another department. The charge for these services is determined by the other provider department. Sometimes the charge is above the market price because the in-house service is based on a standard *full cost* of the department service center. This means that the department providing the service to the unit must balance their budget by charging all services to other departments. To the nurse manager this can be frustrating, especially if the service is available by outside contracting. Although money could be saved by buying the service outside the organization, it is usual for administrators to limit this option and encourage optimum use of in-house resources.

In addition, decisions based on external prices may not be supported or allowed within the institution. In union houses, union contracts may dictate a closed-shop approach. An example that clarifies this dilemma is based on the budgeted repair and maintenance of unit defibrillators. The in-house fee is $42 an hour, while the fee of an independent contractor (the manufacturer) is $30 an hour. Some transfer services may intentionally be priced way above market value to discourage excessive use by other cost centers. An example would be paying double time to the cleaning department for window washing beyond the thrice-annual scheduled services. If the windows require more frequent cleaning because they separate patient care areas, this inflated price would be budgeted and paid.

Sunk costs are monies that have already been spent on an item; because this money was spent originally, the organization is encouraged to invest further in the system. Often nurse managers will be asked to defend or budget additional monies for sunk costs. For example, if the hospital installs special racks to hold a syringe disposal system at each bedside, money to buy the syringe system is budgeted annually. If the nurse manager finds a syringe disposal system that will better meet unit needs, she may be encouraged to stay with the current brand based on the sunk money already invested.[3]

Some costs within the budget are called *proportional costs*. These refer to high volume items that are purchased in proportion to a particular type of service rendered. For example, in an open-heart postoperative unit, the money allocated for pacemaker batteries could be proportional to the number of annual cases.

Controllable costs are those that the nurse manager has some control over. Conversely, the nurse manager has no input into noncontrollable costs. *Noncontrollable costs* include the cost of providing some aspect of care that is both needed and ordered, such as a pacing thermodilution catheter for an open-heart patient. An example of controllable costs includes money spent on incidental overtime of less than four hours.

BUSINESS CONCEPTS

A summary of budgetary expenditures is sent to each cost center monthly or quarterly depending upon the institution. This document compares budgeted figures with actual expenses. The difference between the two expressed as a percentage is the *variance*. Most institutions determine an acceptable or allowable variance and require the nurse manager to justify expenditures over or under this variance. For example, when analyzing the budget, the institution determines that a variance less than 2 percent or expenditure within $500 of the budgeted amount requires no action.

Cost-benefit analysis is used to compare the benefits of a proposed program with the anticipated costs. Alternative ways to reach the same objective may be included. The cost-benefit analysis assumes a causal connection between costs and benefits. The idea is to demonstrate that the benefits match the resources used. For example, the nurse manager wants to add Advanced Cardiac Life Support (ACLS) certification as a unit requirement. The cost of training in-house ACLS instructors to teach staff plus the in-house certification program should be compared with the cost of sending the staff elsewhere for certification; this is done in the project's cost-benefit analysis. The prudent nurse manager would calculate the costs for both approaches and present the analysis with the most cost-efficient method. In this example, the cost of training in-house instructors and certifying staff is found to be higher than the cost of sending staff to an outside agency. However, the nurse manager might suggest the more costly in-house approach if ACLS certification will be instituted in other areas, such as the emergency department and the cardiac arrest team. In this instance, up-front costs would benefit long-range goals.

REVENUE BUDGET

In the true meaning of the word, budgeting is the annual balancing of revenues and expenses. Because nursing has limited control over census and acuity, most nursing budgets are expense budgets that reflect what the unit spends, not what the unit generates in income. Revenue for the unit is usually hidden in the room rate. For baseline calculations, the nurse manager can multiply the average daily census by the charge for the room per day. This approximates the general revenue generated by the unit.

One of the most difficult aspects of budget planning is finding the best method for determining nursing service costs. This can be achieved by per diem costs, by DRG category, or by some type of nursing workload measure. The per diem approach is most commonly used. With this method, the average costs per patient per day is calculated by dividing the total nursing costs by the number of patient days. This is usually done annually. Because resource consumption varies greatly with different patients, these methods do not reflect true costs of care. Therefore, they are not fully reliable. With the current economic constraints, DRGs and nursing workload measures are being explored to find a method that identifies true nursing costs of the individual patient.

Case Study: Budgeting

You have recently accepted the nurse manager position in a 9-bed medical intensive care unit (MICU). You have five years of critical care experience, two of which are in this unit, and you have had a fair amount of charge experience. However, you dread working with the budget because you know nothing about it. The director of the surgical service says that you will learn, but you remain insecure.

As the new manager, you have just returned from a conference and realize that monitoring ST-T wave changes is realistic and practical. You discuss this with your supervisor who suggests that you and the nurse manager of the CCU work on this together. Both of you want to plan capital purchase of this new technology. After a discussion with the medical directors of both units, it is decided that this enhancement is justified.

Table 17-1 lists the capital item justification that was prepared and submitted. Note that the elements listed down the left side of the capital budget form identify the relationship of the item to be purchased to other significant costs, as well as to the reason the item is needed. Although this item was developed for demonstration purposes, the language and explanation are easily understood.

As you start to work with the personnel budget, you develop a table of organization that identifies the number of employees, their categories, and the number of hours each works during the year. Table 17-2 represents the regular staffing table of organization for this 9-bed MICU. The upper part of the table is variable staff, the lower is fixed staff. Note that the salary for the one half-time clinical nurse specialist (CNS) and one quarter-time director is budgeted and accounted for. Using this as a guide, you can establish staffing patterns based on patient classification data.

As the nurse manager, you receive the attached partial budget, labeled as Table 17-3, for costs incurred over the past nine months. This represents the actual expenses charged to the MICU budget. The director requests that you annualize this portion of the budget and make projections about whether the unit will come in under budget (have enough budgeted funds) or come in over budget (not have enough budgeted funds). Table 17-4 depicts the mathematical calculations you completed to provide this data. Since the YTD expenses are for nine months, the spending factor to project annual costs is 1.33.

Finally, you put the projected expenses together with the YTD totals and calculate the difference between what was budgeted and was actually spent. This is called a variance and is simply the percentage over or under the amount budgeted. A negative sign is placed before the variance when it is below the budgeted cost. Table 17-5 represents the comparison of the projected costs to those originally budgeted. Note that most of the variances are negative. This means the better part of this portion of the budget reflects underspending the original budget.

As the nurse manager, you then determine why this budget is underspent. A low census, a decline in patient acuity, or a change in service may be responsible. Better yet, the decreased expenditure may be due to cost-saving efforts.

The budget process is now becoming meaningful. You know how to plan and complete capital purchase requests, relate the table of organization to staffing patterns and patient classification, and interpret annualized expenses to find out why the variance reflects unit underspending.

CONCLUSION

Building a budget takes time and experience. A nurse manager gains much by simply evaluating all expenditures each month until she starts to see patterns and trends. In this way, sporadic or unexpected costs can be clearly identified, and action can be taken to explain or justify them. The best way to proceed is to analyze carefully what has gone on before. The nurse manager who approaches budgeting in this way is relatively assured that future budgets will address past practice.

Table 17-1. CAPITAL ITEM JUSTIFICATION

ST-T Wave Measurement

Description	ST-T wave measurement reads and records the amount of electrical variation in part of the heart cycle. When patients have heart disease, ST-T wave changes indicate heart damage. Patients with large variation in ST-T wave may be experiencing further heart damage.
Cost	Each = $1800
	Number ordered = 9 $16,200
Delivery fee	None.
Installation fee	Each $400
	Number ordered = 9 $3,600
	This includes installation of new computer board and a hardwire connection of each terminal to the central computer.
Maintenance	12-month warranty, then $800 for the second year.
Vendor	Great Star Monitoring Company
	Houston, Texas
Use	This is an enhancement of the current software package that is part of the existing cardiac monitoring system and arrhythmia package.
Nature	Replacement or Renovation or <u>Addition</u>
Year needed	1991
Priority	1 = must have <u>2 = needed</u> 3 = can defer
Benefits	This enhancement to the existing monitoring system will <u>improve patient care</u> and provide a greater degree of <u>patient safety</u> by alerting staff when ST-T wave changes become more significant and thus help prevent more heart damage.
Added personnel	None.
Training	Company will provide on-site training to RNs for application and bioclinical engineers for maintenance and troubleshooting with no additional fee.
Other	None.
How, when to be used	This will be used 100% of the time for all occupied beds in the MICU.
Who will use	RN will add ST-T wave measurement to routine assessment of cardiac rhythms.
Justification	This enhancement will make the discovery of worsening heart damage easier. When the monitor detects changes in ST-T size, it rings an alarm. This tells the nurse to assess the patient's rhythm. If significant, the nurse informs the physician, who can order medication to prevent further damage. This is needed to provide state-of-the-art cardiac monitoring for medical patients. All patients are monitored in the 9-bed MICU; patients with existing heart disease represent 68% of the patient mix; there is an 89% occupancy rate in the MICU.

Table 17-2. TABLE OF ORGANIZATION

	TOTAL HOURS	NUMBER FTES	NONPRODUCTIVE HOURS/YEAR	PRODUCTIVE HOURS/YEAR
Variable Staff				
RN	2080	21	336	1744
LPN	2080	8	256	1824
NA	2080	8	256	1824
Fixed Staff				
Clerk	2080	5	256	1824
Manager	2080	1	336	1744
Assistant	2080	2	336	1744
Instructor	2080	1	336	1744
CNS half-time	1040	0.5	168	872
Director quarter-time	520	0.25	84	436

Table 17-3. NONPERSONNEL OPERATING BUDGET: THIRD QUARTER REPORT MICU

	THIS QUARTER		YEAR-TO-DATE	
EXPENSES	ACTUAL	BUDGET	ACTUAL	ANNUAL BUDGET
Bioclinical Engineering	789	1,000	2,900	4,000
Central Service	1,100	1,500	2,300	4,500
Dietary	275	300	735	1,200
General Stores	3,874	3,000	11,900	12,000
Housekeeping	110	300	710	1,200
Pharmacy	5,742	5,000	13,457	20,000
Respiratory Care	0	200	259	800

Table 17-4. ANNUALIZED EXPENSES TO PROJECT EXPENSES: MICU 9 MONTHS YTD

EXPENSES	YEAR-TO-DATE ACTUAL	SPENDING FACTOR	PROJECTED AMOUNT
Bioclinical Engineering	2,900	(1.33)	3,857
Central Service	2,300	(1.33)	3,059
Dietary	735	(1.33)	978
General Stores	11,900	(1.33)	15,827
Housekeeping	710	(1.33)	944
Pharmacy	13,457	(1.33)	17,989
Respiratory Care	259	(1.33)	344

Table 17-5. COMPARISON OF PROJECTED TO BUDGETED EXPENSES: MICU

EXPENSES	YEAR-TO-DATE ACTUAL	PROJECTED AMOUNT	ANNUAL BUDGET	VARIANCE
Bioclinical Engineering	2,900	3,857	4,000	− 4
Central Service	2,300	3,059	4,500	− 32
Dietary	735	978	1,200	− 11
General Stores	11,900	15,827	12,000	32
Housekeeping	710	944	1,200	− 21
Pharmacy	13,457	17,989	20,000	− 10
Respiratory Care	259	344	800	− 57

Budgeting is done to allow the nurse manager and institution to adjust staffing as needed, to have the resources available to pay staff, to insure that supplies and equipment are readily available, and to justify all expenditures based on the effective and efficient use of resources that match patient care needs. Planning for next year, developing financial projections, and fixing problems before they become unmanageable are expectations of nurse managers who use budgets wisely. This chapter has introduced the basic concepts of capital, personnel, and nonpersonnel operating budgets.

REFERENCES

1. Health Care Education Associates: (1987). Basic budgeting for nurse managers. St Louis, 1987, The CV Mosby Co.
2. Levine-Ariff J, Hartmann M, and Wojcicki T: Budgeting and resource allocation. In Sullivan EJ and Decker PJ, editors: Effective management in nursing, ed 2, New York, 1988, Addison-Wesley Publishing Co.
3. Stevens BJ: The nurse as executive, Rockville, Md, 1985, Aspen Systems Corporation.
4. Strasen L: Key business skills for nurse managers. New York, 1987, JB Lippincott Co.

SUGGESTED READINGS:

1. Edwardson SR and Giovannetti PB: A review of cost-accounting methods for nursing services, Nursing Economics 5(3):107-17, 1987.
2. Hoffman FB: Projecting supply expenses, Journal of Nursing Administration 15(6):21-24, 1985.
3. Kaufman K and Hall ML: Capital planning can mean life or death of the healthcare provider, Healthcare Financial Management (4):31-34, 1987.
4. Poteet GW and Goddard NL: Issues in Financial management. In Henry B, Arndt C, Di Vincenti M, and Mariner-Tomey A, editors: Dimensions of nursing administration. Boston, 1989, Blackwell Scientific Publications.
5. Sheridan DR: Nursing management skills: a modular self-assessment series; module I: economics, accounting and finance. New York, 1989, National League for Nursing.
6. Villemaire M and Lane McGraw C: Nursing personnel budgets: a step-by-step guide, Nursing Management 17(11):28-32, 1986.

Chapter 18

ANALYZING AND FORECASTING BUDGETS

Gayle R. Whitman

Recently major initiatives aimed at constraining the cost of health care have been launched by governmental and private health care organizations. Driven by health care costs that accounted for 13 percent of the gross national product, the government abolished the retrospective payment system and instituted prospective reimbursement. Quickly following suit, major third-party payors began to prospectively negotiate fees for client services. Reimbursement limitations to hospitals quickly placed tremendous focus on financial management. The department of nursing, which traditionally represented a major portion of the hospital's budget, was greatly affected by these events.

As we move through the 1990s, nursing continues its major role in the hospital's fiscal health. Each nurse manager who has responsibility for managing a portion of the nursing budget must have the knowledge and skill required to perform that task effectively. This chapter is designed to help the manager obtain these requirements, for it focuses on analyzing and forecasting budgets. Although these are performed concurrently in practice, for clarity they are presented separately in this chapter. A case study will be used in order to illustrate the key points and to relate theory directly to practice.

ANALYZING THE BUDGET

Budgeting is the process of converting organizational plans and objectives into monetary terms. There are two major functions in budgeting: planning and controlling.[13] Planning refers to that part of the process where decisions are made about what service will be provided, how much of the service will be available, and at what volume and fee the service will be offered. It is during the planning that forecasting plays an important role.

Controlling the budget relates to the issue of whether the goals were met; and if not, why? In health care, these goals are related to positive patient outcomes. Therefore, budget analysis must first address the issue of patient outcomes. Data for this can be obtained from a number of sources, including quality assurance reports, mortality and morbidity reports, and patient mix information from patient classification data.

When negative patient outcomes are identified, the manager must analyze the situation and determine the cause. Specifically, do personnel have a knowledge or skill deficit? Is it related to the newness of a technique or procedure? Is it related to lack of personnel or equipment? Some of these causes can be remedied by financial means; therefore part of the manager's analysis centers on determining the nature of the solution. One cause that may not have a financial solution is a nurse with the appropriate knowledge and skills who lacks the ability to act with a sense of urgency, thereby delaying interventions. Even with extensive goal setting and counseling, which incur additional costs, the nurse may never be able to assume this behavior. Placement in another clinical setting would perhaps be the best solution. The following case study gives an example where financial support can be an effective remedy.

Case Study: Cost Effective Data Analysis

You are a newly appointed nurse manager in a 10-bed mixed adult medical-surgical critical care unit at a large urban hospital. One patient group managed here consists of patients undergoing percutaneous transluminal coronary angioplasty (PTCA). The management of these patients has recently changed. The nurse must now titrate a heparin infusion so that a specific partial thromboplastin time (PTT) is maintained. During clinical rounds you notice an increased incidence of bleeding and hematoma. This subjective perspective is validated by the objective morbidity report with data on complications in the critical care unit, which you receive monthly. The incidence of bleeding and hematoma formation has increased from 3 percent to 10 percent since the introduction of heparin titration. Discussions in staff meetings and with the medical director reveal a prolonged turnaround time for obtaining PTT results as problematic, because excessive anticoagulation levels cannot be known immediately. The turnaround time for the laboratory to obtain and produce PTT results is 30 minutes.

The medical director and you, the nurse manager, determine that activated clotting time (ACT) could be used to monitor the degree of anticoagulation. The ACT can be performed at the bedside by a small machine — with immediate results. You begin to explore a number of issues. How much does the machine cost? How many are needed? Who will operate the machine? How much training does it require? Is ongoing training required? Who will service the machine? What supplies are required to use the machine and what do they cost? How much time is diverted from direct patient care to perform the test? Will using the machine decrease the incidence of bleeding and hematoma formation?

In order to fully answer these questions, you, as the nurse manager, conduct a pilot for one month, during which costs, time, and complication rates of patients are compared for PTT- and ACT-based monitoring. Bleeding and hematoma rates returned to 3 percent in the group monitored with ACT, and their lengths of stay decreased by 1 day. Nursing time was the same in both groups because the increase in time required to perform the ACT corresponded to the increase in nursing time required by PTT-monitored patients who developed bleeding. ACT-group patients' cost decreased slightly because the cost of performing a PTT by the laboratory was higher than the cost of performing an ACT at the bedside. You, as nurse manager, determined the cost of the ACT by adding the cost of the required materials to a depreciation on the machine. This charge will generate sufficient revenue to cover purchase of materials, maintenance, repair, and ultimate replacement of the device.

This is an example of how analyzing subjective and objective negative patient outcome data can help the nurse manager identify instances where practice changes and expenditures for resources can be a solution. Quite often patient outcome data are not negative, and no red flags exist to attract the manager's attention. However, positive outcomes are generated by adequate, competent staff, as well as by physical and environmental resources. The key to achieving and maintaining staff and resources is in developing a well-planned, controlled budget. Therefore, even with positive patient outcomes, constant and ongoing budget analysis is essential for maintaining the resources and personnel that contribute to these positive outcomes.

ANALYZING THE OPERATING STATEMENT

Many reports cross the nurse manager's desk. Perhaps the most useful for budgetary analysis is the monthly operating statement. Because the operating statement provides an accumulated estimate of operating revenue and expenses for the month, it is the ideal document with which to start, whether the manager is new to the area or is conducting an ongoing review.[4,14] A systematic analysis of this report can help the manager identify specific problem areas. Once they are identified, the manager can focus on specific reports related to them. A typical example of a critical care unit's operating statement can be found in Table 18-1. The purpose of the monthly operating statement is to provide the manager with a summary of the current revenues and expenses for her area, as well as a cumulative report for the year. To accomplish this, most operating statements have columns detailing monthly and year-to-date (YTD) activity on the following major categories: revenue, salaries and related expenses, and other expenses. In each

Table 18-1. MONTHLY OPERATING STATEMENT: CRITICAL CARE UNIT

	CURRENT MONTH				YEAR-TO-DATE		
	ACTUAL	BUDGET	VARIANCE (%)		ACTUAL	BUDGET	VARIANCE (%)
Revenue							
Inpatient	425,000	391,000	8.0		1,800,000	1,825,000	−2.0
Salaries and Related Expenses							
Regular earnings	81,300	76,000	−6.9		362,000	372,500	3.0
Shift differential	1,500	1,700	12.0		7,200	8,000	10.0
Unit differential	2,100	2,500	16.0		9,500	11,300	16.0
Overtime earnings	16,000	7,800	−105.0		57,300	34,370	−67.0
Unscheduled paid–time off	4,100	3,100	−13.0		11,500	14,000	18.0
Paid time off earnings	7,600	7,700	3.0		37,500	41,800	10.0
Extended leave earnings	0	400	100.0		1,500	1,500	0.0
Health care	6,800	7,400	8.0		30,000	37,000	19.0
FICA	7,600	7,000	−8.0		38,000	36,000	−5.0
Other benefits	700	900	23.0		2,800	4,900	43.0
Annuities	1,500	1,500	0.0		3,000	3,000	0.0
Total salaries	129,200	116,000	−11.0		560,300	564,370	1.0

Other Expenses						
Hospital pharmacy requisitions	1,400	300	−366.0	6,300	4,000	−57.0
Storeroom requisitions	19,400	14,700	−31.0	97,000	87,000	−11.0
Central service requisitions	61	60	0.0	200	450	55.0
Tuition Reimbursement	250	250	0.0	1,000	3,000	66.0
Purchase: Maintenance & repair	200	200	0.0	800	4,200	81.0
Medical Supplies	270	2,300	98.0	5,600	10,700	47.0
Books/Subscriptions	0	0	0.0	60	200	70.0
Forms/printing	1,300	1,400	7.0	1,400	1,500	7.0
Travel	400	400	0.0	800	1,000	50.0
Registration	100	100	0.0	200	800	75.0
Total other expenses	23,381	19,710	−18.00	113,460	126,950	10.0
GRAND TOTAL	272,419	255,290	6.7	1,126,240	1,137,750	−1.0
Contribution margin (%)	(67)	(60)	(11.6)	(64)	(65)	(−1.0)
Additional Information						
Facilities Expenses	4,000			8,000		
Contractual Allocations:						
Medicare contractual	40,000			80,000		
ABC Insurance Co. contractual	3,000			10,000		
Miscellaneous contractuals	2,000			4,000		
Uncollectables	1,000			3,000		
Totals	50,000			105,000		

section actual and budget figures are listed; there is also a variance column. Because both monthly and YTD activity are listed, the nurse manager can assess immediate- and long-term data. Monthly data alone could cause the nurse manager to overreact to a short-lived seasonal trend. On the other hand, responding only to YTD data may cause the nurse manager to apply interventions too late. For analyzing each item, the variance column should be used as a "red flag" to indicate where further investigation is necessary. The variance column in Table 18-1 indicates the percentage difference in what was budgeted compared to what actually happened. A negative percentage indicates that either less-than-expected revenues were generated, or greater-than-budgeted expenses were incurred. A positive variance in the revenue section indicates that more revenue was generated than budgeted. A positive variance in the salary and expenses section indicates that less money was spent than budgeted. Generally, any large positive or negative variance should be reviewed. Specific techniques used to analyze the variance will be presented shortly.

Analyzing the Revenue

The revenue or income section of the operating report reflects the amount of patient billing each unit generates. Charges in this category generally include room and board rates and nursing care charges. In many institutions, nursing care charges are included in the room and board rates, and are not charged separately. Other charges, such as air ambulance services, may also be included. The usefulness of this section is limited for the nurse manager, because she has little control over the number of patients in the unit, and no control over the price those patients are charged. In addition, these amounts reflect what is billed, not what is actually paid to the hospital: Bad debts and contractual adjustments can significantly alter this amount. However, the revenue section can provide a sense of the volume of revenue, the patient activity, and the nursing care generated by the unit. As such, a significant positive or negative variance can direct the manager to review the level of patient activity in the *patient days activity report* (Table 18-2). This report is generated monthly and yearly, compares projected or budgeted patient days with actual patient days, and supplies a variance. A patient day is a unit of measurement used to describe a single day of hospitalization for a patient. It is a measure of the patient activity. Returning to the case study as an example, if your 10-bed unit was 80 percent occupied (8 patients per day) for a month (30 days), it would have had 240 patient days of activity. Patients are billed for each patient day in the hospital. A decrease in billed revenue usually coincides with a decrease in patient days. Identifying upward or downward trends in patient days is necessary for both short-term and long-range unit planning. By reviewing the operating statement and the patient days activity report, you, as nurse manager, can see that the 8 percent variance increase in current month inpatient revenue from Table 18-1 corresponds with an 8 percent variance increase in the current month's projected patient days from Table 18-2. Specifically,

Table 18-2. PATIENT DAYS ACTIVITY REPORT: CRITICAL CARE UNIT

	MONTHLY			YEAR-TO-DATE		
MONTH	BUDGET	ACTUAL	VARIANCE (%)	BUDGET	ACTUAL	VARIANCE (%)
January	250	200	−20	250	200	−20
February	230	230	0	480	430	−11
March	210	210	0	690	640	−7
April	200	208	4	890	848	−5
May	255	275	8	1145	1123	−2
June	255					
July	225					
August	270					
September	220					
October	280					
November	200					
December	175					
TOTAL	2,770					

an 8 percent increase in patient activity generated an 8 percent increase over budgeted revenues. However, although May exceeded projected patient activity, YTD inpatient revenue (Table 18-1) and patient days still remain 2 percent behind projections. Table 18-2 provides a good example of the importance of trending and balancing monthly with YTD data. On Table 18-2, January's variance for patient days was 50 days below projected. A 20 percent decrease is significant and might lead the manager to consider trimming some costs, perhaps by reducing overtime or limiting per diem agency nurses. Major cutbacks, such as elimination of full-time employees, could have created problems when patient days resumed their normal trends in February and March. Other temporary approaches to this scenario might have been to decrease hours worked by floats and PRN nurses, offer unscheduled vacation days, delay filling unfilled positions, and decreasing the amount of supplies available on the unit. However, eliminating staff positions or not ordering supplies that take a month to be delivered would not be appropriate strategies. These would be used only for long-term trends of decreased activity and, ultimately, decreased revenue.

Analyzing Salaries and Related Expenses

FIXED AND VARIABLE COSTS

The expense portion of the monthly operating statement (Table 18-1) consists of a "Salaries and Related Expenses" section and a "Other Expenses" section. Within both of these sections are fixed and variable costs. *Fixed costs* or *indirect costs* are those that do not vary with the volume of patient activity. They reflect the costs of salaried personnel, such as the nurse manager, or support personnel, such as the unit secretary, who are present regardless of census. Other indirect costs include taxes, insurance, rent, and parking lot pavement.

Variable costs are those that fluctuate with patient activity. A high census generates a larger use of supplies and an increase in personnel utilization. Staff nurse positions are variable costs, because the number of nurses required varies with the patient census and acuity. A critical care unit with 100 percent occupancy and a high acuity will require more nurses than one with 50 percent occupancy and a low acuity. It should be pointed out that fixed costs are fixed only over a relevant range.[6] For example, during a nursing shortage or strike, the fixed positions of head nurse or clinical instructor may become variable positions to assist with staffing.

SALARY AND RELATED EXPENSES

The salary and related expenses portion of the operating statement account for about 70 percent of the total expenses, and thus requires careful attention. Direct payroll costs for both exempt and nonexempt staff are listed. *Exempt* status refers to those employees receiving a fixed salary. *Nonexempt* status refers to employees on hourly rates of pay that fluctuate with overtime and differentials. Overtime, shift and unit differentials, scheduled and unscheduled paid–time off, health care, FICA, annuities, and benefit expenses are all reported in this portion. Most of these are considered noncontrollable by the nurse manager, because wages and benefits are not decided at that level. However, there are a number of useful data the manager can look for and analyze in this section. The first deals with unscheduled paid–time off, also known as sick time. As is seen in Table 18-1, line 5 in the "Salaries and Related Expenses" section there is a 13 percent budget overrun in the current month for unscheduled paid–time off. Monies budgeted for sick calls was $3,100, while the actual expense was $4,100. In assessing the causes for this, the manager might consider the effect of the increase in patient days on staff workload and stress. An obvious increase in staff workload is demonstrated by the dramatic increase in overtime (Table 18-1, "Salary and Related Expenses," line 4) for the current month. Other causes, such as the cold and flu season taking its toll, should also be considered. The YTD unscheduled paid time off must also be reviewed. Here the manager notices that the unit is 18 percent under budget (Table 18-1, "Salaries and Related Expenses," line 5). In general, this would indicate that there is not a trend of increased sick time. The manager would probably make a point to reevaluate the data from next month's operating statement, and continue to observe staff for signs suggesting that sick time is due to stress or fatigue.

PRODUCTIVE VS. NONPRODUCTIVE TIME

The areas that a manager can somewhat control are the overtime categories and the split between productive and nonproductive time. Productive time refers to time spent directly involved in patient care activity, while nonproductive time refers to time spent involved in activities not directly involved in patient care, such as conferences or orientation time. The following box depicts a staffing productivity analysis tool that allows comparison of actual versus recommended staff hours, and includes an analysis of productive versus nonproductive time.

In Part A of the tool, the difference in actual and recommended staffing hours can be determined. In this example, the unit still required 160 more staff hours to meet their recommended staffing level for that pay period. Since a pay period consists of two weeks or 80 hours of work for one FTE, the unit requires 2 more FTE positions. Persistence of this trend would be evidence of a need to increase staffing positions. Critical to evaluating the data in Part A are the reliability and compliance of the classification tool. *Reliability* refers to how accurately the patients are categorized in the classification system. *Compliance* refers to how often they are classified according to the established standard frequency. For example, if the standard is to classify patients daily, but the unit only classifies

---

STAFFING PRODUCTIVITY ANALYSIS TOOL

Part A Pay Period _____

Actual staff	290 × 8 hours = 2,320 hours
Recommended staff variance	310 × 8 hours = 2,480 hours
	−160 ÷ 80 = −2.0 FTEs

Classification tool
  Reliability   100%
  Compliance   100%

Part B

Productive Hours		Nonproductive hours	
Regular Hours	1,769	+Unscheduled paid time off	32
Overtime Hours	333	+Extended leave	80
No Lunch	3	+Workshop	10
Less than 4-Hour block	30	+Orientation	80
Greater than 4-Hour Block	300	+Office Day	8
+PRN hours	40	+Limited Duty	0
+Agency hours	40		
+Float-in hours	0		
−Float-Out hours	0		
−Orient. hours	80		
−Workshop hours	10		
−Office day hours	8		
−Limited duty	0		
TOTAL	2,320	TOTAL	210

Productive hours   2320 = 92%
+Nonproductive Hours   210 = 8%
TOTAL PAID HOURS   2530

half of the time, the compliance rate is 50 percent. Over or underclassifying patient acuity can dramatically alter the recommended staffing numbers. In the example, the reliability and compliance scores add credence to the staffing shortage, since both are 100 percent (See previous box, Part A, lines 5 and 6).

Part B of the tool assesses productive and nonproductive time. The productive time includes regular hours, overtime, PRN and agency hours, and float-in hours. Float-out hours, orientation, workshop, office, and limited duty hours are subtracted from the productive numbers, because they reflect hours paid, but not hours of direct patient care. Limited duty hours refer to those hours worked by an employee who is not involved in patient care because of an injury or illness. For example, after wrist surgery, an employee may return to work unable to deliver direct care to patients for weeks. During this time, the manager may have the nurse assist in quality assurance or educational activities. Orientation and workshop hours are also considered nonproductive—even though they enhance patient care—since they are paid hours not spent at the bedside. These hours appear in the productive column, and they are counted as actual staff hours on the staffing report, because they are hours that staff were on-site and available. The categories considered nonproductive time are also listed in the tool. Although some nonproductive categories cannot be affected by the manager, such as unscheduled paid–time off, extended leave, or limited duty, other nonproductive categories can be controlled, such as office time for staff members, workshop or continuing education time, and the length of orientation. Control of these areas can be achieved through a number of mechanisms. To optimize the orientation program, the clinical instructor, the preceptors, and the nurse manager develop a competency-based orientation program that allows faster orientation of experienced nurses compared to that of inexperienced nurses. To optimize educational activities without increasing the amount of time spent in attendance, you institute a system in which a nurse attending a conference is required to present the content to the rest of the staff. This prevents the need for the entire staff to attend every educational opportunity.

Total paid hours is the sum of productive and nonproductive hours, and the manager has the responsibility to maintain a balance between these categories. Generally each department of nursing determines what it would consider an appropriate ratio; for example, 85 percent productive, 15 percent nonproductive.

The areas that the manager can analyze and affect in Part B are the controllable nonproductive hours, such as office time and overtime. As illustrated, overtime can be broken down into a number of smaller categories. By assessing staffing sheets and time cards, a manager can determine exactly where the overtime occurs. Returning to Table 18-1, the monthly operating statement for the current month shows that overtime was 105 percent over budget ("Salaries and Related Expenses," line 4). The breakdown on the staffing productivity analysis tool seems to support that most of the time was for shift coverage, because 300 hours were attributed to "Greater than 4-Hour Block." If 300 hours had been used in the "Less than 4-Hour Block" the manager might need to investigate why this incidental overtime was occurring. Perhaps such practices as saving all charting until the end of the shift were being practiced. Again, time management might need to be addressed.

Analyzing Other Expenses

The next section of the operating statement deals with other expenses incurred in managing a unit. Again, some of these are noncontrollable by the unit manager, including tuition reimbursement (Table 18-1, line 16) or the cost of supplies. To some extent, however, this category can be proactively controlled: During forecasting, the nurse manager can determine monthly or yearly usage estimates of certain items. The manager can also examine the monthly list of stock drugs purchased by the unit, identify drugs whose status could be changed from floor stock to patient chargeables, and decrease the unit's pharmacy expenses.

The nurse manager watches for significant values in the variance column when analyzing the operating statement. The manager must also be alert for small variances that represent large dollar sums. This is particularly important where large amounts of dollars are assigned, as in the revenue and salary section (Table 18-1, line 1). An illustration of this is seen when reviewing the YTD regular earnings line (Table 18-1, "Salaries and Related Expenses," line 1). A 3 percent variance is equivalent to $10,000. If the nurse manager only looked for large variances, this would have been missed. On the other hand, the 366 percent variance under the current month's pharmacy expenses (Table 18-1, "Other Expenses," line 1)—clearly a large variance—represents only $1,100, the difference between the $300 budgeted and the $1,400 actually spent.

Analyzing the Variance

The identification of a significant variance can either be performed by looking for variance greater than 2 percent or by identifying large dollar amounts differences between actual and budgeted columns. Once identified, the variance needs to be further analyzed. There are three general components of variance: volume, price, and quantity.[5] A *volume variance* develops when the actual workload or volume is different from what was budgeted. A *price variance* develops when the actual price paid is different from the budgeted price. A *quantity variance* develops when the output of resources actually required is different from that budgeted. For an example of price and quantity variance, we shall return to the case study:

> On the operating statement you, as nurse manager, notice a red flag in the variance column for the current month storeroom requisitions. The variance indicates that the unit is overbudget by 31 percent or $5,300 for that month (Table 18-1, "Other Expenses," line 2). From a list of monthly storeroom purchases, you

determine that the number of chest tube systems exceeded the number budgeted. This constitutes a quantity variance. In addition, you also notice that the price paid for the systems was $10 more than budgeted. This constitutes a price variance. Your response is to continue following the usage trend, and then cost and reset the budget appropriately next year. Since most budgeting systems do not allow the budget to be reset within the year, this variance will continue. However, since its cause has been found, this variance will no longer require concern or analysis.[5,11]

This is an example of a *static* budget, which is one that cannot be adjusted throughout the year to reflect actual costs or activity. Even though the actual cost and quantity are higher, the nurse manager cannot recalculate the budget, and thus the variance remains. A *flexible* budget allows recalculation so that the budget reflects the actual workload, price, and quantity, and thus is more accurate.[5,14] It is a helpful tool for the manager called upon to explain and justify budgetary variances. The box on the next page highlights the formulas that can be used to calculate a flexible budget variance analysis of salaries. In this example, the static budget amount calculated for this particular unit was $264,000. This reflects a budgeted number of 16 hours of care per patient day; $15 per hour salaries and 1100 patient days (line a). However, the actual regular earnings were $320,850 and exceeded budget by $56,850, or 21 percent. The manager's task is to justify this $56,850 budget overrun. To calculate the specific composition of the $56,850 variance, the equations listed are used. To determine the volume variance, first multiply the budgeted patient hours by the budgeted hourly salary and by the *actual* patient days (line b). This sum is $276,000. By subtracting the static budgeted value of $264,000 from $276,000, the volume variance (line c) of $12,000 is attained.

To determine the price variance, first use the equation on line d, in which the budgeted patient days are multiplied by the *actual* hourly wage and the *actual* patient days. By subtracting equation (b) from (d), the specific price variance of $9,200 is attained (line e).

Finally, the quantity variance can be calculated. In this calculation, the sum from the equation on line d ($285,200) is subtracted from the total actual costs, which represents actual patient hours, wages, and patient days. Since equation (d) includes wages and patient days, which reflect price and volume variances, the difference between equation (d) and the actual costs represents the quantity variance. Specifically in this example, it accounts for $36,650 (line f).

The final analysis of the regular earnings variance then is as follows:

$12,000	Volume (Patient Days)
$ 9,200	Price (Hourly Wage)
$36,650	Quantity (Patient Hours)
$56,850	Total Variance

Once the specific variances are determined, the nurse manager must interpret them. At first glance, the increase in volume or patient days seems to be a positive aspect. However, it may not coincide with an increase in revenues, particularly if

FLEXIBLE BUDGET VARIANCE ANALYSIS

Static YTD Budgeted Regular Earnings = $264,000
YTD Actual Regular Earnings = 320,850   (21%)
Variance = $ 56,850

Volume Variance

Static Budget					(a)
16 hrs/PD (budgeted)	×	$15/hr (budgeted)	× 1100/PD (budgeted)	= $264,000 (budgeted)	= Regular Earnings
Flexible Budget					
16 hrs/PD (budgeted)	×	$15/hr (budgeted)	× 1150/PD (actual)	= $276,000	(b)
		$276,000			(b)
		−264,000			(a)
Total Volume Variance		$12,000			(c)

Price Variance

16 hrs/PD (budgeted)	×	$15/hr (budgeted)	× 1150/PD (actual)	= $276,000	(b)
16 hrs/PD (budgeted)	×	$15.50/hr (actual)	× 1150 PD (actual)	= $285,200	(d)
		$285,200			(d)
		−276,000			(b)
Total Price Variance		$9,200			(e)

Quantity Variance

16 hrs/PD (budgeted)	×	$15.50/hr (actual)	× 1150 PD (actual)	= $285,200	(d)
18 hrs/PD (actual)	×	$15.50/hr (actual)	× 1150 PD (actual)	= $320,850	
		$320,850			
		−285,200			(d)
Total Quantity Variance		$36,650			(f)

Total Variance

Total Volume Variance	$12,000		(c)
Total Price Variance	9,200		(e)
Total Quantity Variance	36,650		(f)
Total Variance	$56,850		

it reflects longer lengths of stay. (If a length of stay is longer than prospectively approved, either limited reimbursement or no reimbursement will be received for those days over the approved length of stay.) If there are increased lengths of stay, the nurse manager should collaborate with the medical staff to control this. If, however, this increase reflects an increase in unit admissions, then concurrent revenue should be appreciated.

A variance increase in price or salaries can generally be accounted for by agency or PRN nursing hours, overtime hours, or salary adjustments. In this example, regular earnings were singled out; thus this price variance represents differences in regular staff salaries. The fifty-cent-an-hour variance could be due to a new increase in hourly wage, or it could reflect a higher-than-average salary for the unit compared with the rest of the nursing department. For example, the budget calculations may have used a wage of $15 per hour because it represented the halfway point on the salary scale. If the unit had a significant percentage of its staff in tenured positions, the average hourly wage might be $15.50 rather than $15. Average hourly wages less than $15 would most likely be seen on other units with less-experienced, newer staff. It is generally not a common practice to calculate differently budgeted salaries for different units. In order to justify variances, the unit manager needs to include these factors.

Finally, the quantity variance, or the increase in patient care hours, needs to be interpreted. This increase in hours can reflect an increase in patient acuity, which can be validated by the patient classification system. If increased acuity is not present, the manager needs to look further. Possible causative factors include inefficient time utilization, and insufficient supervision of inexperienced or ancillary staff. Calculating a flexible budget can show specific details and help justify variances from the static budget.

Analysis of the Margins and Other Information

The final sections of the monthly operating statement (Table 18-1, p. 290) deal with contribution margins and additional contractual and reimbursement information. The *contribution margin* is the difference between the fee charged for a service and the variable costs; that is, the revenue minus variable costs.[11] (Variable costs are those that fluctuate or are dependent on activity.) This margin of difference is generally assigned to cover the fixed costs of the organization such as the housekeeping, administrative, and maintenance departments. Each cost center is assigned a budgeted contribution margin for the current month. In the example in Table 18-1, the budgeted contribution margin is 60 percent. The actual margin, 67 percent, was higher because of the increase in revenue that month. While not the case here, salaries and expenses that are underbudget can also alter the margin favorably. However, although the current month's margin is favorable, the YTD margin is under budget by 1 percent. This is attributed to the −2 percent variance seen in YTD revenue (Table 18-1, "Revenue," line 1). Again, the revenues listed reflect only the billed revenues. Actual reimbursement will most likely be more than the −2 percent variance in YTD revenue, because generally patient charges are not 100 percent reimbursed. Controlling the budget to meet the budgeted margin is an institutionalwide issue. However, when faced with negative margins the nurse manager must clearly assess whether any inefficiencies in utilization of salaries and expenses are occurring and, if they exist, correct them.

As was mentioned, the revenues listed reflect only the billed revenues. Actual institutional reimbursement will most likely be less, and occurs perhaps months later. Therefore, operating statements are not precise financial tools. In order to help to improve their precision concerning actual cash flow, some institutions now provide an "Additional Information" section on the operating statement (Table 18-1, "Additional Information" section). In this section, monies that will not be reimbursed, or will be lost because of charity or some other reason, are estimated and included in the financial picture. This estimate is usually based on historical information: The amount previously remaining after reimbursement. The estimate can also be based on current information. For example, to return to the case study, the hospital was only able to negotiate payment of 85 percent of patient charges with ABC Insurance Company. Because of this, the hospital knows it will only collect 85 percent of their charges. In Table 18-1, $3,000 for the current month will be deducted from actual revenues to reflect uncollected charges from ABC Insurance. Generally, these uncollectables are not individually reallocated to each specific department budget, but are spread evenly across all. Notice that the largest line item is Medicare contractuals. With Medicare reimbursement continuing to shrink, the nonreimbursable sections related to those patients will continue to increase. Hospitals with the highest percentage of those patients will have the largest nonreimbursable sums.

Again, as with all the sums on the operating statement, these are approximations. The purpose of the operating statement is to provide the nurse manager with information for explanation, understanding, and interpretation of financial data, which in turn enables control of expenses and a rationale for changes to facilitate better budget control.

FORECASTING THE BUDGET

Forecasting or planning the budget for the next year is an ongoing process. As the manager analyzes the current budget, clear unexpected trends become easier to identify. This ongoing information and a sufficient data base are the tools necessary to plan a new budget. (Data bases more than two years old are not helpful, since they do not reflect current trends.) In addition to trends and data bases, the context of the internal and external environment should be assessed and incorporated into the planning. Examples of external forces include Medicare reimbursement, contractual arrangements, and referral status. Internal forces include the philosophy and objectives of the nursing department, the care delivery system employed, new research being conducted, and expansion and cutback plans.[13] Each department of the institution involved in planning will incorporate various aspects of these assessments into its budget. The importance of thorough and precise planning can not be overemphasized: The success of the budget is linked to adequate planning.

Forecasting the Revenue

The first step in forecasting the revenue is to forecast the expected number of patient admissions and average length of stays. In the past, this was based on historical data or predictions generated by department heads. With the advent of prospective payment, case mix strategies are now used.[3,10] With this method, the number of cases in each DRG the institution expects to care for that year are determined. This data is obtained from physician utilization, historical analyses, projection of trends in the population, and other factors. Returning to the case study for an example, coronary artery bypass without cardiac catheterization, (DRG 107, with an allocated length of stay of 8 days) was performed on 1,000 patients last year. That totaled 8,000 patient days. Since the hospital has just been awarded preferred provider status by XYZ Insurance Company, it anticipates performing 200 more bypasses this year. This amounts to a total of 9,600 projected patient days for this group.

Calculation of patient days by this method for all DRGs may be too cumbersome. To simplify it, the *80-20 rule* can be used. The 20 percent or less of the DRGs that account for 80 percent of the units' activity is determined. From these data, projected admissions and length of stay are calculated to produce patient days per nursing unit. Once room rates and nursing care charges are added into these projected patient days, unit revenue forecasts are generated. An example of projected patient days can be found in Table 18-2 on p. 293, where the total of patient days is projected to be 2,770. Projections are as fine-tuned as possible and are made on a monthly basis for each unit. From reviewing the projections in Table 18-2, the manager can identify that the months of March, April, November, and December are predicted to have a lower census. The summer months are predicted to have the highest census. By using these projections, the manager would schedule summer vacations for staff appropriately.

If the institution is expecting to implement new services, new subspecialties, major technological changes, or major shifts in volume, an impact analysis should also be conducted. *Impact analysis* is a management information tool that helps estimate costs associated with proposed changes.[7] By conducting an impact analysis, not only will potential revenues be identified, but direct and indirect expenses will be identified. All affected departments should be involved in the analysis. For example, an impact analysis would be beneficial when there are changes in surgical staff. Perhaps one cardiac surgeon is retiring and another is being hired. The new surgeon has a subspecialty practice in surgical ablation for dysrhythmic patients. The direct and indirect costs associated with this new physician can be significant—most likely, they will include specialized equipment, longer surgery times, and use of personnel from the electrophysiology lab. Knowing this information ahead of time can assist other department

Table 18-3. DETERMINATION OF VARIABLE STAFF

1.	$\dfrac{10}{\text{Bed Capacity}}$	×	$\dfrac{88\%}{\text{Projected Occupancy}}$	=	$\dfrac{8.8}{\text{Projected 199\_ Census}}$
2.	$\dfrac{8.8}{\text{Projected Census}}$	×	$\dfrac{4.5}{\text{Budgeted Acuity}}$	=	$\dfrac{39.6}{\text{Projected Workload}}$
3.	$\dfrac{39.6}{\text{Projected Workload}}$	×	$\dfrac{4.1}{\text{Target Hours/Workload}}$	=	$\dfrac{162.36}{\text{Total Care Hours/24 hours}}$
4.	$\dfrac{162.36}{\text{Total Care Hours 24 hours}}$	÷	8 hours	=	20.3 Variable Staff Needed/ 24 hours

managers, as well as the critical care nurse manager, in budgeting for necessary equipment and continuing education time as the staff learns to care for these patients.

Forecasting Salaries and Related Expenses

The nurse manager's role in forecasting salaries and related expenses is quite critical. In this step in the budget process it is important that accurate staffing mixes and rotations are determined so that salary calculations are precise. To initiate this salary forecasting portion projected occupancies, target hours and acuities need to be obtained from the financial department and the patient classification data.[8] Projected occupancies are determined by the calculation of patient days as was described in the previous section. These days are then allocated to specific patient care units as is illustrated in Table 18-2. Target hours refers to the number of hours of nursing care various categories of patients are budgeted to receive. Patient classification systems are methods of categorizing patients according to acuity. Once a level of acuity is determined, the number of nursing care hours required for care can be calculated. With this information, calculations can be performed to determine the total number of variable staff required to care for the specific types of patients admitted to each unit.

Each patient classification system provides different methods of computing this. In the case study, the Medicus Patient Classification System is used. Table 18-3 illustrates how you, the nurse manager, plan for staffing the unit. According to the hospital's projections your 10-bed unit will have a 88 percent occupancy for the upcoming year. This means that the average census in the unit will be 8.8 patients (line 1). Using the Medicus Classification Tool, patients in this unit have historically been identified as having an acuity of 4.5 on a scale of 2.0 to 5.5, where a 5.5 ranking indicates the highest acuity. When this acuity weighting of 4.5 is multiplied by the average projected census of 8.8 a product of 39.6 is obtained (line 2). This is referred to as the workload index in this system, and it

304 Chapter 18

Table 18-4. DETERMINING SHIFT ALLOCATIONS

Days:	20.3	×	.34	=	6.9	Staff on Days
Evenings:	20.3	×	.33	=	6.7	Staff on Evenings
Nights:	20.3	×	.33	=	6.7	Staff on Nights
	Total Variable Staff/24hrs.		Percentage Mix			

represents not only the census, but the acuity, or the average workload for the unit. Next, nursing care hours are assigned to this workload. The number of hours of nursing care per workload index unit generally ranges from 2.5 to 4.5.

In this instance, the target for nursing care hours was set at 4.1 hours of care for each projected workload index unit. Multiplying the unit's projected workload of 39.6 by the 4.1 hours produces an average need for 162.36 care hours per day, or every 24 hours (line 3). The 162.36 care hours required is divided by 8 hours (each staff works an 8-hour shift) for actual staffing requirements (line 4). Thus 20.3 variable staff are required every 24 hours. Once this value is attained, the manager next needs to determine how the shift breakdowns will occur. Table 18-4 illustrates this. The total variable staff (20.3) is multiplied by the percentage of staff needed for each shift. Shift allocation percentages are generally determined by unit activity. For example, in your critical care unit, the activity is relatively consistent throughout the day so you, as nurse manager, decide to use a 33 percent split. On a busy surgical unit, a nurse manager may allocate a higher percentage of staff for the evening shift when the fresh postoperative cases are returning and requiring more care.

The next step is to determine the skill mix of the staff. This is depicted in Table 18-5. In these calculations, the number of variable staff by shift is multiplied by the skill mix the manager desires for the unit. A skill mix refers to the percentages of professional and nonprofessional staff the nurse manager desires to provide care. You decide to use RNs and nurse aides in a 75%/25% ratio over the three shifts. The final desired staffing numbers for each shift are listed in the last column of Table 18-5. Specifically, 5.2 RNs and 1.7 nurse aides would be scheduled on days for the average 8.8 patient population.

Given the projections for what the manager feels will be required for rotation and mix, the next step is to calculate the total number of full time equivalent (FTE) requirements for the unit. This is shown in the box on the next page where the total number of registered nurses and aides for all shifts is listed. This number is multiplied by a percentage or in this case a factor (1.61) that accounts for sick, vacation and holiday time. The resultant number is the total number of FTE for that category.

The total variable staffing requirements for this unit is 24.5 registered nurses and 8.2 nursing aides. Fixed positions for the unit are 4 secretaries and 1

Table 18-5. DETERMINING SKILL MIX

DAYS	6.9	×	% RN	.75	=	5.2 RN days
	6.9	×	% AIDE	.25	=	1.7 AIDE days
EVENING	6.7	×	% RN	.75	=	5 RN evenings
	6.7	×	% AIDE	.25	=	1.7 AIDE evenings
NIGHTS	6.7	×	% RN	.75	=	5 RN nights
	6.7	×	% AIDE	.25	=	1.7 AIDE nights
	Variable Staff by Shift		Skill Mix Goal			Staff by Shift by Mix

Nurse Manager position. The total table of organization (TO) for the 10-bed unit is as follows:

Manager = 1.0 FTE
RN = 24.5 FTE's
Aide = 8.2 FTE's
Secretary = 4.0 FTE's
Total positions = 37.7

Each FTE is assigned to a designated rotation such as day/evenings, day/nights, straight evenings or nights. Once each employee is assigned a rotation, the financial department can calculate regular earnings as well as shift and unit differentials for the entire year. It is important that as much detail as possible be reported since 3 FTE positions working a day/night rotation will cost more than 3 FTEs working a day/evening rotation if the institution has different shift differentials. In some institutions, employees working straight nights or weekends are paid different rates for these hours. These as well as any special programs, such as 12 hour weekend shifts, need to be separated out so precise calculations can occur. Again, the success of this step of planning for the budget is a vitally important one requiring unit manager participation.[1,2]

Forecasting the Expenses

Forecasting the costs under the expense section is also a critical function for participation by the manager. Two techniques can be used: the zero-based approach and the budgeting-by-exception approach. In the zero-based approach, no precepts from current or past years are included. Rather, all activities are reevaluated, and decisions about their elimination or continuation are made. Funding is determined and activities are prioritized by top management such as the chief executive or financial officers.[9] A manager could use this same zero-based approach to budget equipment and supplies, but it is rather time-consuming. The zero-based approach requires rebuilding equipment and supply lists from scratch, and revising previously made decisions. However, the advan-

Table 18-6. PROPOSED TABLE OF ORGANIZATION

VARIABLE STAFF
   Total RNs all shifts $\underline{15.2}$ × Paid time off factor $\underline{1.61}$ = RN FTE's $\underline{24.5}$
      RN Rotation D/E   =   6.5 FTE's
      RN Rotation D/N   =   6.0 FTE's
      RN Straight Evenings   =   3.0 FTE's
      RN Straight Nights   =   3.0 FTE's
      RN Weekends   =   6.0 FTE's (equals 10 nurses since each nurse is only .6 FTE)

   Total Aides all shifts $\underline{5.1}$ × Paid Time off factor $\underline{1.61}$ = Aide FTE $\underline{8.2}$
      AIDE Rotation D/E   =   2.2 FTE's
      AIDE Rotation D/N/   =   2.0 FTE's
      AIDE Straight Evenings   =   2.0 FTE's
      AIDE Straight Nights   =   2.0 FTE's
      AIDE Weekend   =   0 FTE's

Fixed Staff
      Unit Secretaries   =   4.0 FTE's
      Head Nurse   =   1.0 FTE's

Proposed 199__
Unit Table of Organization
HN — 1
RN   — 24.5
Aide — 8.2
Sec. — 4.0

---

tage of revising decisions about equipment, supplies, and techniques can also be helpful.

The budgeting-by-exception approach builds on previous data and performance. In this approach, the nurse manager only actively investigates and projects changes in costs for new and deleted items or services. For example, the zero-based technique would require the nurse manager to start at the beginning and calculate the number of dressings, rolls of tape, and sets of IV tubing the unit will need for the next year. In the budgeting-by-exception approach, increases in those items would simply be accounted for by increasing or decreasing them by the percentage increase expected in patient days. The nurse manager would focus more on adding new types or quantities of chest tube drainage systems because a new thoracic surgeon is starting, or deleting the old gravity drainage urinary system and replacing it with a new one. The emphasis then is only on the exceptions from the previous years projections. Regardless of the method used, the result is the same: a budget is built every year.

Once the list of the types and quantity of supplies, medicines, and equipment are determined by the nurse manager, it is forwarded to the financial department, where prices are attached. Most departments use a report similar to that of the Hospital Purchasing Services Corporation published by the Joint Purchasing

Corporation. This report provides projections for the year on industry trends and expected changes. For example, one projection for 1989 was that the price of latex gloves would increase by approximately 30 percent. This projection was based on the expected utilization increase resulting from body substance precautions, and on the limited availability of raw latex.[12] Knowledge of this would lead the nurse manager not only to budget more monies for these gloves, but also to change utilization patterns. For example, the nurses in the unit may be using surgeon's gloves for dressing procedures, rather than generic sterile gloves. And the difference in price can be as much as $2 a pair. Reviewing these purchasing guides can be very helpful to the manager in assessing trends and changing practices.

CONCLUSION

Controlling health care costs continues to be a major challenge facing health care providers. Central to meeting this challenge in the 1990s is the critical care nurse manager with the knowledge and ability to forecast and manage the unit budget.

REFERENCES

1. Althaus JN, Hardyck NM, Pierce PB, and Rodriguez MS: Decentralized budgeting: holding the purse strings, part I, Journal of Nursing Administration 12(5):15-20, 1982.
2. Althaus JN, Hardyck NM, Pierce PB, and Rodgers MS: Decentralized budgeting: holding the purse strings, part II, Journal of Nursing Administration 12(6):34-38, 1982.
3. Carey S and Oahes JL: Hospital budgeting in the case mix environment, Computers in Health Care 5(6):38-40, 1984.
4. Dillon RD and LaMont RP: Financial statement analysis, Clinical Management 3(3):36-39, 1983.
5. Finkler SA: Flexible budget variance analysis extended to patient acuity and DRGs, Health Care Management Review 10(4):21-34, 1985.
6. Kerschner MI and Rooney JM: Utilizing cost accounting information for budgeting, Top Health Care Financing 13(4):56-66, 1987.
7. McCutcheon DJ: Impact analysis reduces the guesswork in budgeting, Dimensions Health Service 65(8):24-25, 1988.
8. Porter-O'Grady T: Programming for the human resources budget in nursing finance: budgeting strategies for a new age, Rockville, Md, 1987, Aspen Publishers.
9. Porter-O'Grady T: Supply and operating costs in nursing finance; budgeting strategies for a new age, 1987, Aspen Publishing.
10. Schmitz V, Masters GM, and Delts W: Better forecasting ensures profitability, quality of care, Healthcare Financial Management 43(1):60-66, 1989.
11. Sonstegard L: Health care costs: every nurse's problem, American Journal of Maternal/Child Nursing 10(2):87, 1985.
12. Souhrada L: Annual forecast shows where to beef up budgets, Hospitals 63(14):68, 1989.
13. Stahl LD: Demystifying critical care management, Journal of Nursing Administration 15(11):14-20, 1985.
14. Tower RB: Analyzing accounting reports, Nursing Management 13(9):13-16, 1982.

Chapter 19

LABOR RELATIONS

Patrick E. Kenny

The issue of labor relations and collective bargaining arouses debate by professionals in many fields. Nursing is a newcomer to the world of labor relations, specifically to collective bargaining.

The health care industry, as the fourth leading industry in the United States, is one of the largest employers. The American Hospital Association estimates 5,721 acute care hospitals in the United States, and 854,554 RNs employed in various settings.[1] The state nursing associations are collective bargaining agents for 139,000 health care employees, and other unions represent an additional 102,000.[3] These numbers include all members of a given collective bargaining unit that may include RNs, licensed practical nurses, pharmacists, and other health care professionals as permitted by the state labor relation board when the collective bargaining unit was established. Given the competitive nature of health care and the decreasing memberships of unions, health care is increasingly becoming a union target.[1,3]

Nursing is one of society's most important groups, considering the service provided. Recent nursing activism, however, indicates that mere lip service is given when nurses face wage compression, image problems, and lower wages than other professions. Many are leaving nursing for the higher salaries of other fields, and fewer people are entering the field of nursing. Nursing has moved into the modern era, and career-oriented professionals are concerned with quality-of-life issues for themselves and their patients. Serious questions arise whether a balance can be struck between service to the public and the rights of those who serve.

This chapter will outline sound labor management policies that are applicable in both union and non-union settings. The critical care nurse manager is responsible for implementing fair labor practices, regardless of personal opinions on collective bargaining in a professional setting. Through use of a case study, the nurse manager will be able to apply theoretical content to the practice setting.

Case Study: Labor Relations

> As the new nurse manager for a 10-bed mixed medical-surgical critical care unit, you have never been a manager in a union setting before. A new contract has just been ratified, and you will be responsible for implementing the provisions contracted.

THE BASICS

Labor relations affect every health care provider in every health care facility that employs nurses. The relationship between employment laws, employee needs, professional standards, and legal rights is complex because they all combine to further complicate care provision.

Health care is viewed as a social issue, and the right to health care is strongly debated. The health care system touches every American at some point; therefore, governmental involvement is inevitable. Thus, governmental bodies regulate the delivery of health care to guarantee safe, effective care.

Labor relations are impacted when those governmental interventions shape the boundaries and the relationships between the employee and employer in health care. Labor relations is a study of the balance of power between the employee, the employer, and the regulatory bodies.

Health care institutions of the past comforted the sick; cure was merely a concept, not a possibility. The administrators did what they felt was necessary, and the employee carried out their orders. The administrator was the authority to be obeyed. The nature of the health care industry was perceived by governmental bodies as charitable, and thus exempt from labor relations laws.

Today comfort and concern are important, but new technology has resulted in increased ability, skill, and education. Today's practitioners demand more than a good feeling from altruistic humanitarianism; they expect economic and personal satisfaction. When these needs go unsatisfied, action by management is required. If the action is felt to be inadequate, the perceived imbalance in the power relationship may result in discontent, and collective action may ensue.

ORGANIZATIONAL FRAMEWORK

Ideally, each institution has a defined organizational hierarchy, and each level has clearly defined role expectations and performance standards. Job descriptions are developed in conjunction with the staff, and periodic review is expected. The job description is behavioral in nature and is used in the criterion-based performance evaluation.

Employees who fully understand the scope and breadth of their duties and the institution's expectations provide better services and are more content within their role. It is simply not enough to give the employee the job description without following through with rating the employee.

> As the new critical care nurse manager, you note that the current job description does not provide a clear definition of expected critical care practice. You realize this is an area that you will have to address by working with staff.

PERSONNEL POLICY

Good personnel policies are well thought out, and recognize the needs of all parties—the institution, the employee and the patient. All the policies to be implemented will affect existing employees and those new to the collective bargaining setting. These effects and the employees' perception of the policy must be considered. This is a management responsibility.

Personnel policies identify employment categories and requirements for employment. The policy often includes a prehire physical, drug screening, length of probationary period, performance and behavior standards, grievance procedure, performance evaluations, benefits, compensation, and safety and security procedures. Each employee receives a hard copy of the policy and acknowledges this receipt in writing, which protects the employee and the hospital.

Policies developed with staff input are effective, workable, and unlikely to cause future difficulties and differences of opinion. Thus, participative management in employee relations receives constant emphasis and reinforcement.

> You, as the nurse manager, review existing personnel policies and realize some of the contract language is unclear. You discuss this with your supervisor, who suggests that you meet with the Director of Human Resources.

WORKMAN'S COMPENSATION

All states regulate workman's compensation to ensure that employees are adequately compensated for losses due to on-the-job injuries. Statutes provide legal definitions of terms such as *employee* and *injury*, and delineate payment for specific injuries. Most employers are subject to statutory law, although some states allow exceptions. In those instances, the employee may take the claim to the state commission to determine liability.

Where workman's compensation laws do apply, the employee is prohibited from bringing suit against the employer for the injury. Sometimes an employee will sue the employer for negligence rather than accept the compensation package awarded him. However, an appeal process through the court system is possible, and considerable litigation can occur when differences of opinion arise over whether the injury was indeed out of and in the course of employment. This is considered a key characteristic for qualification for workman's compensation. Further distinctions are made for deciding whether the injury was related causally to an accident or was the result of a particular job. Preexisting conditions and injuries unrelated to employment are excluded.

A well-defined procedure is needed for reporting, processing, and settling workman's compensation claims. When an employee is injured, the employee is informed of the proper sequence of activities to be followed for legitimate claim to be considered. The employee gives written notice of the injury to the employer. This notice and the report of treatment and medical findings constitute the basis for a legitimate claim.

Employees are also told that the claim is not legitimate if the employee was intoxicated with alcohol or drugs, or the injury was caused by the willful intent to harm self or others. Employers have placed significant attention on these exceptions, and they have been upheld by workman's compensation referees and the courts. Many claims have been denied when it is determined that substance abuse played a causative role.

The intricacies of workman's compensation are great, and this is a key area of difficulties between labor and management. In a facility with a bargaining unit, these issues may come under the agreement for resolution. In noncollective bargaining facilities, continued problems with workman's compensation claims may be one issue that leads to collective action.

Great care is taken to ensure that the workman's compensation guidelines and procedures are logical, fair, and approved by legal counsel in accordance with federal, state and local labor laws. An explicit procedure for informing the employee of workman's compensation rules is provided during orientation and periodically, and is available to the employee, and is posted prominently.

> As the nurse manager, you have just discussed workman's compensation with the risk manager, and have determined that in the past, staff who sustain needle stick injuries have not been encouraged to go to health services. As the manager, you realize this is an unacceptable risk and plan a staff meeting to discuss your concerns with your staff.

JOB SECURITY

Few issues raise the concern and ire of employees more than job security. In the absence of due cause and provisions in the facility's rules, the employees may feel that they do not have secure jobs, and that their employment may end subject to an employer's whim. To alleviate unnecessary anxiety, a written statement outlining the length and terms of employment after the probationary period should be given to the employee during orientation, and the employee should sign a receipt. The next box provides an example of a written statement about the probationary period. Putting it in writing constitutes a contract between the employee and the hospital, which gives the employee security and still allows the hospital to terminate an unsatisfactory employee.

> **TERMS OF EMPLOYMENT**
>
> *Probationary Period*
>
> The first three months of your employment with the hospital are considered a trial period. If your supervisor or department head evaluates your performance and other factors, and determines that you are not suitable for the job, you may be terminated at any time during this period. Although you accrue benefits and service credit, no benefits are available for your use until the probationary period has been satisfactorily completed. The hospital reserves the right to extend the probationary period for new employees, as needed, in order to determine satisfactory performance more adequately. The probationary period applies to all categories of employees.
>
> Assuming that you satisfactorily complete the probationary period, your employment with the hospital will be continued for an indefinite period, although the hospital may end your employment for good cause at any time. *Good cause for termination* is when you cannot or will not complete work according to established standards.

A job security enhancement program is instituted so that employees have a feeling of belonging. Ongoing review and refining of the discipline discharge procedures ensures the procedures' fairness. An integral part of this program includes a review of practices to improve management communication to staff about changes that are imminent, anticipated, or envisioned. Nurses are aware of the problems facing health care. Nurses are more likely to work with management if they are informed about the hospital's future, especially in areas that affect their own well-being. A good personnel planning policy, which anticipates nurse shortages or surpluses to avoid sudden staffing changes, provides the employee with a sense of job security. This is a vital part of a job security enhancement program.

MANAGEMENT PRACTICES

Managers ideally are groomed from within the institution for the future. Grooming is achieved by granting increasing responsibility, observing communication skills, and encouraging successful leadership endeavors. A management practices program increases employee satisfaction with advancement opportunities, prepares the employee for a management position, and reduces frustration and turnover in new managers.

A management training program can be instituted to familiarize the employee with what a manager does. Specific skills taught include planning, organizing, delegating, dealing effectively with conflict, giving constructive criticism, handling difficult employees, counseling, and providing feedback. A management practices program is imperative, not only for new managers, but for seasoned managers who need to periodically review and update their own skills. A well-designed review program improves the managers' leadership, planning, and decision-making skills. Institutions with management training programs focus on skill development for managers; this is proactive, not reactive. Thus, crisis management is avoided.

Whether the manager is new or well-established, certain management practices are necessary for a smoothly operating institution. The basic techniques include fair disciplinary practices and timeliness when dealing with problems.

Fair Disciplinary Practices

Few managers enjoy taking disciplinary action. But the cost of avoiding necessary action is high to the institution, the manager, and the employee. When a manager disciplines an employee, the manager operationalizes the institution's philosophy about fairness and equity. If the manager gives only lip service to fair labor relations, employees view the organization and its philosophy as mere rhetoric. However, if management acts and holds to the philosophy, the employees see that management truly strives for fairness.

Identifying tenets that facilitate positive employee relations helps cement working relationships between managers and employees. The box below provides a working list that can be used as a framework for developing a philosophy of fairness unique to the institution.

TENETS OF EMPLOYEE RELATIONS

Most employees respect fairness.
Most employees want to do a good job.
Most people do not like uncertainty.
Most managers have at least one problem employee.
Discipline is corrective, not retaliatory. Employees work better in an environment where there is constructive discipline and when they have respect for the supervisor who administers discipline.
Corrective discipline satisfies the goal for equal treatment when rules, regulations, safety practices, and job expectations, are applied and enforced equally among personnel.
The right to discipline or discharge employees for just cause, and the right to make rules and regulations regarding performance, are primary management prerogatives.
Employees have the right to fair and equal treatment, and when discipline is administered, to grieve the action.
Always get the employee's version of an infraction. This is essential when using a problem-solving approach.

Timeliness of Dealing with Problems

Infractions are dealt with immediately after the event occurs, or as soon as the nurse manager has knowledge of the incident. The nurse manager gathers facts calmly, quickly, and efficiently. Remember, just the facts are gathered. They are recorded, and all notations are based on objectivity and facts, not gossip or surmise. Note the who, what, when, where, how of the infractions. What reason did the employee give for committing the infraction? What merits are there to her reasons? What are the employee's record, past performance, and past incidents of the same type? Do they have bearing on this action or are they unrelated? What were the consequences of the action on work? On the patient? What were the potential results? What policies were violated? Did the employee know it was an infraction?

The burden of proof of an infraction lies with the employer. The manager will find it useful to answer the seven key questions about the infraction in the following box before making decisions.

All of these questions provide a framework that can loosely identify fair management behavior. Remember that labor laws provide excellent guidelines for disciplinary actions, and thus protect both managers and employees. A good rule of thumb for dealing with a difficult decision is to review and discuss the infraction with the director of human resources. Erring on the side of the employee is humane, but this can result in precedent-setting that sends the message to other employees that this type of infraction is acceptable. This is very problematic and inconsistent with effective management.

At your first staff meeting as the nurse manager, you discover that three days ago there was an unreported narcotic discrepancy. The charge nurse then stated she thought the count would be corrected over time. Based on your knowledge of statutory law and institutional practice, you realize this type of behavior is unaccept-

---

SEVEN KEY QUESTIONS ABOUT LABOR POLICY INFRACTION

1. Can it be demonstrated that the employee knew what was expected and the consequences of the infraction?
2. Are the rules, regulations, and directives reasonably related to the efficient and safe operation of the institution?
3. Before disciplining, were the facts thoroughly investigated?
4. Was this investigation demonstrably fair, objective, and impartial?
5. Does the investigation yield clear, convincing evidence that the employee committed the infraction?
6. Are rules, regulations, and discipline fairly and consistently administered throughout the hospital?
7. Is the discipline appropriate based on the proven offense and the past record of the employee?

able, and inform staff that narcotic discrepancies are fully reportable. You ask three senior staff to review policy and confer with the shop steward about this problem, and ask them to report the findings at the next staff meeting.

UNIONIZATION

Collective bargaining is not a product of modern times. The concept dates back to Horace Greely, who published editorials in the *New York Times* about the need for improved working conditions. Collective bargaining as it is known today evolved over a fifty-year period. The historical impetus for collective bargaining arose out of the severe unemployment problems of the 1920s and 1930s. The National Labor Relations Act was implemented in 1935. This law, known as the Wagner Act, gave workers federal protection in their efforts to form unions and organize for better conditions. The National Labor Relations Board (NLRB) was created to ensure that the conditions of the act were carried out. In 1947, the act was amended through the Taft-Hartley Act. Hospital management successfully lobbied to exclude nursing and hospital personnel from collective bargaining rights and protection. In 1962, federal legislation enabled employees in health care institutions to participate. Further legislation in 1967 encompassed investor-owned hospitals and nursing homes. It was not until 1974 that employees in nonprofit hospitals were allowed to bargain collectively.[5]

Unions are more likely to be formed when workers feel frustrated and helpless. Unions are not formed by people that feel that they have been treated justly and fairly. In today's rapidly changing health care field, collective bargaining is viewed as a necessity by those who want and need unions. Wages are still inadequate in most of America, at least considering the knowledge base, technical skills, and work load demanded of the professional. Lack of respect by peers, management, and medicine contributes to the genesis of ill-will and unhappiness. Cavalier attitudes of management that see work schedules, hours, and benefits as things that can be manipulated at will further alienate the professional. Changes in the payment delivery system to hospitals have occurred, and economic chaos is resulting from attempts at cost containment. Employee uncertainty and unrest increases, and hospitals have begun to lay off all levels of employees. Sources in the *Pennsylvania Nurse*[5] said that concern about job security and the perceived unfairness of health care administrators contribute to the continued need for collective bargaining.

Collective bargaining in nursing continues to focus on issues discussed in 1950. The three major issues are:

1. The effective application of professional standards in daily hospital routine
2. Improvement in the dignity, status, and economic welfare of individual nurses
3. The recruitment and retention of sufficient numbers of properly qualified personnel to meet nursing needs[2]

These issues remain unresolved because of the limited gains nursing has made towards professionalism, the lack of autonomy in practice, and the financial constraints resulting from economic cutbacks affecting the health care industry. Until these issues are resolved, many professionals will continue to need collective bargaining.

Collective bargaining is a symptom of problems within the system, and therefore, institutions usually get the kind of union they deserve. If an administrator develops sound policies, provides good working conditions, supports employees, and has supervisors who understand the relationship between employee and employer, the likelihood of collective bargaining is minimal. If all of these conditions exist, what could the union offer? The question is not whether nurses join unions, it is whether management does its job.

Management is clearly responsible for addressing problems, resolving wrongs, and implementing fair labor practices. When these responsibilities are abrogated, unionization is the consequence.

Collective bargaining as defined by S. H Slichter is

> a process and a technique whereby employees participate as a group or bargaining unit in determining jointly, with employers, the conditions of the employment relationship. This means much more than just negotiating salary terms and hours of work. Collective bargaining is also a continuous process whereby the countless day-to-day problems of working relationships can be handled in an orderly and democratic manner. Collective bargaining is not unionism. But unions clearly are ready, willing, and able to serve as the representative for the group.[4]

Labor-management relations do not have to be adversarial. A cooperative approach and attitude by management and labor fosters an attitude of mutual respect and a willingness to work together for the improvement of patient care and equity for all concerned.

The zero-sum–relationship view of labor management relations leads to an antagonistic, negative relationship. When the belief is that when one side wins, the other loses, neither side wins, and unwanted effects such as strikes often occur. Win-win negotiations offer an alternative, and provide tangible rewards for both labor and management. Cooperation is basically a matter of each side being willing to consult with the other.

> As the nurse manager for the critical care unit you have the ability to foster this collegial relationship on your own unit by recognizing and respecting the opinion and views of the shop steward who is one of your senior staff.

Closed Shop and Open Shop

There are pros and cons to both closed- and open-shop local units. Closed-shop arrangements are the result of contract negotiations, and may not be allowed in states with right-to-work laws. In a closed-shop agreement, an employee must join the local unit within a specified period of time of hire to maintain employment. The advantage of the closed shop is that the local unit has sufficient income to provide services to all employees, and has strength in numbers—they literally represent all employees. This provides a bargaining lever in contract negotiations, and allows the local unit to present a unified front. The disadvantage is that some employees join because they have to, and might resent this rule. Some may join the union but not participate in local unit activities, thereby weakening the unit. Lack of commitment can provide a focus for a decertification election prompted by management or a raid by a competing union.

The advantages to an open-shop arrangement are that the members who join are there because they genuinely want to be a part of the unit. This provides strength in purpose and commitment to the ideals of the local unit. There are disadvantages, however. By law, the local unit must represent all eligible employees whether they are members or not. This may be a financial drain on the local unit, and is perceived by union members as patently unfair. Some states have remedied this problem by passing fair-share legislation, meaning that an employee may choose not to join a local unit, but must pay a representative share of the dues to the local unit or professional association. When the employee's religion prohibits participation, the employee donates that portion to charity. Other disadvantages to the open-shop arrangement is that management may notice a small number of employees belong to the local unit. They might infer that the local unit is susceptible to a decertification election or other union-busting techniques.

Union Busting

The term *union busting* means the legal and illegal activities used to prevent or eliminate a union. Activities such as decertification elections, use of management consulting firms, and antiorganizing activities by management are classic examples. Delaying tactics, which prevent or slow organizing activity, are often used. The facility may attempt to decrease the number of eligible employees by challenging the number and titles of employees in the bargaining unit. For example, management may challenge the inclusion of team leaders in the unit, on the grounds that they are management. Tactics include quoting contract language out of context and using strike fear; that is, preying on nurses' feelings about strikes and professionalism.

Administrators frequently feel betrayed by employees when a collective action begins, and may react rather than act. Employers may attempt to talk employees out of unionizing, and they may use subtle or not-so-subtle threats of job loss to prevent organization. These activities are violations of labor law, illegal, and they usually backfire. Proof of these violations often gives the union organizers more ammunition in their efforts to organize.

Management typically resists what is seen as efforts to restrict the prerogatives of management. Managers fear that a negotiated contract restricts their ability to accomplish objectives. Thus they believe that the organization becomes less effective. Resistance results in illegal activities, intentional or not. Top management understands that these reactions are common, anticipates them, and helps the management team avoid the pitfalls.

Signs that management is utilizing a union-busting approach include frequent meetings of first-line management at the head nurse and supervisor level, comments by first-line personnel that they feel the unionizing activity is aimed against them, messages from management to employees that "we're all family," management consultation teams brought in to help tighten things up, and small, informal meetings on the floor by the director of nursing with staff nurses, where none had occurred previously. Nurse managers are responsible for examining personal feelings about this approach and deciding what their expected or actual role is with respect to union-busting.

Union-busting, as a tactic, requires close scrutiny before being employed, with the pros, cons, payoffs, and risks examined in detail. Union-busting is not an easy tactic to employ. Fearing unionization is like admitting that management has not done a good job. It also suggests that management is more concerned about the possibility of a successful election than the issues at hand. Rather than dealing up-front and fairly with employees, union-busting is a sign that preservation of the status quo is important to management—and the employees aren't. In general, it is not advisable to engage in union-busting. Nurse managers usually choose not to be a part of union-busting tactics.

Catching the Worm of Discontent

An ongoing, planned process of open communication and problem solving is the best preventative method. Employee access to the manager, willingness to listen, and openness to ideas and suggestions are the best steps to prevent the widespread discontent that leads to collective bargaining activity. A desire for collective bargaining does not arise overnight and is often the culmination of a long period of discontent and unhappiness. Ongoing use of the problem-solving process, rapid identification of problems, and resolution of those problems is imperative. The problem-solving process is a logical sequence of activities.

As the nurse manager you must recognize your responsibility in this area. By planning regular monthly staff meetings on all three shifts, you can deal with issues identified by staff and build cooperation and trust. Actions and behaviors demonstrating commitment to open communication provide the best strategy to catch the worm of discontent before collective bargaining occurs.

REASSESSING MANAGEMENT PRACTICES

Management circles, quality circles, or other mechanisms for participative problem-solving assists the manager in consistently evaluating the effectiveness of management techniques. Peer review, as well as input from subordinates, is invaluable in anticipating problems, correcting problem areas, and addressing planning issues. By reviewing, assessing, and revising management practices, issues that arise can be quickly identified and resolved. The result of this type of proactive leadership is employee satisfaction, open channels of communication, and a more open work climate.

DEALING WITH UNIONS

Often mistrust and resentment exist before the unionization activity occurs. This mistrust is compounded by the normal sequence of activities that occurs during the unionization process, with management resisting unionization and labor fostering adoption of a union. All the techniques used to promote or reject the union come into play and further increase the distrust and animosity. The manager's attitude toward the local unit has a significant impact on the relationship with the union.

When an adversarial mind-set occurs, or when the manager takes personal offense at union activity, relationships can only go from bad to worse and increase the day-to-day tension. However, if the manager is cooperative, both parties benefit. The manager must be aware of her feelings about unionization in general, and unionization at the facility specifically, before being able to work effectively with the union. Two key concepts that help the manager work with the union are recognizing the role of delegates and shop stewards and knowing the contract.

RECOGNIZING THE ROLE OF DELEGATES OR SHOP STEWARDS

The delegates, or shop stewards, are elected by peers to represent them to management, not only during the negotiation process, but also during the time of the contract administration. Shop stewards *are* employees, duty-bound and obligated to work for peers. Union delegates and shop stewards insure the management's adherence to the contract. The goal is to achieve a satisfactory outcome for the employee. The manager that recognizes the contribution of the shop stewards and union delegates creates allies in the quest for quality care and cooperation. However, managers are aware that union representatives consider the preservation of jobs and viability of the union as paramount.

Under normal circumstances, unions do not intentionally harass management. When management is perceived as unfair, administering or interpreting the contract incorrectly, or proceeding illegally, the shop steward is obligated to take action.

KNOWING THE CONTRACT

The manager's best option is to know the contract (see box on pg. 321). As a manager, you are aware that the union members and shop stewards know what is in the contract and are ready to enforce it. This means that differences in interpretation may arise. Resolution of issues can be achieved through the grievance process. The contract is legally binding and *must* be adhered to by all parties. If you were not part of the negotiating team and are unsure of the contract provisions or what those provisions mean, ask the negotiating representatives or

> **STANDARD CONTRACT PROVISIONS**
>
> *Agreement*
> This agreement made and entered into as of this first day of July, 1990, between the County Hospital (agency) and State Nurses Association (bargaining unit) acting for and on behalf of the Professional Staff Nurses (local unit).
>
> *Witnesseth*
> Whereas, the parties hereto recognize that the enlightened participation of the public, management, and labor is needed if County Hospital is to make its maximum contribution to the community, and recognizing that complete and uninterrupted patient care is of vital importance to the health, welfare, and safety of the community, and desiring to establish conditions of employment under which members of the bargaining unit shall work during the term of this agreement; and
>
> Whereas, the parties hereto are in further accord that effective employee-management cooperation in the public service requires a clear statement of the respective rights and obligations of labor and management, and
>
> Whereas, the parties hereto desire to regulate relations between the parties with a view of securing harmonious cooperation, thereby averting interruptions and interferences with services to patients,
>
> Now therefore, in consideration of the mutual promises herein set forth, it is agreed by and between the parties as follows in the articles below.

legal counsel to clarify the provisions. Countless hours and money are saved when a manager seeks assistance first. Agreements are couched in legal terms and are not easily understood. When in doubt, check the interpretation of the contract with human resources. A minor delay in response or in taking an action is better than creating a problem or a grievance that results in a settlement in favor of the union. Beware of setting precedent in your actions and in your efforts to be fair. Precedent-setting causes difficulties down the road if management allows a certain action once or under a certain set of circumstances. This can and will be used as justification for the same outcome under precedent, or past practice. Be aware of the effect that action and inaction have on the work of the unit or institution, and seek guidance from the labor relations director, personnel manager, or human resource director.

Managing Staff after a Strike

Returning to productivity and workable relationships with staff is difficult under the best of circumstances. A strike engenders many strong feelings on both sides, and those feelings will take significant efforts to resolve. The success or failure of a strike as a bargaining tool will have long-lasting implications for both union and management. The actions of management during the strike will be remembered and referred to throughout the contract period. If management retaliated by firing staff, bringing in replacements, and emphasizing the abandonment of patients in media, then working relationships will be strained at best and management can anticipate problems. When the strike is over, some indicators of discontent occur such as increased sick-time usage, work slowdowns and insubordination. Effective managers deal quickly with the underlying problem.

In a similar manner, managers will remember the actions of staff during the strike, and may display mistrust and anger. Union members and leaders will look for this to use as justification for the strike or the continued unrest. A neutral third party may be needed to resolve bitterness and anger. Managers are well advised to heed the issues that led to the strike and seek corrective action if the issues have not already been corrected by the negotiated settlement.

Contract Language

All contracts are products of negotiation, and thus are agency-specific. The contract recognizes the unique issues, opportunities, and problems of that agency. The contract is a binding guideline of the who, what, when, where, and why of employee and management behavior. The following example is a compilation of several actual contracts that provides an overview of a standard contract. Not all clauses are included. Specific aspects are included to help the new nurse manager understand basic language.

Reading the standard contract provisions provides the nurse manager with insight and promotes a cooperative tone for the binding nature of the contract. Note that both parties recognize the mutual benefits to ongoing positive negotiations relating to conditions of employment and practice.

Management Rights and Responsibilities

As you read the box on the next page on management rights you realize that this empowers management to change the care delivery model, and the scope and conditions of care. Management retains the right to creatively explore future options as health care delivery evolves and adapts to change. For example, to remain competitive in recruitment, management can consider shared governance, clinical ladders, or differentiated practice.

The box on p. 323 identifies those responsibilities management has to the collective bargaining unit. Note that this contract represents a closed shop and that the union can keep track of position control by mandating information from management to maintain the security of the local unit.

Please note that discrimination is very clearly addressed in this contract in the box on p. 324. Professional nurses were instrumental in negotiating a discrimination clause in their contracts to prohibit and prevent exclusion of certain individuals or classes of individuals from bargaining representation. Contract

ARTICLE II MANAGEMENT RIGHTS

1. The management of County Hospital and the direction of the working force is vested exclusively with the Board of Trustees. Except where expressly abridged by a specific provision of this Agreement, County Hospital retains the sole right to hire, discipline, or discharge for due cause; to layoff, promote, transfer, and assign its employees; to determine or change the starting and quitting time and numbers of hours worked; to assign duties to the work force; to establish new job classifications; to organize, discontinue, or reduce a department, function, or division; to carry out the ordinary and usual functions of management whether or not possessed or exercised by County Hospital prior to the execution of this agreement.
2. County Hospital may introduce a change in the method or methods of cooperation, which will preclude a change in job duties and a reduction of personnel in any department. Nothing contained in this Agreement shall prevent the implementation of any program to be hereafter undertaken by County Hospital.
3. State Nurses Association and County Hospital agree to work cooperatively together to attain and maintain maximum patient care and full efficiency.

ARTICLE III ASSOCIATION SECURITY AND CHECK OFF

1. Within sixty (60) days of the effective date of this Agreement, all present employees who are covered by this Agreement must become and remain members of this State Nurses Association in good standing as a condition of employment, and all employees who are hired after the effective date of this Agreement shall as a condition of employment become and remain a member in good standing after ninety (90) days of the date of hire. Any employee who fails to comply with this requirement shall be discharged from his/her position with County Hospital within twenty (20) days after written notice from the association.
2. County Hospital agrees to furnish State Nurses Association each month with the names of newly hired employees, classifications of work, dates of hire, and social security numbers; names of terminated employees; and names of employees on leaves of absence.
3. Each month County Hospital will remit to State Nurses Association all deductions for dues made from the wages of all employees for the preceding month, together with a list of all employees for whom dues have been deducted.

language now prohibits the type of discrimination that historically limited who was represented. These historical controlling activities circumscribed union activity and allowed industry to select the members of the union. The influence of the civil rights movement had a profound impact on the growth, expansion, and acceptance of unions in the professional world.

> **ARTICLE V DISCRIMINATION**
>
> County Hospital and State Nurses Association agree that they will not discriminate against any nurse applicant or any nurse employee because of race, color, national origin, religious or political affiliation, sex, handicap, age, sexual preference, or for lawful association activity.

Mutual Responsibilities

No strike or *lockout* provisions resulted from strike tactics of management and labor in the past. The box on the next page gives an example of contract language that details the prohibited activities. Both management and labor have an obligation to continue to work in good faith with each other during the terms of the contract.

Grievance Procedure

The box on p. 325 defines *grievance* and provides an abbreviated step-by-step procedure. Grievance procedures provide a mechanism for resolving conflict in an orderly and impartial way. The nurse manager recognizes that the employee's rights are protected through these contract provisions. Grievances often arise out of misunderstandings associated with contract interpretation. Employees sometimes grieve everything to test the knowledge and managerial backbone of a new nurse manager. The savvy nurse manager accepts this as a ploy in the power struggle, not as a personal attack or affront of individual employees. In addition, grievances are used to demonstrate to members that the union is working for them.

When the grievance proceeds to Step 3 and beyond, decisions no longer rest with the nurse manager. The director of human resources may decide to settle on behalf of the employee based on a decision that the time and cost for further appeal is not justified. This is particularly true if management's case is not clearly documented, despite verbal assurances that the infraction occurred as stated by the nurse manager. When a decision is made to move to Step 4, this is called *binding arbitration.* This decision is not made lightly by either the union or top-level management.

The arbitrator is selected according to the rules of the American Arbitration Association and can entail lengthy, costly judicial procedure. The decision of the arbitrator is final and binding upon the parties.

Contract Savings Clause

The contract savings clause protects both parties from claims that particular items were not open for discussion or negotiation. The statement assures the contract

ARTICLE VI   NO STRIKE OR LOCKOUT

1. No employee shall engage in any strike, sit-down, sit-in, slow-down, cessation, or stoppage, or interruption of work, boycott, sympathy strike, or other interference with the operation of County Hospital for any purpose whatsoever, including actions in support of other labor organizations. Any employee who participates in or engages in such activity shall be subject to disciplinary action including discharge.

2. State Nurses Association, its officers, agents, representatives, and members shall not in any way directly or indirectly authorize, encourage, participate in, or sanction any strike, sit-down, sit-in, cessation or stoppage or interruption of work, or boycott, or ratify, condone, or lend support to any such conduct or action.

3. In addition to any other liability, remedy, or right provided by applicable statute, should strike, stoppage, sit-down, sit-in, slow-down, boycott or interruption of work occur, the State Nurses Association shall immediately upon request by County Hospital:

    a. Notify employees that such action is a violation of this Agreement and instruct such employees to cease action immediately.

    b. Post notices at appropriate locations advising that such action is in violation of this Agreement and instructing employees to return to work immediately.

4. County Hospital agrees that it will not lock out employees during the term of this Agreement.

ARTICLE XIV   GRIEVANCE PROCEDURE

A Grievance shall be defined as any complaint, dispute, controversy, or disagreement involving one or more employees and County Hospital, or between State Nurses Association and County Hospital, which may arise concerning the application, meaning, or interpretation of this Agreement. Grievances shall be processed and disposed of in the following sequence:

Grievance Procedure

Action	Time Frame
Step 1. Employee meets with Immediate Supervisor.	7 days
Supervisor reviews Grievance and responds.	5 days
If not settled satisfactorily then	5 days
Step 2. The Grievance is put in writing.	5 days
Department Head meets with Grievant.	5 days
If not settled satisfactorily then	5 days
Step 3. Grievance is submitted to Human Resources.	5 days
If not settled satisfactorily then	5 days
Step 4. Impartial Arbitrator	months

parties that every opportunity was afforded both parties to add, discuss, and attempt negotiation on any topic so chosen. See the box below on savings clause.

Other Elements of a Contract

The box below includes a list of other elements that are commonly negotiated with contracts. Because of the specific nature of these items to each institution,

---

ARTICLE XXVI   SAVINGS CLAUSE

County Hospital and the State Nurses Association acknowledge that during the negotiations which resulted in this Agreement, each had the unlimited right and opportunity to make demands and proposals with respect to any subject matter not removed by law from the area of collective bargaining, and that the understandings and agreements arrived at by the parties after the exercise of that right and opportunity are set forth in this Agreement. Therefore, County Hospital and the State Nurses Association, for the life of this agreement, each agree that the other shall not be obligated to bargain collectively with respect to any subject matter referred to or covered in this Agreement or with respect to any subject matter not specifically referred to or covered in this Agreement, whether or not such subject matter was within the knowledge or contemplation of either or both of the parties at the time they negotiated or signed this Agreement.

OTHER ELEMENTS OF A STANDARD CONTRACT

Article I	Exclusivity of Bargaining Agent
Article IV	Hiring of Employees-Probationary Period
Article VII	Wages and Hours
Article VIII	Overtime
Article XV	Seniority
Article XVI	Layoff-Recall
Article XVII	Unpaid Leaves of Absence
Article XVIII	Discharge and Penalties
Article XIX	Personnel Files
Article XX	Association Activities and Information
Article XXI	Inservice Education
Article XXII	Postings and Transfers
Article XXIII	Temporary Reassignment
Article XXIV	Tuition Reimbursement
Article XXV	PRN Nurses and Agency Nurses
Article XVII	Termination

sample language was not addressed. However, there are several other key points that provide basic information about contracts. Most contracts have a clause known as a reopener clause, usually related to wages or specific topics, that allows one or both of the parties to initiate negotiations that prove beneficial to the parties. Otherwise they would need to wait until the end of the contract to readdress these. This occurs when management wishes to raise salaries, adjust wage, overtime, or differential scales, or change conditions of employment (to allow for latch-key or swing-shift hours) after negotiation. This allows the parties to negotiate specifics while the remainder of the contract remains untouched.

Some contracts may encourage and allow for contract extensions; that is, the terms of the current contract are extended for a specific period of time (often one to two years) with negotiated clauses for such things as adjusting salaries. This is particularly true in times of good relations between management and labor, or when reopening or going into full contract negotiations may not prove helpful to one or both parties. For example, when the institution or community has economic difficulties, one or both parties may initiate a contract extension. This is also used as a tactic when antilabor or antimanagement sentiments in the state, nation, or locality could result in bad provisions, give-backs, or higher-than-anticipated benefits. Both parties agree to the contract extension for a specific period of time.

CONFLICT RESOLUTION AND PROFESSIONALISM

Most managers and nurses do not deal well with conflict and confrontation. Avoiding conflict only tends to foster the problem and, in the long run, to take a heavier toll on the nurse manager, other employees, and patients.

Managers give several reasons for avoiding conflict resolution. Social repercussion are foremost. Statements like "I won't be liked," "I won't be perceived as a nice person," or "I don't want to cause an unpleasant experience" are made. Nurse managers fear a bad-guy image because nurses are sensitive to meeting needs in others. Part of the job of manager entails dealing with problems and issues as they arise. If the conflict remains on an objective plane, however, the employee will know that corrective action is focused on outlining expectations for performance, which helps goal achievement.

Managers can fear physical repercussions from the union. Statements heard include, "I'm afraid conflict may be dangerous," or "The union may strike back at me because of the decision." Fortunately the union's bark is usually worse than the bite. Rarely does physical retaliation occur. In the event an employee does lose control, management deals with this immediately before physical escalation can occur. Union scare tactics, such as threatening phone calls and property damage, are intimidating. Each nurse manager decides how much will be tolerated before capitulating or choosing to end employment at that setting.

Fear of Loss of Control

New managers are reluctant to confront problems because they fear loss of control. The best way to deal with this fear is by planning a strategy to deal with the conflict and work toward resolution. By setting the time, place, and agenda of the meeting, the manager is in control.

There are several methods available for use in conflict resolution, all of which have been successful. The fact-finding conference is where the manager lists the facts on both sides of the issue, listens attentively, and gives employees the benefit of the doubt. If possible, have a third, neutral party there to help sort out the issues. An astute manager can use the problem-solving process to her personal advantage to keep control.

By following prudent labor relations principles in all employee interactions, the nurse manager demonstrates accountability for her actions. Nurses are accustomed to being held legally and ethically accountable for their actions in their practice. When clear expectations for performance and practice are set, success can be achieved.

Focus on performance standards. Job evaluations that are criterion and performance based help the nurse manager retain control—if the criterion are valid and fair, and the standards have been developed with input from the staff. Nurses are accustomed to being evaluated and respond positively to realistic, measurable tools that remove subjective elements. Nurses want to perform well. The nurse is usually aware of instances when performance was less than expected, and she will understand performance-improving measures.

Identify positive outcomes. Always focus on the positive aspect of a performance or a relationship. This is especially true for the positive outcomes engendered by a contract and the leadership skills developed by an employee's role in the union. Accent the positive.

CONCLUSION

This chapter has provided a theoretical basis of the knowledge needed by a nurse manager to deal positively with employees in a collective bargaining setting. Emphasis was placed on the responsibility of the nurse manager to keep the relationship collaborative and professional, and to avoid adversarial no-win situations. This will help make labor relations an asset to the nurse manager, the institution, and the employee.

REFERENCES

1. American Hospital Association: Personal communication about 1989 statistics, Chicago, 1990.
2. American Nurses Association: Braving new frontiers; ANA's economic and general welfare program 1946-1986, Kansas City, Mo, 1986, American Nurses Association.

3. American Nurses Association: Personal communication about 1989 statistics, Kansas City, Mo, 1990.
4. Berlow L: Are unions the answer to collective bargaining for nurses? Hospital Topics, May 1961 (reprint).
5. Pennsylvania Nurses Association *Labor Relations.* Harrisburg, Pa, 1986, Pennsylvania Nurses Association.

SUGGESTED READINGS:

1. Adams-Ender C: Developing and promoting managerial talent, Today's OR Nurse 12(3):33-35, 1990.
2. American Hospital Association: Hospital statistics, Chicago, 1987, American Hospital Association.
3. Arch M: Work satisfaction, unionism and military amongst nurses, Community Health Studies 13(2):177-85, 1989.
4. Benesch K, Abramson NS, Grenvik A, and Meisel A: Medicolegal aspects of critical care, Rockville, Md, 1986, Aspens System Corporation.
5. Fought SG: Educational approaches in critical care, Critical Care Quarterly 7(1): June 1984 (editorial).
6. Fiesta J: The law and liability; a guide for nurses, ed 2, New York, 1988, John Wiley & Sons.
7. Ginzberg E: Nursing 1987; a look back and a look ahead, Journal of Nursing Administration 17(12):3-5, 1987.
8. Julius DJ: Managing in a unionized setting; the discipline process, Part I, AORN-J 48(5):919, 922,924-27, 1988.
9. Kruger D: Labor management issues for the future, New York, 1979, National League for Nursing Pub No 20-18-1.
10. Labor management issues in the health care field: New York, 1976, National League for Nursing Pub No 21-1624.
11. Lee B and Parker J: Supervisory participation in professional associations; implications of North Shore University Hospital, Industrial and Labor Relations Review 40(3), 1987.
12. Nierenberg GI: (1983). Fundamentals of negotiating, New York, 1983, Hawthorn/Dutton.
13. Pohlman KJ: Against nursing advice? Focus on critical care 17(1):57-58, 1990.
14. Powills S et al: Hospitals learn to deal with unionization, Hospitals 63(13):44-49, 1989.
15. Shaffer F, editor: Patients and purse strings, New York, 1986, National League for Nursing Publication.
16. Southwick K and Leberto T: Nurse shortage provokes strikes, more organizing, Health Week 2 (16):1, 16, 1986.

Chapter 20

ETHICAL AND LEGAL CONSIDERATIONS

Kathleen E. Powderly

This chapter discusses ethical and legal issues in critical care and the factors that contribute to increasing awareness of these issues. Prominent cases that have affected the legal climate of critical care decision-making are summarized, and intervention strategies for the nurse manager are offered. A case study at the end of the chapter applies the concepts described.

ETHICAL AND LEGAL ASPECTS

Technology has an important influence on ethical and legal health care issues, especially in the critical care unit. The critical care unit is a product of midtwentieth century technological advances. In the nineteenth century, the tools available to health care providers were very limited. In fact, many available therapies were more harmful than helpful; for example, bleeding and purging.[10] Much of what was beneficial to patients would now be known as nursing care. During the twentieth century, dramatic technological advances influenced the delivery of health care and raised some important questions: Is it indeed beneficial to use every available technology on every patient? Can society afford to do so? How should practitioners decide what is helpful and what is futile for the individual and for society? Artificial ventilation and feeding sometimes leads to a prolonged "living" or "dying" of unresponsive, comatose, and vegetative patients. The issues raised with organ transplantation best illustrate the ethical and legal dilemmas of technology. Practitioners and society must ask, "When is the donor *really dead?*"

Traditionally, medicine was a paternalistic practice.[10] The physician made the decisions and the patient (and the nurse, for that matter) abided by them. Patient autonomy is now raising ethical and legal dilemmas. The patient—the health care *consumer*—is assuming a much more prominent role in health care decision-making. The consumer is now demanding information and the right to make decisions for himself or herself. The arrival of the *Patient's Bill of Rights* illustrates the prominence of autonomy in health care. Interestingly, the *Patient's Bill of Rights* merely returns the basic human rights denied to patients in the past. As the consumer asks more and more questions, health care providers become more introspective, which can be seen by the discussions about the rationale of health care decisions and about ethical and legal issues.

High-technology critical care is extremely expensive. Until recently, health care providers in the United States functioned as if financial resources were infinite. Despite expenditures on health care (11.5 percent of our gross national product), statistics do not reflect a healthy society.[3] We are finally realizing that we cannot afford to provide all available modern technological health care to everyone.[2] Although individual health care providers function at the bedside as if cost were not a factor, cost is a factor. In addition, what the health care system spends on unreimbursed care affects the system's health. This major societal issue stresses the clinician at the bedside and the health care manager trying to balance the budget.

We spend a lot of money on providing care, especially acute care to the elderly. Most of Medicare's budget is spent on old people, and our society is increasingly aging. Some suggest that age could be considered in limiting access to high technology interventions.[2] Others feel that many elderly citizens have good quality of life and are entitled to whatever health care interventions they desire. This is an issue that society will increasingly grapple with in the next century.

Although nursing may not yet have the degree of autonomy in practice it wishes, it is certainly no longer a profession of handmaidens. Ethical and legal issues are increasing in critical care nursing practice. Patient advocacy is fundamentally a part of nursing. Because of their relationships with patients and families, nurses have much to offer the decision-making process. When faced with decisions with ethical and legal ramifications, nurses have a professional responsibility to contribute to the process. Although the physician is responsible for the order to stop ventilation, most physicians would appreciate input from those who have worked with the patient and family in the decision-making process—the nurses. Even when the nurse's input is not solicited, nursing must remain in the role of patient advocate.

The nurse-patient relationship is fundamentally different from the physician-patient relationship. The Code of Ethics of the American Medical Association states, "A physician may choose whom he will serve."[8] Most physicians, except house staff, have primary contractual relationships with their patients. This means that the contract can be broken by either party. If the patient does not like the physician's advice, he or she may seek another opinion and change health care providers. If the physician feels the patient is noncompliant, the physician may break the contract.

On the other hand, nurses, who are almost all employed by institutions, must contend with their values, the ANA Code of Ethics, the patient's values, *and the institution's values* in the usual nurse-patient interaction.[7] In addition, the ANA Code[1] states,

> The nurse provides services with respect for human dignity and the uniqueness of the client unrestricted by considerations of social or economic status, personal attributes, or the nature of health problems.[7]

The nurse lacks the physician's option to choose patients. If the institution's primary value is economics, some nurses and nurse managers may function within the institution under great ethical stress.

It is easy to see why these issues are important in critical care nursing where the nurse's role is very important and very autonomous. This is "rescue nursing." However, when rescue fails, but does prolong expensive and futile therapy, the patient, family, and staff suffer. Nowhere are the dilemmas caused by technology felt more acutely than in the critical care unit. In addition, the critical care unit has a tremendous economic impact on an institution. A significant number of patients who can not afford expensive technology and care can be an economic burden to society. The critical care nurse manager must be able to help alleviate the ethical and legal stresses of critical care practice on staff. Some strategies for intervention are at the end of this chapter.

MAJOR CASES INVOLVING WITHDRAWING OR WITHHOLDING TREATMENT

How aggressive should treatment be? Some believe that their units give overaggressive treatment; others believe that treatment is not aggressive enough. Some feel that patients are singled out for more aggressive or less aggressive treatment. Who should decide the aggressiveness of treatment? Sometimes the patient and the physician make the decision. Sometimes the nurse and the family give suggestions. Even more controversial is the problem that occurs when the patient is incompetent and cannot contribute to the decision-making process—which happens frequently in the critical care unit.

Table 20-1 outlines the major cases related to withdrawing and withholding treatment. Important ethical and legal principles will be explained in this section's discussion of these cases. Although the cases all involve the *legality* and *ethics* of withdrawing treatment, it is important to note that there is no *moral* difference between withdrawing and withholding treatment.[9] In addition, there is no legal difference once treatment has been deemed futile. However, the definition of *futility* and the desires of previously competent patients make these end-of-life decisions very complex and stressful for patients, families, and staff.

Table 20-1. MAJOR CASES INVOLVING WITHDRAWING OR WITHHOLDING TREATMENT

CASE	DECISION	IMPLICATIONS FOR PRACTICE
Karen Ann Quinlan	Karen's father (guardian) granted the right to make decision to withdraw ventilator based on her right to privacy and previously indicated wishes; mandated use of institutional ethics committee.	Aggressive life-sustaining measures could be withdrawn in certain cases; ethics committees could be used as resource.
Joseph Saikewicz	Negative factors (burdens) of treatment exceeded benefits; no further chemotherapy for this mentally retarded man with no capacity for consent; all supportive and comfort measures to be provided.	Aggressive life-sustaining measures not required for individual unable to consent; comfort and support to be provided.
Paul Brophy	On appeal, Massachusetts courts allowed removal of gastrostomy tube from man in vegetative state who had indicated he would not want to be maintained in such a state.	Gastrostomy tube (food and fluids) could be removed in certain cases; benefits and burdens of treatments should be considered.
Nancy Cruzan	U.S. Supreme Court upholds Missouri court; no *clear and convincing* evidence that Nancy would not want to be maintained in vegetative state with a gastrostomy tube; parents' request to remove tube denied.	*Clear and convincing* evidence of wishes required; living wills and surrogate decision-makers acknowledged; food and fluids viewed as any other treatment.

Karen Ann Quinlan

For unknown reasons, Karen Ann Quinlan, age 22, ceased breathing for at least two 15-minute periods while at a party. On admission to the hospital, her temperature was 100 degrees, her pupils were unreactive, and she was unresponsive even to deep pain. She was diagnosed as comatose with evidence of decortication, and required a ventilator to assist her breathing. She later required a tracheostomy. Extensive detailed neurological examinations were performed.

The EEG was characterized by her examining physician as "abnormal, but it showed some activity and was consistent with her clinical state."[1] The brain scan, angiogram, and cerebrospinal fluid were normal. The physician testified that

> Karen has been in a state of coma, lack of consciousness, since he began treating her. He explained that there are basically two types of coma, sleep-like unresponsiveness and awake unresponsiveness. Karen was originally in a sleep-like unresponsive condition but soon developed 'sleep-wake' cycles, apparently a normal improvement for comatose patients occurring within three to four weeks. In the awake cycle she blinks, cries out, and does things of that sort, but is still totally unaware of anyone or anything around her.[1A]

It was determined that she was in a *chronic persistent vegetative state* — defined by an expert witness as the state of a "subject who remains with the capacity to maintain the vegetative parts of neurological function but who . . . no longer has any cognitive function."[1A]

Karen's parents went to court to obtain the right to disconnect the ventilator sustaining her, since they believed she would not have wanted to be maintained by artificial means. The New Jersey Supreme Court ultimately granted her father, as her guardian, the right to make this decision in conjunction with her attending physicians. The court also mandated consultation with the institution's ethics committee. The ventilator was disconnected, and Karen continued to breathe on her own; but she remained in the vegetative state for another ten years. It is interesting that the Quinlan decision used both *comatose state* and *chronic, persistent vegetative state* to describe Karen. Clearly she was vegetative — an important distinction for the critical care practitioner to make. Dr. Ronald Cranford,[5] a recognized expert in this area, differentiates as follows:

> *Brain death:* cerebral functions cease (consciousness and awareness); all brain stem functions cease (eye movements, pupillary responses, cough, gag and swallowing, and spontaneous respiration); although heart beat and other vegetative functions may persist because they are less dependent on brain stem integrity.
> *Persistent vegetative state:* the brain stem, including the ascending reticular activating system, is relatively intact; most neurological destruction is in the cerebral hemispheres, and is usually the result of asphyxia; generally, patients lapse into a "temporary" coma lasting two to four weeks, after which their condition is one of eyes-open unconsciousness (periods of wakefulness and sleep occur, the eyes wander without purpose, pupils respond to light, patients are completely unconscious and unaware).
> *Coma:* sleeplike (eyes-closed) unarousability due to extensive damage to the reticular activating system; often with impaired reflexes (cough, gag, and swallow).

The "awake and unaware" behavior of the vegetative patient can be extremely disconcerting to clinicians and family members. It is important to remember these distinctions when making decisions about life-sustaining treatments in these situations.

Joseph Saikewicz

Joseph Saikewicz was a 67-year old resident of a state school with an IQ of 10 and a mental age of approximately 2 years and 8 months. He was suffering from acute myeloblastic monocytic leukemia. The court case revolved around the issue of medically indicated chemotherapy in a patient who could not consent and could not be made aware of the adverse, painful side effects. In this case, the court determined that the negative factors of treatment exceeded the benefits and ordered that no further treatment for the leukemia be administered. In addition, the court ordered that all reasonable and necessary supportive measures (medical or otherwise) be taken to safeguard Mr. Saikewicz's well-being and reduce his suffering and discomfort.[1] This case is noteworthy because it weighs the benefits and negative factors of treatment of a patient who has never had the capacity to make health care decisions.

Paul Brophy

Paul Brophy was a 43-year old firefighter who had had experience with severely injured people in his work. He had often told his family he did not want to be maintained by extraordinary means if he was ever unable to function. Mr. Brophy ruptured a cerebral aneurysm one morning. While awaiting surgery, he again indicated to his family that he would not want to be maintained if he couldn't function and enjoy life. Mr. Brophy survived his surgery, but he went into a persistent vegetative state. His wife, functioning as his guardian, consented to placement of a gastrostomy tube, and he was moved to a long-term care facility. Several months later, she went to court to have the gastrostomy tube removed, it being clear that he was in a vegetative state. She had the agreement of his mother, siblings, and grown children in this matter. The lower court decision acknowledged that Mr. Brophy had expressed that he would not want to be maintained by artificial, extraordinary means. The relative benefits and burdens of continuing the gastrostomy tube were considered in depth. However, the lower court decided that the burdens did not outweigh the benefits and denied the request to remove the tube. This was reversed on appeal. Mr. Brophy died several days after his feeding tube was removed. This decision was important because it considered the relative benefits and burdens of treatment and death with the withdrawal of food and fluids.

Nancy Cruzan

Nancy Cruzan was the victim of an auto accident. An extended period of anoxia left her in a persistent vegetative state. After approximately five years of hospital and nursing home care, her parents petitioned to have her gastrostomy tube removed. The trial court directed compliance with the request. The court considered her vegetative state, lack of cognitive ability, previous "vivacious, outgoing, active, and independent" state, and wishes expressed to a friend before the accident. The Missouri Supreme Court, however, reversed the decision, on the premises that the gastrostomy tube was not "oppressively burdensome" and that the evidence of her wishes was "inherently unreliable."[6] This case is notable because it was the first "right to die" case to go to the United States Supreme Court, and on June 25, 1990, the court ruled that a person whose wishes were known had a constitutional right to the discontinuance of life-sustaining treatment. The justices differed, however, on how specific the person must be in making his or her wishes known. The court ruled by a vote of 5 to 4 against the Cruzan family, stating that the state of Missouri had a right to sustain Nancy Cruzan's life because the family had not presented "clear and convincing" evidence of Nancy's wishes. The "clear and convincing" evidence standard was already in place in the state of New York. This standard may make it very difficult to withdraw life-sustaining therapy unless the patient left explicit wishes. The decision did acknowledge the importance of living wills, and these will become increasingly important as "clear and convincing" evidence of a person's wishes. The decision also recognized artificially administered food and fluids as a treatment that could be withdrawn. The concept of a surrogate decision-maker appointed by an individual was also raised in this decision. This concept was legitimized for the first time by the New York state legislature on July 1, 1990, when it passed a Health Care proxy bill. This bill, drafted by the New York State Task Force on Life and the Law, combines the concepts of a living will and a surrogate decision-maker. This clear direction from a previously competent patient should make end-of-life decisions much easier for critical care staff and managers.

DO NOT RESUSCITATE ORDERS

Do Not Resuscitate (DNR) orders are often considered for critical care patients, and present controversies and dilemmas to staff. Some believe that DNR patients should be transferred out of the critical care unit. Whether they stay or transfer, however, DNR patients are entitled at least to basic nursing care. In addition, they may still be candidates for other medical therapies. DNR simply means that resuscitation is deemed to be medically futile or that the patient and family do not desire such heroics.

It is often difficult to get physicians to write DNR orders. Sometimes, they are unwilling to risk liability and sometimes they just can't accept the fact that further intervention is futile. Actions to help physicians feel more comfortable about writing DNR orders have been taken: In New York State the Governor's Task Force on Life and the Law drafted a law effective April 1, 1988, providing a legal basis for a properly documented DNR order. The task force also hoped that the legislation would force doctors to discuss with patients at risk of cardiopulmonary arrest their wishes, should this occur.[1A] An appropriate therapeutic exception is included for when this discussion would be detrimental to the patient's condition (for example, a labile cardiac patient in a CCU). This law has helped in many situations, but is bureaucratically cumbersome and misunderstood by many. Hopefully, education in this area will help physicians and nurses deal better with the concept of DNR.

Critical care practitioners are expected to deal with acutely ill patients in a high technology environment. They often find it difficult to admit that nothing can save their patient, and that all they can give is supportive care. And this is especially difficult if the patient has been in the unit for some time, which may lead to overaggressive treatment. If the futility is recognized and a DNR order is written, it may lead to undertreatment, no treatment, or transfer to a medical-surgical unit. From a resource allocation perspective, transfer may make perfect sense. Critical care beds should be used for patients who can benefit from high technology care. However, the patient should not be abruptly transferred because the critical care staff cannot deal with a dying patient who can't be "rescued." If the patient has been in the unit for a long time, abrupt transfer may be very traumatic for patient and family. They may have become quite dependent on the staff, they are familiar with individuals, and they fear that less care is available on the regular medical-surgical unit. Transfer when further aggressive therapy is futile also necessitates patient and family acceptance of that futility. It is important that this type of transfer be explained in a supportive, caring manner to the patient and family. If the critical care bed is not needed immediately, time for this transition is most beneficial. Even if the transfer must be made abruptly, the critical care nurse who has established a relationship with the patient and family can help to ease the transition by visiting the patient and communicating individualized plans of care to the staff on the new unit.

ORGAN TRANSPLANTATION

The ability to transplant organs safely has raised many ethical issues for society and for health care practitioners. The basic definition of death and when it occurs became very important once organs could be successfully harvested and transplanted.

From a societal perspective, vital organ transplants can provide life to someone with no other hope for survival. A cornea transplant can restore vision. However, the cost of organ transplantation and aftercare is steep. In addition, in every organ category, the demand far exceeds the supply. How does society deal with this major resource allocation issue?

The economics of organ transplantation are troublesome, although less so now, owing to the success with newer antirejection drugs. Oregon limits transplants as an expensive therapy which benefits few. Oregon disallows state

Medicaid funds for transplants and puts the money into maternal and child health to benefit more people. In other cases, the decision to perform a transplant is based on the patient's ability to afford aftercare and comply with the therapy.

Many states have passed "required request" acts to increase the number of organs available when the supply of organs decreased as a result of lower speed limits and fewer automobile accident deaths. Required request mandates that families be asked (at the time of the patient's death or impending death) to donate the organs. Many feel this is cruel and ghoulish to a family experiencing an unexpected loss. However, society may become more comfortable with this routine as they did with autopsy requests, and it will become easier. Discussing organ donation is often very stressful for the critical care nurse, who deals closely with the patient and family at this time. It is important to remember that the organs are not useful to the patient anymore, but may benefit several other hopelessly ill people. Respecting the values and wishes of the potential donor is always a priority.

Once the donor is declared brain-dead, care can be very disturbing for the critical care nurse. Life support often must be maintained for hours pending arrangements for harvesting and transplantation. Humane, dignified care of a person declared dead but whose vital functions are maintained by technology can be very stressful for the nurse. Stressful too is turning off the "life" supports after the organs are harvested. Nurses must support each other in these emotionally difficult situations.

A new organ transplantation controversy involves the use of anencephalic infant donors for infant organ transplants. Because there are few potential brain-dead donors of this age and size, the donation of organs from brain-absent infants might help solve this resource allocation dilemma. In addition, it might even comfort parents despondent over the certain demise of their anencephalic infant, because their loss might help another infant and family. However, many people are quite disturbed about using infants who are not brain-dead for transplantation. Most anencephalic infants die within hours or days if they are not supported, but some do survive longer. Before the organ donation issue, families were encouraged to bond during the baby's few hours. If the vital organs are to be donated, aggressive support of these infants is necessary until the organs are harvested. This would disturb family bonding and grieving. In addition, if a suitable recipient was not found within a reasonable amount of time, life support would have to be withdrawn. A unit at Loma Linda University Medical Center has supported these infants for 7 days. No suitable recipients were found for the few infants sustained in this unit. In bioethics and society at large, the controversy still rages. If this practice becomes reality, it will cause tremendous ethical stress for the nurses who care for these mothers and infants. From a management standpoint, this will mean support for these nurses and families, as well as clearly delineated policies and procedures.

EDUCATION

Ethical dilemmas are increasing and are causing a great deal of emotional distress for critical care nurses. In this era of nursing shortage, stress and burnout must be minimized as much as possible.

Ethically difficult decisions often get made by default in an environment of great emotional tension. Ethics education for critical care nurses is needed so they can make decisions in a more positive environment. This should ideally be included in basic nursing programs, and indeed it now is in many schools. Many critical care nurses' educations, however, did not include ethics in the curriculum. Ethics training thus becomes the responsibility of the institution and the nurse manager. Workshops can be conducted in the unit. Articles and basic texts in nursing ethics can be made available. Several excellent audiovisual presentations are available, such as the video *Code Gray*.[4] These resources begin the education of staff in ethics and principles of ethical decision-making.

Ethics Rounds and Case Conferences

Basic reading material does not guarantee that staff will become educated. Interactive discussion is necessary for realization of the material's importance to the staff's work. Nurses need to listen to the views of their colleagues and learn to respect the values of others. Case conferences are often useful. In the beginning, it is often difficult to discuss a current case that is emotionally wrenching for the staff. However, retrospective or hypothetical case review often allows staff analysis of decisions and strategies in a less emotional climate. When options are discussed, staff often realize that the perfect choice doesn't exist and that different staff have different points of view which are also based on sound principles. A good facilitator is important in these sessions. Staff may in time become comfortable discussing current cases. A discussion of the ethical issues of difficult cases may be as important as the clinical parameters in the bedside report. It may take many educational sessions to facilitate a high level of understanding in the staff.

Ethics Consultant

More and more hospitals are employing ethicists, philosophers-in-residence, and consultants to assist staff in dealing with difficult ethical issues. If these resources are available, they should be used as much as possible for ongoing education and case consultation by the critical care nurse manager and staff. The cost of consultation may be justified by the nurse manager who can demonstrate that relief of ethical stress reduces turnover in the unit. If these resources are not routinely available or are totally unavailable, the responsibility for dealing with the ethical stress of the nursing staff may fall to the nurse manager or clinical nurse specialist. Facilitating discussion and providing educational resources should help to reduce some of the stress. This could, in turn, be used as a justification to pursue further resources in this area.

Ethics Committees

Ethics committees are increasingly available in hospitals. They tend to be interdisciplinary; most have at least one nurse member. The critical care nurse manager should be familiar with and have access to the ethics committee if one exists in the institution, and should also inform the staff. Ethics committees serve an educational and a consultative role, and they function to facilitate communication in problematic cases. Nursing input on Ethics Committees is vitally important. In some institutions, nursing ethics committees have been established to deal with issues that relate specifically to nursing or to increase awareness of ethical issues and educational resources for the nursing staff.

Case Study: Ethical Issues and Death

> As the nurse manager for a progressive 20-bed critical care unit in a teaching hospital, you are aware that many experienced staff are undergoing ethical dilemmas as a result of a patient's hospitalization in the unit. Mary is a 42-year old married mother of three. A viral cardiomyopathy has resulted in Mary's advanced congestive heart failure. She came to the unit after an episode of ventricular tachycardia on the medical floor. Despite investigational drug therapy, her arrhythmias continue and require intermittent counter shock.
>
> In the unit Mary was evaluated for a heart transplant; last week it was denied. Apparently her lungs and liver are involved, and the surgeon thought she would not benefit long-term from a transplant.
>
> When Mary and her husband discussed this with her attending physician, she verbalized that without the hope of transplantation, she'd better think about dying. The staff are devastated by this. As the nurse manager you realize that proactive management is necessary.

Mary is the type of patient who raises real ethical issues and increases the stress of the critical care staff. She is a young woman with a family, and staff are likely to identify with her, which makes it more difficult to care for her in an objective, professional way. Staff meetings in which nurses ventilate their feelings and plan for Mary's care are very important. Pastoral care for Mary and her family, and psychiatric liaison services, if available, should help facilitate the grieving of Mary, her family, and the staff. This must be done now because Mary is beginning to verbalize her feelings about dying. Although confronting death and dying is difficult with a young, alert patient and her family, it is better than denying death and avoiding meeting the patient's real needs. Support regarding death, dying, and feelings may be more important than the technical care provided in the critical care unit. This does not mean that Mary's physical care should be neglected. Everything that maintains her comfort should continue to be provided. In addition, Mary's family must be included as much as she wants them to be. Since she is competent and alert, she should be making decisions for herself. As she is dying, her family should be allowed to be with her as much as possible. This may entail a more creative and flexible visiting regime than is usual in the critical care unit.

Mary is terminally ill and dying if she is not a candidate for transplant. Transfer from the unit is a consideration at this point. This should be discussed with Mary and her family, if she wants them to be included. In this hypothetical case, Mary and her family would like her to stay in the unit. They have come to know the staff and feel comfortable with the level of care and their ability to discuss feelings. The medical and nursing managers must consider this request. If it is possible to keep Mary in the unit, this should be communicated to Mary, the family, and the staff. The staff may have to confront their feelings more directly if Mary stays in the unit. Even if Mary is transferred, the nurses who have been caring for her have some continuing responsibility. They must communicate the complete plan of care, especially those elements that deal with emotional support for Mary and her family. They may need to continue involvement with Mary and her family after transfer to provide continuity of care. If the transfer is necessary for appropriate use of critical care resources, this should be explained to Mary and her family in an empathetic manner. They should be assured of continuity of care and continued support. In either case, Mary should be allowed to die as humanely and as much in control over the circumstances of her death as possible.

Aggressiveness of further medical treatment needs to be discussed with Mary and her family. The nursing staff must be involved and informed about these discussions and decisions. Since her condition is irreversible and terminal, resuscitation might be viewed as futile. The alert, competent patient has a right to make that decision, however. It is important that discussions about DNR orders include realistic prognosis for survival, and descriptions of what happens during a resuscitative attempt. The patient and the staff need to decide what a DNR would mean if she had another episode of ventricular tachycardia. The withdrawal of drug therapy already in place may also need to be discussed, as it might be considered futile without the prospect of a transplant.

As stated previously, it is most important that Mary's right to make decisions for herself be respected. Her family should be included as much as she desires and the staff should endeavor to support her wishes regarding dying. The nurse manager needs to support Mary, her family, and especially, the critical care staff in this difficult work. Ongoing staff discussions that allow ventilation of frustrations and feelings and provide educational resources and support are essential to minimize the stress of this situation.

CONCLUSION

There are often no clear-cut solutions to ethical dilemmas. Critical care managers must strive to become more educated about ethical and legal issues so they can facilitate the best decisions and choices for their staff and unit. Understanding personal values and respecting the values of others is an expectation of all professionals. Ongoing education is vital. Particularly stressful cases can be dealt with retrospectively and prospectively. General education is also important to raise the consciousness of critical care practitioners. The creative and responsible critical care manager will strive to provide resources to staff to achieve these educational goals.

REFERENCES

1. American Nurses Association, Code for Nurses. The Association, Kansas City, 1976.
1a. Arras J and Rhoden N: Ethical issues in modern medicine, ed 3, Mountain View, Calif, 1989, Mayfield Publishing Company.
2. Callahan D: Setting limits, New York, 1987, Simon and Schuster Inc.
3. Churchill, LR: Rationing health care in America; perceptions and principles of justice, Indiana, University of Notre Dame Press, 1987.
4. Code Gray (Video), Boston, 1984, Fanlight Productions.
5. Cranford RE: The persistent vegetative state; the medical reality (getting the facts straight), Hastings Center Report 18(1):27-32, 1988.
6. Cruzan vs Harmon: Midwest Medical Ethics 5(1,2):2, 1989.
7. Davis AJ and Aroskar M: Ethical dilemmas and nursing practice, ed 2, Norwalk, Conn, 1983, Appleton-Century-Crofts.
8. Mappes TA and Zembaty JS: Biomedical ethics, New York, 1981, McGraw-Hill Inc.
9. President's Commission for the Study of Ethical Problems in Medicine and Biomedical and Behavioral Research: Deciding to forego life-sustaining treatment, March 1983, US Govt Publishing Office.
10. Starr P: The social transformation of American medicine, New York, 1982, Basic Books Inc.

SUGGESTED READINGS

1. Arras J: Personal communication, 1989.
2. Cohen CB, editor: Casebook on the termination of life-sustaining treatment and the care of the dying, Bloomington and Indianapolis, 1988, Indiana University Press.
3. Fowler MDM and Levine-Ariff J: Ethics at the bedside, Philadelphia, 1987, JB Lippincott Company.

Chapter 21

ON TO THE FUTURE

Jo Anne Bennett

The International Critical Care Teaching Institute is about to begin. About 27,000 critical care nurses and 2,000 other intensivists are expected to tune in the telecast. The keynote presentation is a relatively simple broadcast, compared to the rest of the week's sessions, which include interactive rounds at bedsides in 40 participating medical centers on several continents. Daily practice without satellite conferences is hard to imagine, but the difference between a network of 8 or 9 receiver points and the 250 sites involved in the Teaching Institute seems a little futuristic—even to nurses at Grand Crown Hospital.

Grand Crown is one of the seven United States hospitals participating in the Stellar Project, which is jointly sponsored by the National Center for Nursing Research, the National Aeronautics and Space Administration, AfriEuroCare, and the North American Nursing Diagnosis Association. Of the six current critical-care projects, four are nursing studies. Grand Crown nurses are co-investigators on several studies, and Grand Crown is an affiliation site for almost all the nurses taking courses at the nearby Space Academy. And of course, Grand Crown nurses are the ground crew for the Academy dispensary, more commonly known as the Spaceroom. At first the Spaceroom was practically a closet off the surgical critical care unit, but now it fills two floors in the hospital's east wing. No longer a mere telemetry unit, Spaceroom now provides remote assistance for a myriad of physiologic upsets caused by neutral buoyancy and other routine changes in gravity and energy. Unit staffing includes two float slots to allow nurses from other units to work in the unit. The graduate nursing students doing the two-month practicum in Spaceroom frequently are home care nurses, who increasingly find more applications than their critical care counterparts. In fact, the remote links developed for Spaceroom are making the "ICU without walls" concept of the 1980s into a reality for home care in the 2020s.

The Teaching Institute's closing plenary presentation will simultaneously open the Thirtieth Conference on Nursing in Space, which will be delivered (not by design) from an orbiting space station. Because recent weather has caused numerous delays in shuttle launchings, the cardiovascular nurse who pioneered the introduction of rocketry and space station design into nursing curricula, not to mention nursing into space history, will not be on earth for the anniversary celebrations. Her presentation is expected to be a summary of the decade of multicenter, multidisciplinary research that provided the foundation of the current Stellar programs. People in the past looked to space research for answers to predominantly technologic and kinesiologic questions. But the current research foci are derived from turn-of-the-century chronopsychoneuroimmunology advances. Subjects in one study include healthy adolescents and adults in space and on earth, and also adults on four continents with cancers, allergies, and chronic lung diseases. A different study examines diverse alterations in skin integrity. Laser and sonar technologies and microtechniques have solved many problems, but also have raised new questions about the dynamics of wound healing.

* * *

The *future*. What images does the word bring to mind? Do we imagine real Star Trek possibilities? Or do we envision the not-too-distant future as not too different from today? If pressed, we might admit that despite the changes that may ensue, we expect our immediate world and mundane routines to remain very much the same.

OK, so we're not futurists. We are clinicians and managers firmly grounded in the here-and-now. From the clinician's perspective, critical illness is one of constant, often rapid, potentially devastating psychophysiologic change. The manager works in a bustling environment where innovations become obsolete while they are being implemented. We are constantly planning and revising our plans. We have learned to expect the unexpected: what once was catastrophic is now business as usual. Surely we can face the future, right?

Well, let's consider it: What will our world be like? How different will it be from the world we know now? Will the planet (or the critical care unit) still exist? What choices will we have? What are our expectations? our predictions? The bases for our predictions? The range of possible answers shows that we realize change can be managed but not controlled. This humbling fact should not overwhelm us, but should guide our approach to planning and help us avoid some pitfalls.

This chapter addresses this planning by looking at societal, health care, and critical care trends for a perspective on cycles and new directions (see Figure 21-1). Planned management of change is discussed and ways to assess future possibilities to enable strategic planning are emphasized.

↑ DIVERSITY   ↑ COMPLEXITY

Advances
Nursing science
Medical science
Surgical techniques
Pharmacologic agents
Computer technology

Shifting emphasis in
  community resources
Cost containment
Big business

Δ Values
Legalism
Ethical dilemmas

CRITICAL
CARE
NURSING

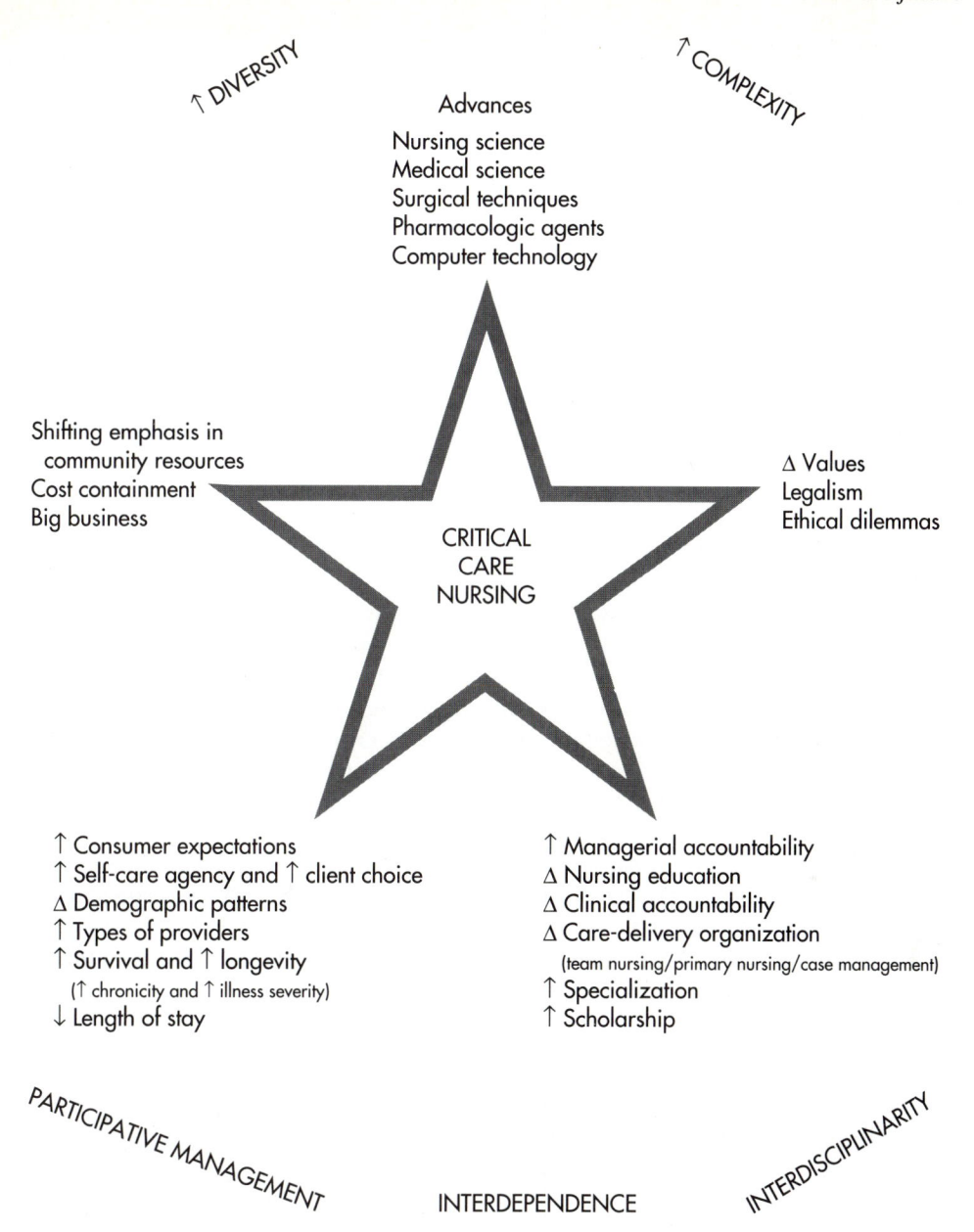

↑ Consumer expectations
↑ Self-care agency and ↑ client choice
Δ Demographic patterns
↑ Types of providers
↑ Survival and ↑ longevity
  (↑ chronicity and ↑ illness severity)
↓ Length of stay

↑ Managerial accountability
Δ Nursing education
Δ Clinical accountability
Δ Care-delivery organization
  (team nursing/primary nursing/case management)
↑ Specialization
↑ Scholarship

PARTICIPATIVE MANAGEMENT   INTERDEPENDENCE   INTERDISCIPLINARITY

FIGURE 21-1. Factors contributing to the future direction of critical care nursing.

BACK TO THE FUTURE

The upcoming turn of the century provides a focus for projections into the future and comparisons with the past. Observing the end of this millenium provides a broad perspective for considering technological advances within ecological and political contexts. History shows us that expanding technologies bring both problems and improvements, and that the actual effects of these advances far surpass their intended purposes, for better and for worse.

Health care in the twentieth century is markedly different from that of previous times. Around 1900, the modern professions of nursing and medicine arose and diverged. The need for formal, standardized nursing and medical education was recognized. Their prerogatives were legally sanctioned. The hierarchy of care delivery emerged from the social politics of male-female roles, from economic competitions, and perhaps to a lesser degree, from qualitative or quantitative differences in services provided by different professional groups.[10]

The advances in health care and the outcomes achieved during the first half of the century (that is, the decrease in morbidity and mortality and the increase in longevity) were largely due to prevention of infection transmission and the improved physical and social environment of the community in general, and the sickroom in particular. The pharmacopoeia at midcentury was only slightly larger than it was in 1900. In 1950, medical art was still more useful than medical science to the clinician, just as nursing art was emphasized over nursing science. The newborn critical care specialty emerged only in the last third of the century, resulting from space age technology as much as from advances in biomedical and nursing sciences. The growth of critical care was part of the burgeoning health care industry that followed the Great Society legislation of the 1960s. The focus was on actualizing and augmenting potential, rather than on cost. Through the 1970s, critical care specialization reflected the increasing specialization and subspecialization throughout medicine and nursing. At the same time, the increase in the number of health care professions changed the perceived boundaries and territorial rights of traditional disciplines. In the 1980s, interdisciplinarity and multidisciplinary teams became commonplace, although collaboration was not always easy and comfortable.

The health care environment (and the social environment of which it is a part) that evolved during the 1980s was very different from what was anticipated in the 1970s. The idea that limits are necessary and that health care providers cannot and should not be the decisionmakers about health care priorities, such as values, goals, and spending, began to be addressed by the public media, as well as by scientific, philosophic, and political journals. Worldwide social and political changes indicated that alternatives would need to be considered when planning health care. All these trends have implications for critical care.

CRITICAL CARE TODAY

The earliest critical care units were defined more by demographics and geography than function: patients with similar problems were placed together in one area to facilitate close observation. Indeed the acronym *ICU* for "intensive care unit" emphasizes "I see you" and what's going on constantly. The goal of continuous monitoring was, of course, the immediate detection of life-threatening changes in a patient's condition and prompt intervention to reverse these changes. The movement away from wards toward private and semiprivate rooms had removed patients from nurses' view, but postanesthesia units (recovery rooms) had remained useful. When the space age provided sophisticated vital sign monitors that allowed continuous assessment, it made sense to keep the equipment on one unit that had specially trained staff. Initially, close monitoring in the critical care unit was used primarily for postsurgical and post–myocardial infarction patients in whom life-threatening but reversible physiologic changes are expected.

Gradually these became larger independent units, rather than de facto extensions of recovery rooms and emergency rooms. Monitoring not only facilitated rapid assessment but eventually deepened the understanding of the complex processes occurring. Intensivists not only became skillful at emergency life-support procedures, but developed more effective interventions, which then often were preventive by design, and required even more specific assessment of physiologic changes. Technology was developed to provide more information; computers enabled complex analyses of diverse parameters and better appreciation of trends. Now critical care units are often extended by adding step-down units.

In the 1980s, the range of medical problems that could be better managed intensively expanded. New medical problems were discovered; some iatrogenic, others the product of expanding scientific knowledge. The availability of critical care increased the feasibility of more complex surgeries, and technology extended surgeons' abilities. New therapies entered the critical care agenda. Some, such as biotherapies, involve patients that previously were not considered ICU candidates; for example, persons with cancer. The youngest patients are increasingly younger and the oldest patients increasingly older. And all types of patients are being subjected to more intensive therapies than ever before.

Thus, the concept of the critical care unit evolved from a place staffed by nurses proficient in emergency procedures (which all nurses knew, but most seldom used) to a practice specialty involving all phases of the nursing process and collaboration with similarly specialized physicians. During the 1980s, the increasing patient acuity and the increasing demand for critical care beds led to discussions of critical care beyond "ICU walls." Indeed, technologies once found only in critical care units are now often found in the home. These developments would certainly suggest spiraling demands for critical care in the future.

PROMISE AND PROBLEMS

In the beginning, critical care units enabled the timely use of the knowledge we already had, which alone improved outcomes considerably. The goals of the past were largely limited by what was technologically feasible. Now it seems that technology is limited only by demand, and demand limited only by supply (and cost). It seems that the most modern unit will soon be obsolete. Since there is no apparent limit to what is possible, our imagination must be guided. We must know what we want, and then plan for it. Do we want everything? Should we do everything we have the capacity for? Others outside of health care have been asking these questions too. The answers will affect the direction critical care takes in the future.

To many people, critical care symbolizes the frontier of today's health care that heralds the commonplace of tomorrow, and the promise of cures and survival not yet achieved. To many others it epitomizes unplanned, nonstrategic, runaway health-care spending. These critics note the deemphasis on public health principles in health care policy planning. To almost everyone, critical care typifies rapid technical, therapeutic, and social change. Some perceive such rapid change as revolution, rather than evolution. Nevertheless it is possible that the trends observed are actually part of a cycle that will become more apparent in the coming decades. In other words, the pendulum may naturally swing back and forth between rapid technologic advance and more tempered application of such advance. Trends in health care delivery and in society should not be overlooked; for example, the public's focus on wellness and fitness, public health efforts at health promotion (rather than disease prevention), retrenched government spending on social services, and recognition of growing social problems that affect individual and community health, such as homelessness and chemical dependency. Trends in nursing are also relevant: personnel shortages and our response to them, education trends, licensure and certification requirements, and availability of funding for research.

Just as we can lose ourselves in day to day details and crisis management, we can look at these trends and think we have no influence on them—or them on us or on our unit. Where do we fit in? What is our role in planning for the future?

PLANNING FOR THE FUTURE—IS THERE A ROLE FOR YOU?

Sometimes we think of planning in terms of laying out a blueprint—a definite, detailed design for the way something will be. This implies control and suggests that we will have the physical force, authority, or political strength to ensure outcomes or, at least, processes. The clinician, the first-line manager, and frequently the middle manager often do not feel they have much control over many aspects of design and implementation, and thus they may resist their role as strategic contributors to the overall plan. When their input is not sought, they are unlikely to assert their views because they are unconvinced of their ultimate effect. However, being overlooked is not usually the result of deliberate rejection by administrators, but is the result of unintended ignorance.

Administrators may assume they have all the available information needed for their decisions. Or they may recognize deficits in their data, but they may also feel too constrained by time or by funding to pursue more data. With insufficient information, some administrators will adopt a wait-and-see approach, for they know that the better their information, the better their decision. Therefore, administrators are likely to welcome the insights of front-line and clinical managers. If this attitude is not readily apparent, it is probably due to a dysfunctional communication system (informal and formal), or a good system obstructed by one or more poor communicators.

Thus, we must first determine the bases for the decisions that affect us and our work: the intended effects (goals) and the information that was considered. This will tell us if data we consider critical were overlooked in planning. It will also give us the opportunity to consider alternatives ourselves. Then we can present cogent arguments for our views, whether they are proposals or disagreements. If possible, we should present alternatives and their potential impacts.

Note how this approach differs from complaining and griping: It is active, not passive; proactive, not reactive. And it is both informed and reflective. By identifying potential solutions and not just problems, we can be counted as problem solvers. By doing our homework before suggesting improvements, we will be considered innovators rather than demanders who beg "Give me, give me." Others will expect ideas from us, not just tales of woe, which will open communication lines. As with any conversation, one person must speak first. We need not wait for others to ask us questions.

THE BIG PICTURE STARTS ON ONE UNIT

Communication is the core of local and global planning. The nurse manager needs a handle on what's happening at the bedside and how it is changing and might change short-term and long-term. Department and hospital administrators need to understand the work of the various units. But the need for understanding care-delivery processes does not stop there. Government regulatory agencies and legislative bodies at local, state, and federal levels need information too. Their information sources must include at least all points in the system that their decisions affect. No one else can provide our perspective, and no other provider has our understanding of our patients' perspective. We must assume the responsibility of communicating to public officials.

Know your unit and your hospital. It is one thing to recognize national trends over a decade, but where is your community in this picture? What is happening and what can be expected in the next six to twelve months? The answers may involve physical renovations, moving to new space, census trends in medical and nursing diagnostic data, severity and acuity. What makes your hospital different from or similar to others? How does your unit differ from others like it in other hospitals? How do these differences relate to hospital differences in demographics, interdepartmental systems, and mission? What are the implications of these differences to specific needs, limitations, and potentials?

What information from outside sources can you use? What is being done elsewhere? What has worked and what hasn't? In what circumstances? Can others' methods be used or adapted to avoid reinventing the wheel? What have others learned that can be applied to making your methods better? What are others studying? Why? Who should you involve in your data gathering?

Involve everyone. Keep the lines of communication as wide open as possible. If we are to facilitate clinical work, we must know clinicians' perceptions, their ideas, their current and foreseeable problems, their wish list for innovations, their unfinished to-do lists, and their observations of and ideas about trends inside and outside the hospital.

Communication is a two-way street. Managers of well-informed staff get useful information and substantive suggestions, rather than rote reports of standard data. Encourage staff consideration of *possibilities*—of improvements, cost containment, increased efficiency and productivity, and clinical excellence. A continuous flow of information should come from those to whom we provide information. This information flow is important because it tells us what staff are currently focusing on, which prepares us for the immediate future and enables us to plan even further ahead. In addition, we can see how staff interpret and use the information we have already provided, and this feedback enables us to correct misinterpretations and to provide additional data. And finally, we can see the big picture from the smaller pictures that others provide.

WINDOWS ON THE WORLD

It is important to keep up with the current trends in the nursing field and related fields. Active participation in professional organizations provides managers and clinicians with the benefits of personal networks for support and data sharing. It also enhances the sphere of influence of the practitioner and the institution. Many employers do value this, but even if they don't, the individual practitioner can gain much from participation. Professional organizations directly influence standards, and often influence funding and regulations that affect us whether we actively participate in them or not. Clearly it is better to know what changes are coming, so that their potential effects can be determined and imminent problems can be prepared for. Proaction is better than reaction for advances, innovations, potential problems, and administrative concerns. Usually education programs sponsored by professional organizations include discussions and evaluations of the latest advances and comprehensive reviews of the state of the art.

Today's research reports herald tomorrow's practice innovations. Presentations at meetings, even national meetings, usually predate publication by at least a year. Pilot studies presented at these meetings may never be published, but they can point to trends and the directions that larger future projects are likely to take. The findings can suggest questions for local study: applied research, quality assurance, or demonstration projects, to replicate, to extend to a different situation or population, or to modify a previously tested protocol. Of course, we could wait for the project's results and let others do the additional studies. But that could mean waiting ten years. And maybe no one else's study would address our most important concern.

It is even a bigger challenge to keep up with related fields, such as nursing outside critical care, critical care medicine and biotechnology, and the allied health fields. Meeting this challenge involves interdisciplinarity, which requires extensive, constant, and substantive communication and collaboration beyond buzzwords about teamwork. This involves taking first steps and firmly expecting cooperation and reciprocity. Personal timidness must give way to risk-taking. Collaborative relationships are neither adversarial nor competitive; they are focused on mutual goals and embedded in interdependence and trust. Assertiveness does not mean power play. If knowledge is power, then strategic use of power means keeping everyone well informed. A manager's role is to promote information sharing and evaluation.

Nursing specialization and subspecialization further increase the need for good information flow. Nursing advances must be brought to the interdisciplinary critical care team. The critical care nursing perspective must be brought to managerial discussions. Critical care concerns must be known by the field of nursing in general, as well as by other nursing specialties. Up-to-date management approaches must be used in unit-level and department-level planning, decision making, and administration. It is also just good to know how others think, experience our shared world, and perceive us in it. This communication can be the basis of new understanding, creative solutions, and valuable innovations.

POSITIONING FOR SUCCESS: USING POWER

Preparing for the future—even for six months from now—is not a one-person job. The information flow alone is difficult for one person to manage. How can one avoid being overwhelmed and immobilized? How does one ensure being part of the solution and not part of the problem?

Management philosophy, leadership style, and time management systems influence the perspective and the plan of action for both a short- and long-range future. Management is operationalization of policies and plans. Even though they don't actually do the job, managers are supposed to ensure that the job does get done. Managers guide, direct, and facilitate. Effective management means successful accomplishment. But who plans? Who makes policies? Where do ideas for innovation and improvements come from? Who identifies the problems and suggests solutions?

The management of professionals, or of people who must use judgment or creativity in their work, involves coordination and facilitation: providing requisite supports, promoting communication, and ensuring a workable environment. The manager is not necessarily always the idea person and the originator of plans and policies, but is often the middle person—the translator, the active two-way conduit for ideas and impressions, and the balancer of competing interests. Rather than exercise authority, the manager regulates energies, efforts, and foci. The fortunate manager has an expert staff (and novices and students) with ideas and enthusiasm that keeps her running. For the fortunate manager finds leadership in her staff.

Nursing and nursing management are indivisible.[2] Participative management and shared governance are relatively newly labeled concepts in managerial and nursing discourse, but in some limited ways they have been underlying realities in nursing environments recognized as centers of excellence. Managers are responsible for effecting the corporate climate; the worker is recognized as an individual within the larger community: "There is no such thing as a good structural answer apart from people considerations, and vice versa."[16] In the professional environment, where even clients are recognized as partners in decision-making, the manager must detect and ignite potential.

Leadership provides vision. Vision emerges from diverse perspectives. Leadership is not the bailiwick solely of managers or bosses. Be prepared for visions to be unsettling. Leaders are not mired in tradition or habit; they embrace change instead of "the way we've always done it." Creativity, innovation, and flexibility are the hallmarks of explorers, discoverers, and the finest clinicians. Leaders are impatient with the status quo and intolerant of empty rhetoric. A leader may be the gadfly that consistently ruins a manager's day. Is it possible that the most future-thinking manager really dreams of working with a staff comprising leaders? On the other hand, could a successful manager be oblivious to the limits of her own vision?

Whence comes vision? How do we get past the rhetoric and the fantasizing? Time management is essential. Of course, it is somewhat easier to measure productivity and efficiency in areas other than planning. To avoid putting off thinking about tomorrow until tomorrow, we first must recognize that thinking about the future is not a luxury done during free time; it is real work. Next, we must stop crisis-mode management. If long-term management is not occurring because crises must always be solved, maybe it's time to address that as the problem. Finally we must actually schedule planning—we need to plan to plan.

What manager does not already spend a lot of time meeting and planning? Let's examine our agendas. How far do our plans project into the future? Are these plans for problem-solving or potential-creating? Whose goals are we addressing, others' or our own? Shouldn't there be a little of everything on the agenda? When we have identified what is missing, then we can include it by scheduling it. We may also find much that could be delegated. And we should look to see if more front-line staff could participate in discussions about the future—discussions which inevitably address current problems and potentials.

If this approach is too participative for the institutional culture, smaller steps can be taken even within a single unit. Invite participation on one issue at a time, one meeting at a time, one project at a time. The initial focus does not have to be too far into the future to start building momentum. For some units it may seem pretty futuristic just to try to implement something that Big Deal Medical Center has been doing for years.

The Power Source

The adage that knowledge is power warrants more consideration in the context of planning for the future. What specific knowledge? What exactly is power? What compromises power?

Barrett[1] defines power as knowing participation in change; that is, intentional action with awareness of choice. This understanding of power was derived from Martha Rogers' Science of Unitary Human Beings,[17] and it provides direction for managers who are planning for the future. It suggests that power is confronting change; it is involvement. Power nurtures diversity and creativity. It is integrative. There is no connotation of resisting change *nor* forcing change *nor* controlling others or the environment. The focus is on interaction, not command. Knowledge sharing, collaboration, and trust are inherent in power.

This view diverges sharply from previous conceptualizations of power, which associate power with exploitative, manipulative, and competitive notions. Although Miller[15] uses these traditional concepts of power in her work, some of her observations are congruent with Barrett's theory:

> The greater the individual's expectation to have control and the greater the importance of the desired outcomes to the individual, the greater the perceived powerlessness experienced when the individual does not, in fact, have control. . . . Power is a resource for living that is present in all individuals. . . . Knowledge and insight about what is happening [enables control of] the anxiety of uncertainty.

Miller thus describes knowledge as a power resource and as an antidote to powerlessness.

Barrett's theories of power need to be tested in organizational and political contexts, but support for them is already evident in the critical care literature. Knaus and colleagues[8] compared thirteen critical care units in major medical centers. They found that units with a high degree of coordination (high levels of communication, respect, and trust between physicians and nurses) have lower mortality. The better units typically had extensive educational programs for staff nurses and nurse managers; they also had ample opportunity for nurse-physician consultation during admission, treatment, and discharge. In a study that specifically used Barrett's theory, Trangenstein[20] looked at power, job diversity, satisfaction, and involvement. Wright[22] uses Barrett's theory to examine the relationship between power and trust in the elected leaders of a professional nursing association. Miller[15] cites numerous studies in which individuals' knowledge about the anticipated possibilities was associated with lower levels of perceived powerlessness. The oft-quoted "magnet study" examined characteristics of hospitals that attract and retain nurses, and found that directors and staff nurses in magnet hospitals convey a lack of powerlessness and recognize others' power:[14]

> These staff nurses have an image of themselves as influencing decisions and being in relative control of their own practice. They can and do make decisions that affect nursing care, [they believe they have] a body of knowledge and expertise of significance to the organization, and [they expect] support in carrying out their legitimate role. . . .
>
> Autonomy . . . is invariably discussed within the context of a freedom . . . to assume and carry out responsibility [i.e. use knowledge]. The ability to establish standards, set goals, monitor practice, and measure outcomes is part of this freedom. . . . Many patient care programs have come into existence in these hospitals as a result of the nurses' ability to function in an autonomous manner. In each instance, innovation and creativity appear to flourish side by side with accountability. . . .
>
> They recognize the power held by physicians in the admission of patients [and] confident of their own competence and concerned that clients receive the best care possible, nurses are changing the balance of power. They know that patients are in the hospital because they need nursing care. [They] no longer accept situations where they do not have a voice.
>
> Directors and staff nurses have become more collegial and collaborative. Both expect to participate in management decisions . . . the staff nurse in all matters related to care of patients and the role of the nurse. . . . Ideas for programs are designed and executed at the unit level. . . . Committees appear to play a strategic role in engaging the nursing staff in the affairs of the hospital and nursing organization.
>
> A positive practice environment. Rather than a matter of strategy, it is a matter of quality.

Thus it appears that skillful management is the artful proficient use of knowledge, not through exploitation or restraint, but through collaboration. Pursuing control, the need to exercise authority over others, may actually drain power: It restricts communication, focuses energy away from productive goals, and denies others' vision. The power of management is exercised through empowering others. Since power rests on knowledge, power for the future depends on the knowledge-seeking activities we employ and promote. These must gather extant knowledge and also extend it.

Knowledge for the Future

What will we be doing? How will we be doing it? How can we prepare? It seems that the answer to the third question depends on the answers to the first two questions. These answers will evolve, perhaps more rapidly than we expect. What we must recognize is that the answers will be created, not discovered.

The quantity of nursing research has grown tremendously in the last decade. Today half a dozen nursing journals are devoted solely to research reporting and theoretical discourse. In addition, reports of research regularly appear in clinical and management journals. Consider that the first nursing research journal *(Nursing Research)* appeared forty years ago and remained the sole research journal for almost thirty years. We have barely begun but we are off and running.

Though it is difficult to keep up with the knowledge explosion, it is relatively easy to recognize findings that we can apply in our practice. It is also easy to identify gaps in the scientific base for what we do. A bigger challenge is choosing what questions to study and to what should we direct our limited research resources. This choice does not belong solely to researchers. As the consumers of research, clinicians must contribute to program planning. Managers can promote this partnership.

PRIORITIES FOR RESEARCH

Florence Downs,[3] the editor of *Nursing Research,* bemoans the sporadic, fad-like scattered interest in nursing research topics, saying that the "'stop-and-go' activity ends in proliferation of isolated findings" that do not further understanding. Among her examples are burnout, job satisfaction, stress, and turnover, which are all considered priorities by managers. Clinicians too have identified these as priorities for nursing research. Critical care nurses, when asked in a Delphi survey to specify topics for nursing research that would help "improve the welfare of the critically ill," included these topics among the top 15 (see the box below).

Clinicians are concerned about managerial issues, and they relate these concerns to patient welfare. Obviously, it is urgent that we address these issues in practice, in pursuing research, and in applying the findings. But Downs points

---

PRIORITIES FOR CRITICAL CARE NURSING RESEARCH[13]

1. Effective sleep promotion; prevent sleep deprivation.
2. Prevention/reduction of critical-care nurse burnout.
3. Effective orientation—cost, safety, long-term retention.
4. Effect of verbal and environmental stimuli on intracranial pressure.
5. Least anxiety-producing methods for maximizing weaning efficacy.
6. Patient classification systems (valid/reliable/sensitive).
7. Incentives for nurse retention in critical care.
8. Effective stress reduction for critical care staff.
9. Effective interventions when communication is impaired.
10. Positioning effects on cardiovascular and pulmonary functions.
11. Effective staffing patterns.
12. Measures for preventing infection associated with invasive procedures.
13. Maximum time a patient receiving PEEP can be off ventilator without significantly lowering paO_2.
14. Effective ways to incorporate research into practice.
15. Effective pain relief in various types of critical illness.

out we do not yet have our research act together since we are not bearing down on a question: our research attention wanders before we have fully answered the initial question and the questions it raises. It is also apparent that management questions are not icing on the cake; they are perceived by clinicians to be vital to, not separate from, good patient care.

Although reviewers[4] have not found evident pursuit of the identified priorities in published research, this may be due to the time it takes to complete the research once the problem is identified. If priorities were indeed pursued in the early 1980s, results will begin to become clear in the 1990s. Most of the work published through the 1980s results from studies begun before the publication of these priorities in 1983.[13] Meanwhile AACN commissioned a second study in 1988, which should enable us to keep our research endeavors on target. It will be interesting to see if and how clinicians' perceived knowledge needs have changed. But we must keep in mind Downs' admonition against nonsynthesizing "stop-and-go" activity, which echoes previous observations of nursing's failure to build a cumulative science. Our inquiry must be systematic. According to Stevenson,[18] more concentrated work on the major phenomena basic to nursing's perspective of health care brings the profession into a second stage in knowledge development. This seems to be our entry into the 1990s. But the first stage—establishment of the environmental structures to facilitate research in academic and clinical settings—is far from complete. For most of us this is a goal for 2000, not pie-in-the-sky, but a concrete expectancy.

The National Center for Nursing Research (NCNR) has attempted to provide a blueprint for knowledge development with a National Nursing Research Agenda (NNRA), which will guide the allocation of federal support. It comprises seven broad priorities organized into three stages.[6,7] Technology dependency across the lifespan, which includes prevention of iatrogenic complications, is one priority directly relevant to critical care.

DISSEMINATING AND USING KNOWLEDGE

Nursing approaches the next century not as a prescientific procedural occupation, but as an increasingly scholarly, research-based profession. Management too rests on a growing foundation in the behavioral sciences. But we have not yet met the challenge of timely transfer of research results into practice. This challenge grows more important as we anticipate more research data in the coming years. Without effective strategies to close the gap between new knowledge and the practical state of the art, the gap can be expected to widen rapidly. Ada Sue Hinshaw,[6] NCNR's first director, presents what is needed:

> In the future, research will be an acknowledged way of life for all nurse professionals. Each will integrate research as a part of professional practice, ranging from the process of utilization or application of information in clinical and administrative decision making to the explicit merger of research into curriculum patterns, both graduate and undergraduate, to the individual whose primary role responsibility is that of conducting and disseminating research information. As

such, research will be a part of all job descriptions. . . . The ability to transfer, use and be comfortable with manipulating and understanding research results will be evident.

Tactics for dissemination of some specific results may begin with the clinician as source of the research question. Research publication in clinical journals is vital. Organized group activities can promote dissemination. Journal clubs have successfully increased interest in and awareness of current research publications. Bulletin boards need not be overlooked. More and more research is being reported at continuing education programs, especially those sponsored by professional associations. These groups are also devoting more meetings solely to research. Some nursing departments have newsletters that contain abstracts of reports deemed relevant.

Information gathering is not sufficient. It needs to be further processed and evaluated, mined for its specific usefulness and limitations. Research reports do not tell us what we should do or where we should go. Hinshaw[6] advised us to glean concepts and principles, not rules and procedures. These news and insights can then guide our continuing assessment and revision of policies, procedures, and attempts to individualize care.

The manager whose clinical staff is proposing changes suggested by research needs a different strategy than the one who must begin by sparking staff interest in new data.

FUTURISTICS AND FUTURCASTING

It is no surprise that there are researchers who specialize in studying the future. *Managing the future* implies planning for possibilities with full recognition that "the operating conditions present during the implementation phase are expected to differ greatly from those present during the planning phase."[11] Futures researchers formulate alternative futures by analyzing information about the past and present. Their goal is to assist decision makers with long-range planning by examining trends and estimating what may happen. These estimates are called *forecasts*. Forecasting is primarily concerned with studying trends to determine their probable and logical outcome. *Futurcasting* is concerned with ways to arrive at desired outcomes and goals; that is, ways to use or steer trends.[9] Futurcasts are attempted because we recognize that

> there is no single, inevitable, predestined future to be predicted and prepared for [as there exist] countless possible futures—some desirable, toward realization of which we may choose to devote present energies, and some undesirable, which we may work to avoid.[5]

Forecasts and futurcasts make uncertainty manageable by promoting anticipation. In other words, they improve our power base by enabling us to move toward the future more knowingly. Undoubtedly there will be surprises: Often even the best, most systematic forecasts and futurcasts are wrong.[9] But future shock[19] is unnecessary.

The term futurology was coined in the mid-forties, but futures research is still in relative infancy. Humanistic futures studies have been slow to develop, and so far, futurology has been dominated primarily by physical and social scientists "who are prone to think of humans en masse rather than as individuals."[12]

Futures Research Methods: Looking for the Future

The basic assumption of forecasting and futurcasting techniques is that

> past behavior of individuals, organizations, and events often can be a useful predictor of future events if analyzed correctly, systematically, and creatively, while keeping in mind the context within which the events take place.[9]

> The trends of history may be likened to a tidal wave that carries all civilizations and cultures rushing in a general direction. [Although there are many temporary divergences,] all people and all cultures travel in the same general direction, at different rates of speed, but with different degrees of comfort on an individual or institutional level. . . .
>
> Humankind has been careless with regard to the future. In most instances it [was assumed] that humans would adapt to any type of change [but] throughout history we have decompensated innumerable times, under various circumstances. We have succumbed to diverse pressures in the form of disease, psychologic stress, and sociologic holocausts. [However, depending on many factors, there are] rare opportunities for improved clarity and understanding of tomorrow's today.[12]

Futurcasting uses both logical and intuitive techniques:

Branching point diagrams (see Figure 21-2) plot the way events may flow through time by branching the possible effects of each change from an initial straight line of action.

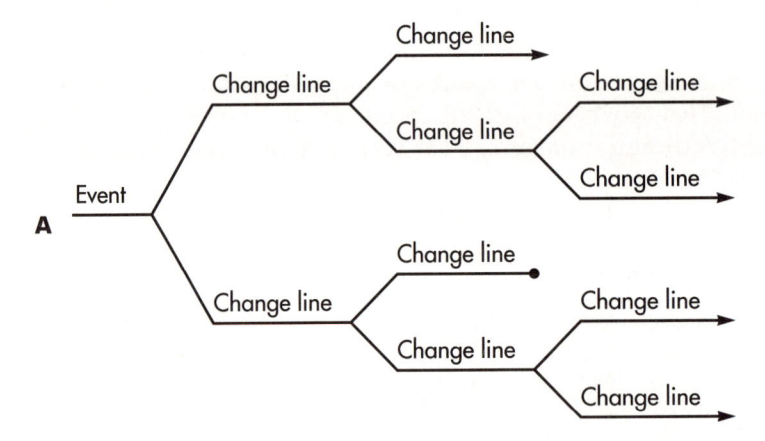

FIGURE 21-2. Branching point diagrams chart the logic of how events change. (A) A branch indicates a change in the line and flow of events through time. If nothing significant happens, the line remains straight. (B) An example of a completed branching point diagram for a nursing issue.

On to the future 361

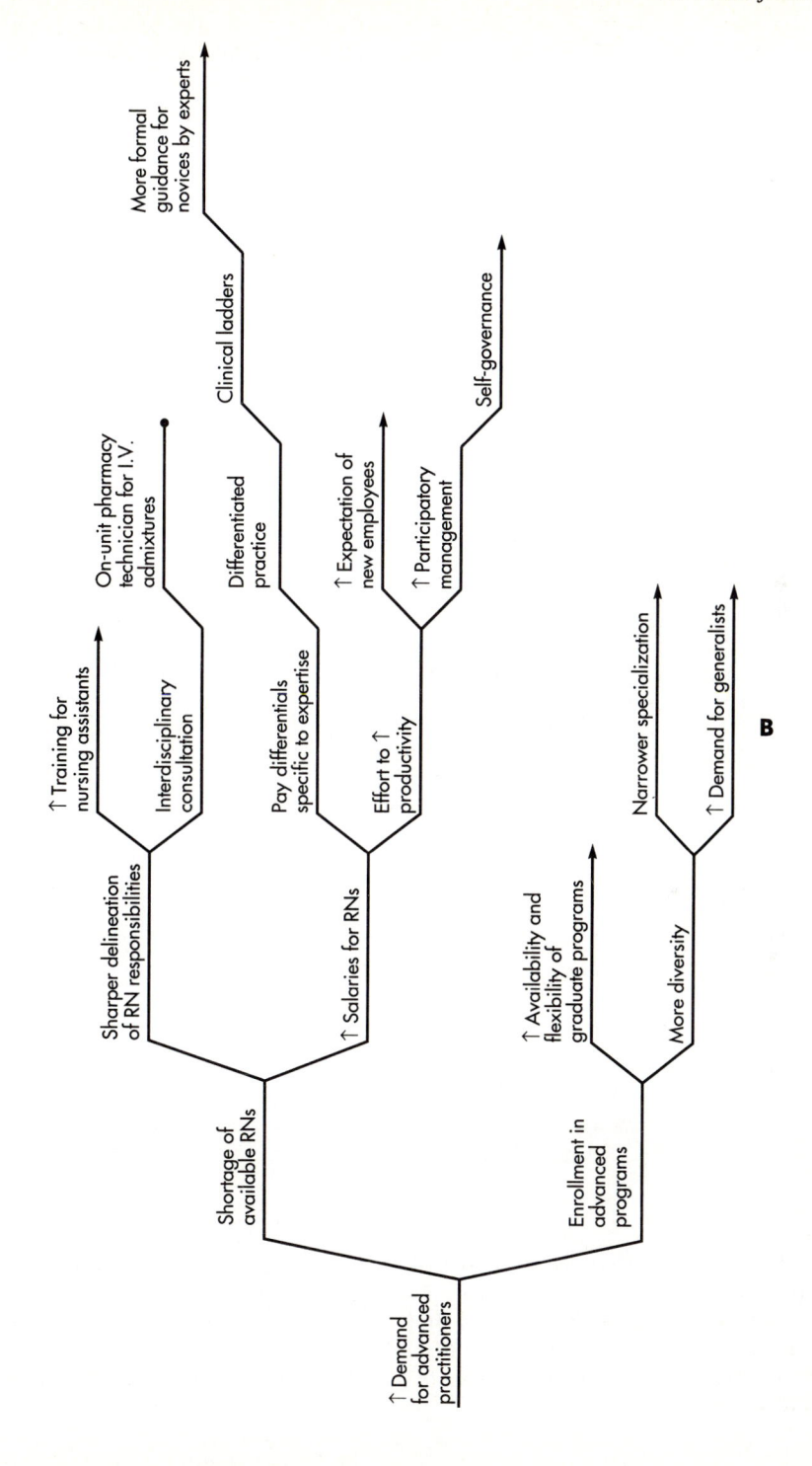

[Tree diagram showing nursing workforce trends, read from bottom to top:]

↑ Demand for advanced practitioners
→ Shortage of available RNs
  → Sharper delineation of RN responsibilities
    → ↑ Training for nursing assistants
    → Interdisciplinary consultation
      → On-unit pharmacy technician for I.V. admixtures
  → ↑ Salaries for RNs
    → Pay differentials specific to expertise
      → Differentiated practice
        → Clinical ladders
          → More formal guidance for novices by experts
    → Effort to ↑ productivity
      → ↑ Expectation of new employees
      → Participatory management
        → Self-governance
→ Enrollment in advanced programs
  → ↑ Availability and flexibility of graduate programs
  → More diversity
    → Narrower specialization
    → ↑ Demand for generalists

B

362 *Chapter 21*

Visioning is the guiding of fantasies to specific and important curiosities. Visioning has been called "daydreaming with a purpose" though without censorship.[9] Some people call it right-brain thinking.

Trees of impact (see Figure 21-3) are used to determine the possible consequences of a decision that is being made or the probable repercussions of an

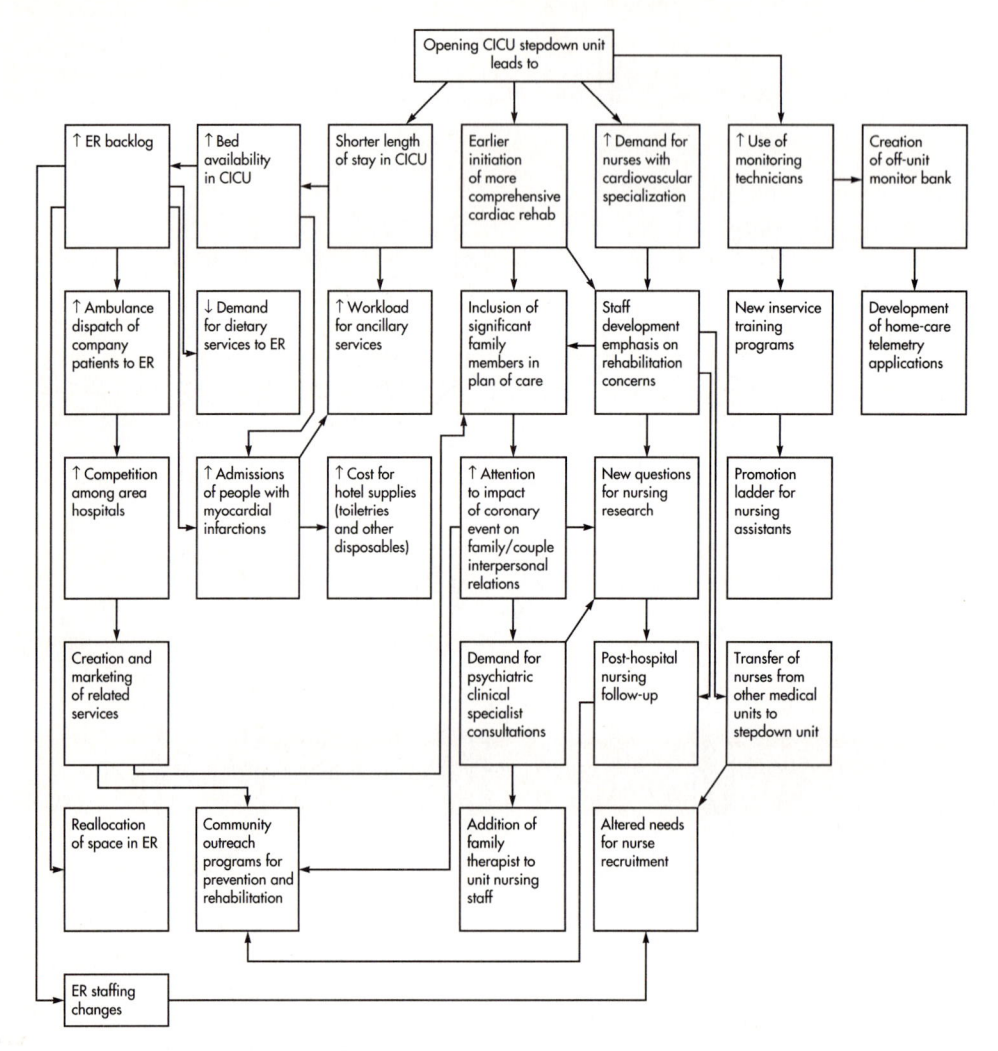

FIGURE 21-3. Example of a tree of impact. The impact of opening a coronary critical care stepdown unit over one year. Note that trees of impact plot *alternative* futures, not *the* future. Without time frames, they are a tool for surveying the extent of an event's impact on related systems. A time frame may be used to limit the period for which projections are plotted (a one-year or five-year impact). They can also be used for contingency planning.

event that is already underway. These trees are surprise-free graphic dry runs used to analyze a particular system's logic of change. The interrelationships suggested rely upon history, logic, and expert consensus. They can be used with or without time frames and are particularly useful for *brainstorming*. They can also be used outside of group work to draw conclusions from what is in the literature. Of course, history, logic, and expert consensus do not guarantee that cause-and-effect logic will determine future events. And we do not have to agree with others' opinions. But we do need to be cognizant of them and whence they come. We also need to consider counterintuitive patterns (responses contrary to what seems plausible).

The example shown in Figure 21-3 is a relatively simple short-term analysis of a simple event. It demonstrates that before attempting any analysis, the would-be futurist must recognize how related processes affect one another. Our example rests on the assumption that demand for coronary admissions will increase beyond what the ER can accomodate, that the demand will continue to increase, and that options other than a new unit will not become available. A tree of impact could become very complex if all the interrelationships of the hospital's subsystems and departments, the community networks of health care providers, and other diverse contingencies are included. Whether the goal is simple or complex, short- or long-term, all analyses begin with

The history of the event (coronary care unit too full to meet immediate demands from emergency room)

The logic of the event

What experts say (epidemiologic predictions, experiences of others who have tried similar approaches)

The analysis can be quantified by using exact calculations, starting with the number of beds that a proposed new unit would have.

Counterintuitive impacts must also be considered. For example, do not assume that everyone perceives the same current problems and consider that some perceive that the purpose of the new unit is for diagnostic work. The anticipated rate of freeing critical care beds or the unit's focus on postinfarct rehabilitation might not be so great.

Extending this analysis for far-reaching future impacts would require expectations of changing standards for coronary care, needs associated with lengthened survival, and other predictions.

Maps of processes extend trees of impact to include a wider context of concurrent and related events. They demonstrate interrelationships between subsystems. With computers, maps of processes can quantify impacts as they spread.

Scenarios are narratives that portray the way the future might be. They use current facts for their background and logic, the most probable facts of tomorrow for their outcome, and recognized interactions of known systems for their driving force.[9] Thus they are based on either reliable or speculative data (see Table 21-1). The key issue in developing a meaningful scenario is specifying the *main theme,* the conditions under which the assessment is being done. The theme

Table 21-1. A SCENARIO

	PARTICIPATORY MANAGEMENT	NURSING RESEARCH	INTERDISCIPLINARITY	APPLICATIONS OF TECHNOLOGY
Best	RN staff self-governance with staff selection of administrative director; quality circles and other committee participation by nonprofessional staff.	Multicenter clinical trials; clinical specialists participate with university faculty in planning applied studies; graduate students use staff-nurse generated questions for school projects; staff development agendas emphasize research dissemination and application.	The discipline of team leader depends on individual patients' specific problems; families' concerns are included in care plan; lay care partners (usually family members) are on hand to assist; joint clinical/technical training and staff development.	Integrated interface: monitors/diagnostics/communications; complete online data management at bedside; minimal downtime for maintenance.
Most likely	Shared governance, with flattened managerial hierarchy, with greater decentralization; staff-nurse committees address issues related to practice; committee membership determined by clinical staff rather than administrative appointment.	Journal clubs are active in different ways (e.g., on different units, or with specific foci); research committees proliferate; more research is reported at meetings and in clinical journals; a greater proportion of nursing research involves intervention trials.	Case-management and integrated charting systems promote coordination and enhance communication; problem-focused rounds review patient progress; committees involve leaders/staff with special interests to address specific problems or goals.	Partially integrated systems; completely computerized data management with limited interface; episodic equipment failures.

Continued.

"forms a kind of background to add a dash of simulated reality to the scenario-generating task."[9] Generating a scenario begins with knowing the present situation well.

Scenarios are probably the most widely used and applicable futurcasting technique.[9] This chapter begins with a scenario. Philosophers, novelists, and science fiction writers create scenarios, but the futures researcher's purpose is a systematic assessment of the facts in a changing context. More complex scenarios

Table 21-1. A SCENARIO—cont'd

	PARTICIPATORY MANAGEMENT	NURSING RESEARCH	INTERDISCIPLINARITY	APPLICATIONS OF TECHNOLOGY
Worst	Hierarchical organization maintains vertical lines of communication; administrators, reporting to director of nursing, are responsible for establishing policies and are principal avenue of communication between clinical and executive staffs; suggestions for new program ideas and solutions to problems are managerial responsibility.	Staff nurses are more aware of ongoing research through professional media & conferences; findings are applied and standards change more quickly to keep pace with changing knowledge; most master nurses and hospitals' research focus is confined to quality assurance; a few clinical specialists attend research conferences.	Nurses/physicians assigned to patients as available; shift reports involving each discipline separately are key communication; planning committees comprising administrators seek clinicians' input for specific issues; unidisciplinary continuing education with occasional guest presentations from other specialty.	Equipment gathered as needed; separate systems used by each department; data-gathering fragmented from data-management systems; manual search required for retrieval of current test results; significant chronic downtime.

Scenario building helps clarify the dynamics of change; it draws attention both to issues that strategic planning needs to address and to details that require deliberate decision making. Scenarios offer ways of studying how the future evolves and suggest where a purposeful interaction will have a desired effect.

The scenario at the beginning of the chapter may seem improbable. To determine alternate scenarios, identify what you consider the most important factors and variables in the present situation that can be expected to change. What might the best, worst, and most likely changes for each of these be? How could these changes interact?

Include as many factors as the final scenario will address; for example, funding sources and ceilings, treatment goals and limits, medical-surgical innovations, public perceptions, social values, specific new projects, allied health personnel availability and training, nursing competencies, social values, technology versus ecology, tertiary versus primary care emphasis, communications technology would be added to the above.

are the grand scenario and the matrix scenario. Although weeks of group work might be used to develop any scenario, a *grand scenario* requires several people, usually experts. Each rates the probabilities of a number of situations in the best, worst, and most likely scenarios (see Table 21-1). Situations with the highest consensus are then tied together to form a single narrative. *Matrix scenarios* also use expert opinion. The matrix scenario blends several scenarios into a larger, more complex scenario showing the interaction of events. Relationships are weighted to show which enhance and which inhibit specific variables or events, or how responsive one element is to another. Matrix scenarios, also called *cross impact matrices,* can be computerized. They are considered "fluid forecasts."[9]

The Delphi technique is a highly structured method for polling experts for consensus on a specific issue. The experts are asked their opinion at least three times. On each turn after the first, each participant is given an anonymous tally of all the opinions so she can reassess and revise her own accordingly. The goal is consensus, not creativity. The results may be reported in a narrative using only the cluster of opinions near the average. The Delphi can be used with questionnaires or by telephone interview. It can also be used in nonanonymous groups. There are many types of Delphis. The Delphi technique has been a popular nursing tool for identifying priorities, most frequently research priorities.[21] It can also be used for policy analysis. *Policy delphis* seek the preferred group choices, however; consensus is not the goal. In futures research (as opposed to planning) it is used to project the timing of possible innovations by surveying experts' expectations (see Figure 21-4). Their use in nursing has not been reported.

Trend analysis is a quantitative explanation of how events move through time, a description of the momentum of a chain of events. The analysis examines the circumstances that enhance or retard momentum and looks for *envelope curves,* or long-term trends that comprise multiple short-term trends.

CONCLUSION

Today's reality encompasses the past and the future. Looking back just fifty years fuels the imagination to think how different it will be fifty years from now. The possibilities that lie ahead can dazzle us. Though critical care will not be nursing's newest frontier then, we will know new critical care frontiers. Meanwhile we have barely begun to explore the territories of our current critical care technology and scope of practice. Over the last decade, much attention was given to nursing's image. Our future image rests in large part on others' seeing *what we say we can do* consistently practiced.

This chapter has addressed preparing for the future. The manager's opportunities in helping to shape the future are extensive. Collaboration—more important and more evident than ever—empowers us and others. Recognizing opportunities is exciting. Needless to say, the future will arrive whether we are well prepared or ill-prepared for it. So how do we measure our success? By not being surprised when the future arrives—by actualizing current potential and fully participating in today. And so, anticipating a wide range of possibilities, we are ready to greet the future and welcome its challenges.

> Whatever the future of nursing may be, it will be within the context of rapid change, diversity, new knowledge, and new horizons.
>
> Martha E. Rogers

	2000	2005	2010	2015	2020	Distant Future
Bedside data management		●				
Transcutaneous blood gases	●					
Noninvasive hemodynamics			●			
Noninvasive diagnostic scanners				●		
"Spare part" transplantation					●	
Bedside MRI			●			

Innovation	Fill in date
Bedside data management	
Transcutaneous blood gases	
Noninvasive hemodynamics	
Noninvasive (total body) diagnostic scanners	
"Spare part" transplantation	
Bedside MRI	

FIGURE 21-4. Delphi survey techniques create a more systematized scenario by tapping the judgment and intuition of a number of well-informed participants. Two ways to use a delphi survey to get experts' estimates of when practice or technologic innovations will have diffused (or will be introduced) are (A) a check-off questionnaire, and (B) an open-ended fill-in-the-blank format. (Of course, the determination of who is an expert and what is the expertise needed to make the best estimates are the major keys to the Delphi's reliability.)

REFERENCES

1. Barrett EAM: A nursing theory of power for nursing practice: derivation from Rogers' paradigm. In Riehl-Sisca J, editor: Conceptual models for nursing practice, ed 3, Norwalk, Conn, 1989, Appleton and Lange.
2. Caroselli-Dervan C: Visionary opportunities for knowledge development in nursing administration. In Barrett EAM, editor: Visions of Rogers' science-based nursing, New York, 1990, National League for Nursing.
3. Downs FS: 1989. New questions and new answers. (editorial). Nursing Research. 38:323.
4. Dracup K: Annual Review of Nursing Research, Critical Care Nursing 5:107-133, 1987.

5. Helmer O: Looking forward: a guide to futures research, Beverly Hills, Calif, 1983, Sage Publications.
6. Hinshaw AS: Nursing science: the challenge to develop knowledge, Nursing Science Quarterly 2(4):162-71, 1989.
7. Hinshaw AS, Heinrich J, and Bloch D: Evolving clinical nursing research priorities, Journal of Professional Nursing 4:398, 458-59, 1988.
8. Knaus WA, Draper EA, Wagner DP, and Zimmerman JE: An evaluation of outcome from intensive care in major medical centers, Annals of Internal Medicine 104:410-18, 1986.
9. Kurtzman J: Futurcasting: charting your way to your future, Palm Springs, Calif, 1984, ETC Publications.
10. Larson M: The rise of professionalism: a sociological analysis, Berkeley, 1977, University of California Press.
11. Lee JL: Futures research. In Sarter B, editor: Paths to knowledge: innovative research methods for nursing, New York, 1988, National League for Nursing.
12. Lesse S: The future of the health sciences: anticipating tomorrow, New York, 1981, Irvington.
13. Lewandowski LA and Kositsky AM: Research priorities for critical-care nursing: a study by the American Association of Critical Care Nurses, Heart and Lung 12:35-44, 1983.
14. McClure ML, Poulin MA, Sovie MD, and Wandelt MA: Magnet hospitals: attraction and retention of professional nurses, Kansas City, Mo, 1983, American Nurses' Association.
15. Miller JF: Coping with chronic illness: overcoming powerlessness, Philadelphia, 1983, FA Davis.
16. Peters TJ and Waterman RH: In search of excellence: lessons from America's best run companies, New York, 1982, Harper & Row.
17. Rogers ME: Nursing science and art: a prospective. Nursing Science Quarterly 1:99-102, 1988.
18. Stevenson JS: Nursing knowledge development: into era II, Journal of Professional Nursing 4: 152-62, 1988.
19. Toffler A: Future shock, New York, 1971, Bantam Books.
20. Trangenstein PA: Relationships of power and job diversity to job satisfaction and job involvement: an empirical investigation of Rogers' principle of integrality, Doctoral dissertation, New York University, 1988.
21. Warnick M and Sullivan T, editors: Nursing 2020: a study of the future of hospital-based nursing, New York, 1988, National League for Nursing.
22. Wright B: Power and trust among nursing leaders (Study in progress).

INDEX

A

AACN; *see* American Association of Critical-Care Nurses
Absenteeism, 42
Accountability, and managed care, 90
ACLS; *see* Advanced Cardiac Life Support
Acquired immune deficiency syndrome, 136, 175
Acquisition knowledge, 173
Acute Physiology and Chronic Health Evaluation, 84, 142, 144-146, 147, 148, 149, 150, 151, 152
Adams, R., 156
Adler, D., 42, 43
Administrative skills, 237-368
    and budget analysis and forecasting, 287-307
    and budgeting concepts, 271-285
    and ethical and legal considerations, 331-343
    and future, 345-368
    and labor relations, 309-329
    and strategic planning, 259-269
    and technology, 239-258
Admission, transfer, and discharge, 160
ADT; *see* Admission, transfer, and discharge
Advanced Cardiac Life Support, 281
AfriEuroCare, 345
Agency nurses, 163-167
AHA; *see* American Hospital Association
AIDS; *see* Acquired immune deficiency syndrome
Alt, J. M., 191
AMA; *see* American Medical Association
American Association of Critical-Care Nurses, 92, 99-111, 146, 182, 206, 210, 221, 231, 239, 358
American Association of Critical Care Nurses Certification Corporation, 14
American Hospital Association, 206, 309
American Medical Association, 332
American Nurses Association, 114, 199, 222, 333

ANA; *see* American Nurses Association
Analyses
    budget; *see* Budget analysis and forecasting
    cost-benefit, 280-281
    impact, 302
    of trends, 366
Ancillary cost center, 133
Ancillary support, 26-29
Anger, 42
Anxiety, 42, 59; *see also* Management by anxiety
APACHE; *see* Acute Physiology and Chronic Health Evaluation
Application knowledge, 173
Appraisal, performance and staff, 62; *see also* Self-appraisal
Arbitration, 324
Assertiveness, and collaboration, 84, 85
Assessment, and CNS, 230; *see* Basic Knowledge Assessment Test *and* Self-assessment
Assignments, making, 23
Assistant director, 11
Assistant head nurse, 11
Associate director, 11
Assurance, quality; *see* Quality assurance
Attitude, 11
Atwood, J., 42
Authoritarian leadership, 70-71
Authority, and CNS, 226-231
Autocratic leadership, 70-71
Automation, 57

B

Bailey, J. T., 40, 44
Bargaining, collective; *see* Collective bargaining
Barnum, B. S., 17

Barrett, E. A. M., 355
Bartz, C., 43
Basic Knowledge Assessment Test, 182, 184
Baylor model, 156
Beecroft, P. C., 222
Behaviors, positive, 62-63
Bevis, E. M., 47
Beyerman, K. L., 224, 225
Bias, 50
Biculturalism, 78
Binding arbitration, 324
Biomedical engineer, 250
BKAT; *see* Basic Knowledge Assessment Test
Blanchard's Situational Leadership; *see* Situational leadership
Bower, K. A., 87, 93
Brain death, 335
Brainstorming, 28, 363
Branching point diagrams, 360-361
Broome, M., 43
Brophy, Paul, 334, 336
Browner, C., 42
Buchanon, B. F., 223
Buddy, 23
Budget; *see* Budget analysis and forecasting *and* Budgeting
Budget analysis and forecasting, 287-307
  analysis introduced, 288-289
  analysis of margins, 300-301
  analysis of operating statement, 289-301
  analysis of revenue, 292-293
  analysis of salaries and related expenses, 293-297
  analysis of variance, 297-300
  fixed and variable costs, 293-294
  and flexible budget, 298, 299
  forecasting of expenses, 305-307
  forecasting introduced, 301-307
  forecasting of revenue, 302-303
  forecasting of salaries and related expenses, 303-305
  productive and nonproductive time, 294-297
  and static budget, 298
  and table of organization, 306
Budgeting, 271-285
  and budget types, 272-279
  and business concepts, 280-281
  and capital approval process, 273-274
  and capital budget, 272-276
  and capital item justification, 283
  and capital planning process, 274-275
  and cost types, 279-280
  and depreciation, 275-276
  and expenses, 284, 285
  and nonpersonnel operating budget, 278-279, 284
  and operating budget, 272, 276-278
  and personnel budget, 277-278
  and revenue budget, 281-282
  and self-evaluation, 60
  and table of organization, 277, 284

Budgeting—cont'd
  zero-based, 278
Burnout, 40, 42, 43

C

CAI; *see* Computer-assisted instruction
Calendar, development of, 64-67
Cameron, E. M., 233
Capital approval process, 273-274
Capital budget, 272-276
Capital item justification, 283
Capital planning process, 274-275
Care
  and competency; *see* Competency-based orientation
  depersonalized; *see* Depersonalized care
  NQA, 115
  patient; *see* Patient care
  self-; *see* Self-care
  special and routine, 133
  standards of; *see* Standards of care
Career development, 3-20
  and advancement, 6
  and career goal, 3-4
  and career moves, 5
  and critical care, 15-19
  and excellence, 14-15
  and job fit, 4
  job interview and preparations, 6-9
  and leadership styles, 12
  and managerial job types, 13
  and managing staff, 13-14
  and mentors, 6
  and nurse manager functions, 9-15
  and nursing management levels, 11-12
  and opportunities, 5
Career goal; *see* Career development
Career ladders, 189-203
  and clinical ladder, 190-192
  and clinical nurse, 192, 197, 200
  development, 190
  and education, 192, 197, 200
  evaluation criteria, 192, 196-198
  implementation, 195-196
  integration into organizational structure, 199-201
  job descriptions, 198-199, 200
  and management, 192, 197, 200
  planning, 193-195
  policy development, 198
  problems, 192-193
  program maintenance, 201-202
  and tracts, 191
Care Plan of the Week award, 17
Care time, 139-141
Caring environment, 21-37
  ancillary support, 26-29
  assignments, 23
  decision making, 23-24

Caring environment—cont'd
  guest and employee relations, 31-36
  mutual recognition, 30-31
  negotiation, 24-25
  networking, 25-26
  unit needs, 21-23
  visiting hours, 33-36
Case mix profile, 131
CBO; *see* Competency-based orientation
CCRN; *see* Critical care nursing
Centralized system, and CNS, 228-229
Cerebral vascular accident, 142-143
Certification, and CCRN, 14
Change, 78, 110, 262-263
Charge nurse, 11
Charges, and DRG, 132, 133-134
Chart, organizational, 74, 226, 227, 228, 229, 230
Children's Hospital of Los Angeles, 210
Christopher, N. F., 260
Chronic persistent vegetative state, 335
Clark, S., 231
Clinical effectiveness, 232
Clinical expert, and CNS, 222-223
Clinical nurse, 192, 197, 200
Clinical nurse specialist (CNS), 199, 208, 209, 221-236, 239
  assessing staff needs, 230
  authority, 226-231
  centralization versus decentralization, 228-229
  and clinical effectiveness, 232
  clinical expert, 222-223
  complementary leadership styles, 230-231
  consultant, 224
  defined, 222-225
  and education, 233-234
  educator, 223-224
  executive, 225
  measuring outcome, 231-235
  organizational development, 225-226
  planning, 231
  research, 224, 231-233
  role of, 221-236
  and standards of practice, 234-235
  trusting relationship, 230
  unit preceptor, 229-230
Clinical supervisor, 11
Closed shop, 317-318
CNS; *see* Clinical nurse specialist
Code Gray, 340
Code of Ethics of the American Medical Association, 332
Code of Ethics of the American Nursing Association, 333
Collaborative practice, 83-96
  and collaboration, 84-85
  and health care provider relationships, 85-93
  model principles, 92
Colleagues, and communication, 18

Collective bargaining, 317
Coma, 335
Comatose state, 335
Commitment, 49; *see also* Moral commitment
Communication
  and groups, 18-19
  and nurse manager, 17-19
  and peers and colleagues, 18
  and physicians, 18
  and positive behaviors, 62-63
  and self-evaluation, 60
  and superiors, 17-18
  and trust, 46
Compartmentalization, 43
Compensation, 311-312
Competency-based orientation (CBO), 169-187
  administrative support, 174-175
  benefits, 172-174
  and competency, 170-171
  and critical care, 175-179, 185
  defined, 171-172
  hospital policies and procedures, 177
  implementation, 174-175
  learning contract, 176
  learning resource development, 179-181
  and lectures, 171
  mandated topics, 175-176
  position descriptions, 177
  time frames, 185-186
  unit-specific DRG statistics, 177-178
  validating learner competency, 182-186
Compliance, 295
Compressed acuity, 134-136
Computer-assisted instruction (CAI), 181
Conference days, 159-160
Conflict resolution, and professionalism, 327-329
Consortiums, 246
Consultant, and CNS, 224; *see also* Ethical and legal considerations
Consumer, 332
Contact person, 13
Content validity, 141
Contracts
  language of, 322, 326-327
  learning; *see* Competency-based orientation
  and nurse intern program, 214-215
  savings clause, 324-326
Contract savings clause, 324-326
Contribution margin, 300
Control, loss of, 328
Controllable costs, 280
Controlling, of budget, 288
Cooperation, and collaboration, 84, 85
Coping strategy, 43-44
Corey, 227
Coronary artery bypass surgery management pathway, 88-89, 91
Cost-benefit analysis, 280-281
Cost center, 277

Costs
    and DRG, 132, 133-134
    fixed, 293-294
    indirect, 293-294
    and nurse intern program, 215-217
    and technology, 246
    types, 279-280
    variable, 293-294
Council of the Society of Critical Care Medicine, 92
Cox, S. H., 10
Craver, M., 207, 208
Creighton, 191
Creighton University, 213
Crimean War, 221
Crisis quicksand, 58
Criteria, NQA, 115
Critical care, nurse manager in, 15-19; *see also* Competency-based orientation
Critical Care Institute, 210, 212, 213, 217
Critical Care National Teaching Institute, 65
Critical care nursing (CCRN), 14
Critical care professionals, 30
Critical thinking, 184
Cross, D., 44
Cross impact matrices, 366
Cruzan, Nancy, 334, 336-337
Cullen, 145
Cutback, 55
CVA; *see* Cerebral vascular accident

D

Data management; *see* Patient data management system
Decentralization
    and decision making, 24
    and participative management, 73, 74
Decentralized system, and CNS, 228-229
Decision making, 23-24, 73, 74
Deines, E., 73
del Bueno, Dorothy J., 169, 184, 194
Delegation, 17
Delphi survey technique, 366, 367
Democratic leadership, 71
Demoralization, 30-31
Department of Health and Human Services, 51
Depersonalized care, and technology, 244
Depreciation, 275-276
Descriptors, 137
Development
    of calendar, 64-67
    and career ladders, 190
    career; *see* Career development
    CNS; *see* Clinical nurse specialist
    learning resource; *see* Competency-based orientation
    of managerial skills; *see* Managerial skills
    of people skills; *see* People skills
    policy; *see* Career ladders

Diagnosis, principal, 132, 142
Diagnosis related group (DRG), 131, 132-137, 143-144, 146, 148, 149, 150, 151, 152, 262
    and CBO, 177-178
    and compressed acuity, 134-136
    and costs versus charges, 133-134
    and impact on practice, 136-137
Direct care time, 139-141
Direct costs, 279
Director, 11
Direct purchases, 246
Disciplinary practices, and labor relations, 314
Discipline, staff, 62
Discontent, 319-321
Discrimination, and labor relations, 324
Distributor purchases, 246
Documentation committee, 106
Donius, M. A., 210
Do not resuscitate (DNR), 136, 337-338
Douglas, S., 233
Douglass, L. M., 47
Downs, Florence, 357
Draper, E. A., 84
Ducette, J., 42, 43
Dyer Tool, 214

E

Education
    and career ladders; *see* Career ladders
    and CNS, 233-234
    and ethical and legal considerations, 340-342
    and technology, 255-256
Education days, 159-160
Educator, and CNS., 223-224
Effectiveness, clinical, 232
Efficiency, 55
Eighty-twenty rule, 302
Emergency Department (ED), 26
Employees, and relations, 31-36
Energy, performance, and time, 55-68
Enthusiasm, 42
Entrapment, 42
Entrepreneur, 13
Envelope curves, 366
Environment
    and job satisfaction, 44-51
    and self-evaluation, 60
Equipment, 272
Essential relationships, 45
Estrogen conjugates, 239
Ethical and legal considerations, 331-343
    and DNR, 337-338
    and education, 340-342
    and ethics committees, 341-342
    and ethics consultants, 340-341
    and ethics rounds and case conferences, 340
    and organ transplantation, 338-339

Ethical and legal considerations—cont'd
　and withdrawing or withholding treatment, 333-337
Ethics committees, 341-342
Evaluation, 56, 57
　APACHE; *see* Acute Physiology and Chronic Health Evaluation
　and career ladders; *see* Career ladders
　managed care, 94
　NQA, 115, 119, 125-156
　product, 245
　and technology, 248-249
Excellence, 14-15, 114
Executive, and CNS, 225
Exempt status, 294
Expenses, forecasting, 305-307; *see also* Budgeting
Expert, 13
Extracorporeal membrane oxygenation (ECMO), 239

F

Factor system, 138-39, 146, 147, 148, 149, 150, 151, 152
Fain, J. A., 10
Fatigue, 42
Favoritism, 50
Fear, of loss of control, 328
Feedback, and technology, 245
FICA, 294
Filmstrip programs, 181
Fixed costs, 293-294
Flexible budget, 298, 299
Flex staffing schedule, 161, 162, 163, 164
Flynn, K. T., 230
Folkman, S., 40
Forecasting, 359; *see also* Budget analysis and forecasting
Frustration, 42
Full cost, 279
Full-time equivalent (FTE), 157-159, 277-278
Futurcasting, 359-366
Future, 345-368
　and futuristics and futurcasting, 359-366
　and knowledge, 356-357, 358-359
　and planning, 350-351
　and power, 353-357
　and research, 356, 357-358, 360-366
　and unit, 351-352
Futuristics, 359-366

G

George Washington University Medical Center, 144
Georgia Nurses Association, 155
Glanville, C. I., 223
Gleason, J. M., 230
Goal, career; *see* Career development
Goals, NQA, 119-121; *see also* Strategic planning

Gore, Bill, 50
Gor-Tex, 50
Gramling, L., 43
Grand Crown Hospital, 345
Grand scenario, 365
GRASP, 138
Great Society, 348
Greely, Horace, 316
Grievance procedure, 324-326
Groups, and communication, 18-19; *see also* Diagnosis related group (DRG)
Guests, and relations, 31-36

H

Hamric, A. B., 222, 231
Hartz, A. J., 63
Head nurse, 11
Health care consumer, 332
Healthcare organizations, JCAHO; *see* Joint Commission on Accreditation of Healthcare Organizations
Health care provider relationships, 85-93
Helplessness, 42
Hersey's Situational Leadership; *see* Situational leadership
Herzberg's Two-Factor Theory, 50
Hierarchy of Needs, Maslow's, 39, 61
Hill, M. N., 233
Hinshaw, Ada Sue, 42, 358
Hiring practice, and nurse manager, 9-10
Hodgman, E. C., 231
Honeymoon stage, 77
Hopelessness, 42
Horn's severity of illness; *see* Severity of illness index
Hospital information systems (HIS) specialist, 251-255, 256
Hospital resources, and technology, 246-256
Hotter, A. N., 231, 232
Houston, G. R., 191
Hughes, L., 206
Human relations management, 73

I

Iatrogenic injury, 243
Illness, severity of; *see* Severity of illness index
Impact analysis, 302
Indicators, NQA, 115
Indirect care time, 139-141
Indirect costs, 279, 293-294
Inequality, 50
Information,
　paths, NQA, 128
　sharing, 46, 47
　systems; *see* Hospital information systems (HIS) specialist *and* Spectra Medical Information System

Injury
  and compensation, 311
  iatrogenic, 243
Inlier, 132
Innovation, 114
In Search of Excellence, 10, 114
Insider, 13
Instrument reliability, 141
International Critical Care Teaching Institute, 345, 346
Interpersonal relationships, 45, 49-51
Interrater reliability, 141
Intervention, TISS; *see* Therapeutic Intervention Scoring System (TISS)
Interview, and preparations, 6-8

J

Japanese management, 74
Javits, Jacob, 95
JCAHO; *see* Joint Commission on Accreditation of Healthcare Organizations (JCAHO)
Job descriptions, and career ladders, 198-199, 200
Job fit, 4
Job interview, preparations for, 6-8
Job satisfaction, 39-54
  and coping strategies, 43-44
  and essential relationships, 45
  and interpersonal relationships, 45, 49-51
  and pride, 48-49
  and stress, 40-44
  and success strategies, 51-52
  and trust, 45, 46-48
  and work environment, 44-51
Job security, 312-13
Job sharing, 163
Job titles, 11-12
Job turnover, 42
Job types, managerial, 13
Johnson, B., 156
Joint Commission on Accreditation of Healthcare Organizations (JCAHO), 103, 114, 115, 116, 121, 124, 137, 156, 175-76, 208, 250
Journal club, 106-7

K

Kansas City Royals, 48
Kaufmann, Ewing, 48
Keane, A., 42, 43
Kelley, R., 64
Kelly, F., 44
Kilmann, R. H., 84, 85
Kirsch, J., 13
Knaus, W. A., 63, 84, 144, 355
Knowledge
  acquisition and application, 173

Knowledge—cont'd
  and future, 356-357, 358-359
  problems, 243-244
  and technology, 240-242
Kramer, M., 10, 77, 78
Kriegel, R., 59

L

Labels, and professionalism, 30
Labor relations, 309-329
  and binding arbitration, 324
  and closed shop and open shop, 317-318
  and contract resolution and professionalism, 327-329
  and contract savings clause, 324-326
  and disciplinary practices, 314
  and discontent, 319-321
  and discrimination, 324
  and fear of loss of control, 328
  and grievance procedure, 324
  and job security, 312-313
  and management practices, 313-316
  and management rights and responsibilities, 322-324
  and organizational framework, 310-311
  and personnel policy, 311
  and staff management after a strike, 321-322
  and timeliness of dealing with problems, 315
  and union busting, 318-319
  and unionization, 316-327
  and workman's compensation, 311-312
Laissez-faire leadership, 71
Laliberty, R., 73
Lamb, L. H., 233
Lazarus, R., 40
Leadership
  authoritarian, 70-71
  autocratic, 70-71
  and CNS, 230
  democratic, 71
  laissez-faire, 71
  and management, 69-70
  situational; *see* Situational Leadership
  styles, 12, 70-72
  and vision, 354
Learning contract, and CBO; *see* Competency-based orientation
Learning resource development, and CBO; *see* Competency-based orientation
Lectures, and CBO, 171
Length of stay (LOS), 132
Levering, R., 42, 45, 46, 47, 48, 49, 50
Levine-Ariff, J., 277
Liability, and technology, 243-244
Licensed practical nurse (LPN), 156
Licensed vocational nurse (LVN), 156
Limited resources, 55

Lockout provisions, 324, 325
Loss of control, 328

M

McBride, A. B., 55, 59, 61
McDougall, G. J., 225, 226
McGregor's Theory X and Theory Y, 12, 39
Magnetic Resonance Imaging (MRI), 27
Main theme, 363
Malila, F. M., 255
Mallard, C. O., 17
Maloney, J., 43
Managed care, 87, 90, 94
Management
   after strike, 321-322
   and career ladders; *see* Career ladders
   and communication, 17-19
   coronary artery bypass surgery pathway, 88-89, 91
   and future, 359-366
   human relations; *see* Human relations management
   Japanese, 74
   job types, 13
   and labor relations, 313-316
   and leadership, 69-70
   MBA; *see* Management by anxiety
   MBO; *see* Management by objectives
   MBWA; *see* Management by walking around
   military workload system, 138
   nursing; *see* Nursing management
   participative; *see* Participative management
   PDMS; *see* Patient data management system
   rights and responsibilities, 322-324
   risk; *see* Risk management
   shift; *see* Shift management
   skills; *see* Managerial skills
   of time, 56-57
Management by anxiety (MBA), 64
Management by objectives (MBO), 64, 72
Management by walking around (MBWA), 64
Manager, nurse; *see* Nurse manager, 9-15
Managerial skills, 97-236
   and career ladders, 189-203
   and clinical nurse specialist's role, 221-236
   and competency-based orientation, 169-187
   and nurse intern program, 205-220
   and patient classification, 131-154
   and quality assurance and risk management, 113-130
   and standards of care, 99-111
   and twenty-four hour staffing, 155-168
   see also Management
Manipulation, 50
Maps of processes, 363
Margins, analyis of, 300-301
Marion Laboratories, 48
Marketing, and nurse intern program, 211

Marquis, B., 10
Maslow's Hierarchy of Needs, 39, 61
Mason, S. A., 260
Massachusetts General Hospital, 145
Master of art (MA), 222
Master of nursing (MN), 222
Master of science (MS), 222
Matrix scenario, 365-366
MBA; *see* Management by anxiety
MBO; *see* Management by objectives
MBWA; *see* Management by walking around
M. D. Anderson Hospitals and Tumor Institute, 191
Measurement, of outcome, 231-235
Medicare, 131, 132
Medicus Classification Tool, 138, 303
Medicus Patient Classification System, 138, 303
Medium, 17
Medoff-Cooper, B., 233
Meetings, and self-evaluation, 60
Menard, S. W., 224
Mentors, 6
Message, 17
Metcalf, J., 222
Meyer, J. S., 233
Military workload management system, 138
Miller, J. F., 355
Mims, B., 208
Minimum competency, 170-171
Mintzberg, 13
Mission statement, 263-64
Monitoring, NQA, 115, 119, 128-129
Moral commitment, 11
Morale, and technology, 241-242
Motowidlo, S., 42
Moves, career; *see* Career development
MRI; *see* Magnetic Resonance Imaging
MS; *see* Master of science
Mutual recognition, 30-31
Myrick, F., 209, 210

N

National Aeronautics and Space Administration (NASA), 345
National Center for Nursing Research (NCNR), 345, 358
National Institute of Occupational Safety and Health, 42
National Joint Practice Commission (NJPC), 92
National Labor Relations Act, 316
National Labor Relations Board (NLRB), 316
National Nursing Research Agenda (NNRA), 358
Nauert, L. B., 141
NCNR; *see* National Center for Nursing Research (NCNR)
Needs
   hierarchy of, 39, 61
   of unit, 21-23

Negotiated prices, 246
Negotiation, 24-25
Networking, 25-26, 49
Neuman System Model, 117-118
New Jersey Supreme Court, 335
New manager, 13
New York Times, 55, 163, 316
Nightingale, Florence, 217, 221
NJPC; *see* National Joint Practice Commission
NLRB; *see* National Labor Relations Board
NNRA; *see* National Nursing Research Agenda
Noble, M. A., 223
Noncontrollable costs, 280
Nonexempt status, 294
Non-nursing time, 139-141
Nonpersonnel operating budget, 278-279, 284
Nonproductive time, 278, 294-297
North American Nursing Diagnosis Association, 345
No strike provisions, 324, 325
NQA; *see* Quality assurance (QA)
Nurse
  agency; *see* Agency nurses
  clinical; *see* Clinical nurse
  CNS; *see* Clinical nurse specialist (CNS)
  intern program; *see* Nurse intern program
  LPN; *see* Licensed practical nurse (LPN)
  LVN; *see* Licensed vocational nurse (LVN)
  manager; *see* Nurse manager *and* Nursing management
  RN; *see* Registered nurse (RN)
Nurse intern program, 205-220
  background, 205-207
  collaboration with school of nursing, 213
  content, 208-211
  costs, 215-217
  criteria and selection, 212-213
  literature review, 207-208
  personal issues and contracts, 214
  recruitment and marketing, 211
  research, 214-215
  retention, 215
Nurse manager, 11
  and calendar development, 64-67
  and communication, 17-19
  in critical care, 15-19
  and excellence, 14-15
  functions of, 9-15
  and hiring practice, 9-10
  and leadership styles, 12
  and leadership versus management, 69-70
  and managerial job types, 13
  and managing staff, 13-14
  and NQA, 122
  self-evaluation, 60
  and staff retention, 10
  and turnover reduction, 11
  see also Nursing management
Nurse of the Month award, 31
Nursing care hours (NCH), 157-159

Nursing Management, 119
Nursing management
  levels of, 11-12
  and managerial job types, 13
  and managing staff, 13-14
  see also Nurse manager
Nursing quality assurance (NQA); *see* Quality assurance
Nursing Research, 356, 357

O

Office of the Inspector General, 51
Open shop, 317-318
Operating budget, 272, 276-278
Operating Room (OR), 26
Operating statement, analysis of, 289-301
Opportunities, career; *see* Career development
Organization, of work, 57-58; *see also* Organizations *and* Table of organization
Organizational chart
  and CNS, 226, 227, 228, 229, 230
  decentralized, 74
Organizational development, and CNS, 225-226
Organizational framework, and labor relations, 310-311
Organizational responsibilities, and self-evaluation, 60
Organizational structure, 70, 71, 75-77
  and career ladders, 199-201
  and participative environment, 75-77
  traditional, 70, 71
Organizations
  healthcare, JCAHO; *see* Joint Commission on Accreditation of Healthcare Organizations
  innovative and excellent, 114
  see also Organizations
Organ transplantation, 338-339
Orientation, CBO; *see* Competency-based orientation (CBO)
Ouchi's Theory Z, 39, 50, 74
Outcome, measurement of, 231-235
Outlier, 132
Overtime, 159-160
Oxygenation, ECMO; *see* Extracorporeal membrane oxygenation (ECMO)

P

Packard, J., 42
Papenhausen, J. L., 222
Paper chase, 113
Participative management, 69-81
  and change, 78
  and decentralization, 73
  environment characteristics, 74-77
  and leadership styles, 70-72
  and manager's role, 79
  and MBO, 72
  and organizational structure, 70, 75-77

Participative management—cont'd
  and reality shock, 77-78
Patient care, and technology, 240-241
Patient care coordinator, 11
Patient care cost center, 133
Patient classification, 131-154
  and compressed acuity, 134-136
  and costs versus charges, 133-134
  and DRG, 131, 132-137, 143-144, 146, 148, 149, 150, 151, 152
  and impact on practice, 136-37
  systems and nursing, 137-144
  systems relationships, 146-152
Patient data management system (PDMS), 251-255
Patient days activity report, 292, 293
Patient's Bill of Rights, 332
Pediatric Intensive Care Unit (PICU), 43-44
Peers, and communication, 18
Pennsylvania Nurse, 316
People skills
  and career development, 3-20
  and caring environment, 21-37
  and collaborative practice, 83-96
  development of, 1-96
  and job satisfaction, 39-54
  and participative management, 69-81
  and performance, time, energy, 55-68
Per diem charges, 133
Performance
  appraisal, 62
  evaluations, 56, 57
  time and energy, 55-68
Persistent vegetative state, 335
Personality types, 12
Personnel budget, 277-78
Personnel policy, 311
Peters, J. P., 261
Peters, T. J., 10, 114
Pforitz, S. K., 6
Pharmacy and therapeutics committee, 250-251
Physicians, and communication, 18
Pinkerton, S., 76
Planning
  capital; *see* Capital planning process
  and CNS, 231
  and future, 350-351
  strategic; *see* Strategic planning
Plant, 273
Policy delphis, 366
Policy development; *see* Career ladders
Political manager, 13
Porter-O'Grady, T., 74, 79
Positive behaviors, 62-63
Post-Anesthesia Care Unit (PACU), 26
Practice, standards of, 234-235; *see also* Collaborative practice
Preadmission tour, 32
Preceptor, unit; *see* Unit preceptor
Preceptor program, 9

Predictive validity, 141
Premarin, 239
Prestholdt, P. H., 11
Price, C., 163
Price, S. A., 6
Price
  negotiated, 246
  variance, 297
Pride, 48-49
Principal diagnosis, 132, 142
Principles, and collaboration, 84
Prioritization, 43
Problem identification tool, NQA, 129
Procedure and policy committee, 106
Product evaluation, 245
Productive time, 294-297
Productivity, 55, 295
Products committee, 246-250
Professionalism
  and conflict resolution, 327-329
  and labels, 30
Professional Recognition System, 210
Programs, intern; *see* Nurse intern program
Property, 272
Proportional costs, 280
Prospective payment system (PPS), 131
Prototype system, 137-139, 146, 147, 148, 149, 150, 151, 152
Purchaser consortiums, 246
Purposes, and collaboration, 84

Q

Quality, 113-114
Quality assurance (QA)
  and CBO, 178
  committee, 106
  and Neuman System Model, 117-118
  and NQA program, 115, 116-130
  and risk management, 113-130, 178
  terminology and concepts, 115
Quality circle, 74
Quantity variance, 297
Quinlan, Karen Ann, 334-336

R

React-and-adapt approach, 260
Readiness, unit, 86
Reality shock, 77-78
Real property, 272
Real time manager, 13
Receiver, 17
Recognition
  mutual, 30-31
  and Professional Recognition System, 210
Recovery stage, 78
Recruitment
  and nurse intern program, 211

Index

Recruitment—cont'd
  and technology, 242
Registered nurse (RN), 156
Reid, R., 74
Reinow, F., 74
Relations, and guests, 31-36; *see also* Human relations management *and* Labor relations
Relationships
  and CNS, 230
  essential, 45
  health care provider, 85-93
  interpersonal, 45, 49-51
Reliability, 140-141, 295
Rescue nursing, 333
Research
  and CNS, 224, 231-233
  and future, 357-358, 360-366
  and nurse intern program, 214-215
Resolution
  conflict, 327-329
  stage, 78
Resources, limited, 55; *see also* Hospital resources
Responsibilities
  management, 322-324
  NQA, 120
  organizational, 60
Result-oriented approach, 260
Retention
  and nurse intern program, 215
  and technology, 242
Revenue
  analysis of, 292-293
  forecasting, 302-330
Revenue budget, 281-282
Revision, career goal; *see* Career development
Rhetoric, 113
Rights
  management, 322-324
  patient, 332
Risk management (RM)
  and CBO, 178
  and Neuman System Model, 117-118
  and quality assurance, 113-130, 178
  terminology and concepts, 115
Robichaud, A. M., 231
Room and board charges, 133
Routine care, 133
Rufo, K., 208

S

Saikewicz, Joseph, 334, 336
Salary
  analysis, 293-297
  forecasting, 303-305
Sanford, R. C., 191
Sashkin, M., 73
Scenarios, 363, 364-366

Schmalenberg, C., 10, 77, 78
Science of Unitary Human Beings, 355
Searle, L., 206
Secretary's Commission on Nursing, 206
Security, job, 312-313
Self-actualization, 61
Self-appraisal, 58-61
Self-assessment, 77
Self-care, 33
Self-concept, 42
Self-confidence, 31
Self-esteem, 31, 61
Self-evaluation, 6, 60, 79, 80
Self-perception, 47, 58
Self-talk, 43
Selye, Hans, 40, 41
Sender, 17
Severity of illness index, 142-144, 146, 147, 148, 149, 150, 151, 152
Shift allocations, determining, 304
Shift management, 11
Shops, closed and open, 317-318
Short staffing, 55
Sick time, 159-160
Simms, L. M., 6
Sinclair, V., 244
Situational leadership, 39, 71
Skill mix, determining, 305
Skills
  administrative; *see* Administrative skills
  managerial; *see* Managerial skills
  people; *see* People skills
Slichter, S. H., 317
Slide programs, 181
Smeltzer, C., 42
Smith, H. L., 74
Social pressure, 11
Special care, 133
Specialists
  CNS; *see* Clinical nurse specialist
  HIS; *see* Hospital information systems specialist
Special orders, 246
Spectra Medical Information System, 156
Staff
  appraisal, 62
  and change, 263
  discipline, 62
  education and technology, 255-256
  and input for CBO, 178-179, 181
  managing, 13-14
  and productivity analysis, 295
  retention of, 10
  and self-evaluation, 60
  and staff position, 227
  and turnover reduction, 11
  valuing, 63-67
  see also Staffing
Staffing
  and self-evaluation, 60

Staffing—cont'd
　short, 55
　twenty-four hour; *see* Twenty-four hour staffing
　see also Staff
Stakeholders, 260
Standards, NQA, 115
Standards committee, 106
Standards for Nursing Care of the Critically Ill, 99
Standards of care, 99-111
　conceptual framework, 99-104
　and critically ill, 101-102
　one year later, 109-111
　process beginning, 104-107
　process standards, 99-100
　progress report, 107-109
　structure standards, 100
Standards of practice, 234-235
Stat, 28
Statements; *see* Mission statement *and* Operating statement
State University of New York, University Hospital, 213
Static budget, 298
Steffer, S. M., 42
Stevenson, J. S., 358
Strategic planning, 259-269
　and change, 262-263
　goal identification, 265-266
　and mission statement, 263-264
　and objectives, 266-269
　overview, 259-261
　and unit culture, 261-262
　see also Strategy
Strategy
　and clinical effectiveness, 232
　coping, 43-44
　and interpersonal relationships, 51
　and pride, 49
　and trust, 48
　see also Strategic planning
Stress
　and coping strategies, 43-44
　and job satisfaction, 40-44
　physical manifestations of, 40, 41
　and technology, 244
　in workplace, 40-43
Stressors, 40, 43
Strike, managing after, 321-322
Structure, and collaboration, 84; *see also* Organizational structure
Styles Stipulation, 84
Sunk costs, 280
Superiors, and communication, 17-18
Support
　ancillary, 26-29
　and CBO; *see* Competency-based orientation systems, 90-93
Sutherland, A., 163

Systems
　HIS; *see* Hospital information systems specialist
　information; *see* Hospital information systems specialist
　PDMS; *see* Patient data management system
　recognition; *see* Professional Recognition System
　and systems support, 90-93

T

Table of organization, 277, 284, 306
Taft-Hartley Act, 316
Talking-head video programs, 180-181
Tappen, R., 56
Team manager, 13
Teamwork, and technology, 241-242
Technology, 239-258
　biomedical engineer, 250
　dependence on, 243
　and depersonalized care, 244
　and education, 255-56
　evaluation checklist, 248-249
　and feedback, 245
　hospital information systems (HIS) specialist, 251-255, 256
　and hospital resources, 246-256
　and iatrogenic injury, 243
　and knowledge, 240-242
　liability increase, 243-244
　and morale, 241-242
　and patient care, 240-241
　and PDMS, 251-255
　pharmacy and therapeutics committee, 250-251
　problems, 243-244
　and product evaluation, 245
　and products committee, 246-250
　and recruitment, 242
　and retention, 242
　and staff education, 255-256
　strategies to maximize benefits, 244-256
　and stress, 244
　and teamwork, 241-242
Termination, 313
Tetronix, 46
Themes, 363
Theory X, McGregor's, 12
Theory Y, McGregor's, 12, 39
Theory Z, Ouchi's, 39, 50, 74
Therapeutic Intervention Scoring System (TISS), 142, 145-146, 147, 148, 149, 150, 151, 152
Therapeutics; *see* Pharmacy and therapeutics committee
Thomas, C., 261, 262
Thomas, K. W., 84, 85
Time
　CBO; *see* Competency-based orientation (CBO)
　and labor relations, 315
　management of, 56-57
　nonproductive, 294-297

Time—cont'd
  performance, and energy, 55-68
  productive, 294-297
  and systems, 139-141
  and time frame, and strategic planning, 269
  and time sheets, preparation parameters, 165
  tyranny of, 56
Tomasik, K., 243
Tour
  hours, 160-163
  preadmission, 32
Tracts, and career ladders, 191
Trangenstein, P. A., 355
Transfer; see Admission, transfer, and discharge
Transfer prices, 279
Transitions, 78
Transplantation, organ, 338-339
Treatment, withholding or withdrawing, 333-337
Trees of impact, 362-363
Trend analysis, 366
Trim point, 132
Trust, 45, 46-48
  and CNS, 230
  and communication, 46
Turnover
  job, 42
  reduction of, 11
Twenty-four hour staffing, 155-168
  and agency nurses, 163-167
  and eight-hour shift, 161
  and flex staffing, 161, 162, 163, 164
  and full-time equivalents, 157-159
  and historical data, 159-160
  and job sharing, 163
  and nursing care hours, 157-159
  and pattern development, 160
  policies past, 155-156
  staff need identification, 156-167
  and tour hours, 160-163
  and twelve-hour shift, 161, 162, 167
Two-Factor Theory, Herzberg's, 50
Tyranny of time, 56

U

Unionization, and labor relations, 316-327
Unit
  climate, 261
  culture, 261-262
  evaluation, 79, 80

Unit—cont'd
  and future, 351-352
  needs, 21-23
  and NQA, 119, 121, 125
  preceptor, and CNS, 229-230
  readiness, 86
University of Texas, 191

V

Validation, CBO; see Competency-based orientation
Validity, and systems, 141
Variable costs, 293-294
Variance, 280, 297-300
Vegetative state, 335
Video programs, 180-181
Vision, and leadership, 354
Visioning, 362
Visiting hours, 33-36
Volume variance, 297

W

Wabschall, J. M., 233
Wagner, D. P., 84
Wagner Act, 316
Wallace, 227
Wantland, Earl, 46
Watch dogs, 113
Waterman, R. H., Jr., 10, 114
Webber, J. B., 261
Weddle, 63
Withdrawing or withholding treatment, 333-337
Work
  environment and job satisfaction, 44-51
  organization of, 57-58
Workman's compensation, 311-312
Wowk, P., 58, 64
Wright, B., 355

Y

Year-to-date (YTD), 279

Z

Zero-based budgeting, 278
Zimmer, J. J., 191
Zimmerman, J. E., 84

Perfect Complements.

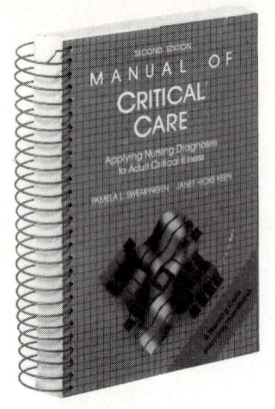

NEW!
MANUAL OF CRITICAL CARE: APPLYING NURSING DIAGNOSES TO ADULT CRITICAL ILLNESS
2nd Edition
Pamela L. Swearingen, RN;
Janet Hicks Keen, RN, MS, CCRN, CEN
1991   (0-8016-5084-4)

This comprehensive, up-to-date care-planning manual provides an excellent clinical reference to critical care disorders and dysfunctions. Focusing on nursing care of clinical patient problems, each chapter begins discussion with a brief review of pathophysiology, followed by discussions of assessment data, diagnostic tests, medical management/surgical intervention, nursing diagnoses/interventions, rehabilitation, and patient and family teaching.

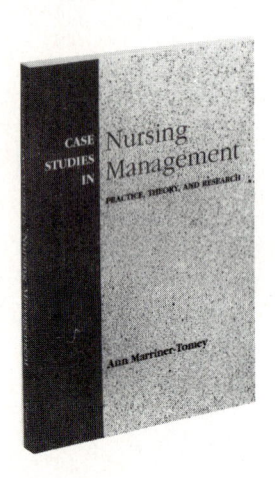

CASE STUDIES IN NURSING MANAGEMENT: PRACTICE, THEORY, AND RESEARCH
Ann Marriner-Tomey, RN, PhD, FAAN
1990   (0-8016-5848-9)

This useful text helps nursing students and nurse managers apply management theory to all levels of nursing management by using theory to analyze case studies. Each chapter begins with a case study, presents a theory, and then analyzes the case using the theory. The chapter concludes by presenting nursing and non-nursing research related to the theory. The text is organized according to the management process of plan, organize, lead, motivate, and evaluate.

To order ask your bookstore manager or call toll-free 800-426-4545. We look forward to hearing from you soon.

Mosby Year Book

NMA-051